DESIGNING PARTIAL DENTURES

DESIGNING PARTIAL DENTURES

David M Watt PhD FDS DRD RCS(Edin)

Professor (Emeritus) of Restorative Dentistry, University of Edinburgh. Formerly Consultant in Restorative Dentistry, Lothian Health Board. External Examiner Universities of London, Belfast and Singapore. Visiting Professor University of New York at Buffalo and Royal Dental School, Copenhagen
Recipient of the Research in Prosthodontics Award of the International Association for Dental Research and of the Medal Award of the British Society for the Study of Prosthetic Dentistry

and

A Roy MacGregor PhD FDS DRD RCS(Edin)

Professor of Prosthodontics, University of Glasgow. Consultant in Prosthodontics, Greater Glasgow Health Board. External Examiner Universities of Wales and Edinburgh. Formerly External Examiner Universities of London, Belfast and Lagos. Formerly Visiting Professor University of Michigan in Ann Arbor

WRIGHT
Bristol
1984

Published by John Wright & Sons Ltd, 823–825 Bath Road, Bristol BS4 5NU, England

British Library Cataloguing in Publication Data
Watt, David M.
Designing partial dentures.
1. Partial dentures
I. Title II. MacGregor, A. Roy
617.6′92 RK664

ISBN 0 7236 0810 5

Library of Congress Catalog Card Number: 84–51164

Typeset by
Severntype Repro Services Ltd,
6 Market Street, Wotton-under-Edge, Glos. GL12 7EA

Printed in Great Britain by
John Wright & Sons (Printing) Ltd,
at The Stonebridge Press, Bristol BS4 5NU

To

Janet

and

Nancy

Preface

Show a patient requiring partial dentures to any group of dentists and each dentist will design the prosthesis in a different way. This is because many desirable features of design are mutually exclusive and the process of designing is a journey through a maze of compromises. In this book we aim to help dental students and general dental practitioners find their way through this maze by a better understanding of the principles of designing partial dentures.

When making partial dentures, dentists quite rightly put more emphasis on preserving what remains than on replacing what is lost, but from the patient's point of view a partial denture should have three qualities: it should look good, it should feel good and it should do good to the remaining teeth and supporting structures. The patient's priorities are usually allocated in that order and if the denture does not look good or feel good the patient will not wear it. Several surveys show that an unduly high proportion of partial dentures are not worn by patients and that many dentures damage the oral structures. In this book we examine some of the reasons for these problems and suggest designs of dentures that are not only acceptable in appearance and comfortable to wear, but also avoid damage to the tissues. As far as possible we have identified causes of failure and commented on how to avoid unsuccessful dentures.

In the first four chapters we discuss the assessment of partially edentulous patients, the oral changes following loss of teeth and how these changes affect the design of partial dentures. We then consider the retention of partial dentures by clasps and prefabricated attachments, and deal with connectors and the principles of design. In the following five chapters specific designs for partial dentures are discussed and the last chapter is devoted to the factors that affect appearance. Throughout the book we emphasize the importance of streamlined designs that increase the patient's comfort and we indicate the designs that are very often rejected by patients. We omit much of the routine technology of partial dentures and we assume the reader has a working knowledge of laboratory and clinical procedures. Techniques that are useful for understanding the text are to be found in the appendices, so that the general theme of the book is not interrupted. The appendices comprise the preparation of the mouth for partial dentures, the maintenance of oral hygiene, a step-by-step approach to surveying, and a historical review of partial denture classifications. A glossary of terms used in the book is also provided.

We are particularly indebted to Josephine Buchanan for editing and typing the script. We are very grateful to John Davies, Anne Harrow, Gail Drake, Robert Renton and Ian Goddard, all of whom did the bulk of the photography, and to Paul Geissler for many of the clinical photographs. We also thank Ruth Swan who drew *Figs.* 2.3 and 10.7, and Anne Hughes for *Figs.* 9.12 to 9.14. Many members of the staff of both our departments in Edinburgh and Glasgow contributed their special skills and we owe a special debt of gratitude to Arthur Craig, Grant Miller, Ian Mack, Harry Howie and Ronald McCarron. We are very conscious that many others provided clinical and technical help and we are deeply grateful to them all.

DMW
ARM

Contents

Chapter 1

Assessment of partially edentulous patients

Before any steps are taken to make partial dentures for patients, two questions must be asked:

1. Is a partial denture really necessary?
2. Is the patient willing and able to keep the mouth sufficiently clean to ensure that a partial denture does not damage the remaining tissues?

From the patient's point of view, the reasons for making partial dentures are:

1. To restore the appearance
2. To restore the occlusion of the natural teeth

The restoration of appearance is very important as far as the patient is concerned. Some patients who have had many posterior teeth missing for years may request a partial denture only when an anterior tooth is lost. From the dentist's point of view, the restoration of occlusion and the preservation of the remaining teeth are of the greatest importance, but the dentist must be aware of the patient's priority—a good-looking, comfortable denture.

In the preliminary examination attention must first be directed to the patient's periodontal health and oral cleanliness. The measures that should be taken to improve oral hygiene are discussed in Appendix I. Only after patients have demonstrated their ability to maintain very clean mouths should they be accepted for partial denture treatment. Concurrently with oral hygiene and periodontal assessment (Miller, 1938; Russell, 1956; Laster et al., 1975; Lindhe and Nyman, 1975; Hibberd, 1981), the dentist should assess the patient's occlusion. Study casts should be made and mounted on an adjustable articulator so that the tooth relationships can be examined.

Over-erupted and Misplaced Teeth

Patients requesting partial dentures often have over-erupted, tilted or misplaced teeth. Each of these irregularities presents problems that must be solved before the final impressions are taken for the partial dentures.

Over-erupted Teeth

Over-erupted teeth cause two types of difficulties:

1. If they over-erupt into a gap, they leave insufficient room between their mesial or distal borders and the abutment teeth of the gap. The over-erupted teeth may slide on the mesial or distal surfaces of the opposing teeth, rather like scissor blades crossing each other (*Fig.* 1.1). These contacts cause a postural adaptation of the mandible (Watt, 1981), and even after they have been ground to provide room for occlusal rest connectors the contacts may re-establish themselves because of a change in the mandibular/maxillary relationship after the occlusion has been freed from the premature contacts. Thus, although adequate room has been provided before taking final impressions, the dentist may find that the contacts have returned by the time the denture is fitted. Before taking impressions for partial dentures it is of the greatest importance to establish a stable occlusion in which no sliding sounds on occlusion or disocclusion can be detected with a stereostethoscope.

2. The over-eruption of posterior teeth sometimes leaves insufficient room for teeth to be placed on the opposing partial denture (*Fig.* 1.2). Even if very short teeth are used, the marked step on the occlusal surface interferes with lateral and anteroposterior movements of

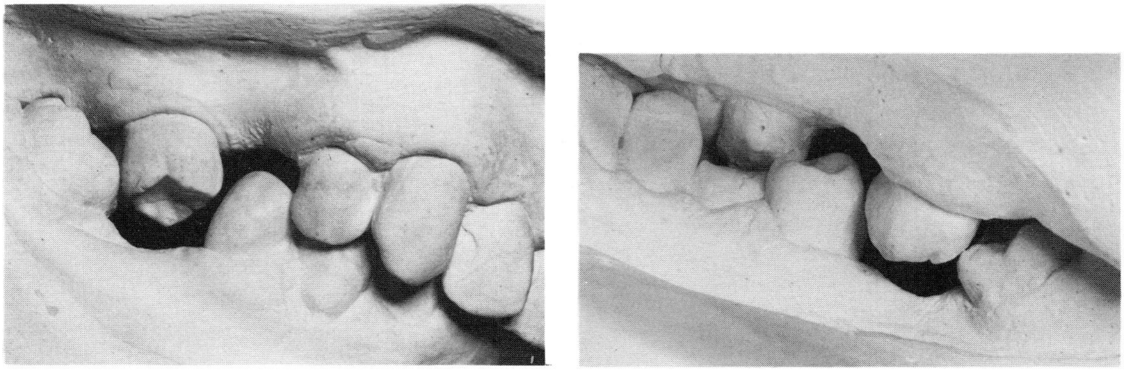

Fig. 1.1. Buccal and lingual views of the right posterior teeth on articulated casts. The loss of teeth allows over-eruption of the opposing teeth and produces sliding contacts and disrupted occlusion.

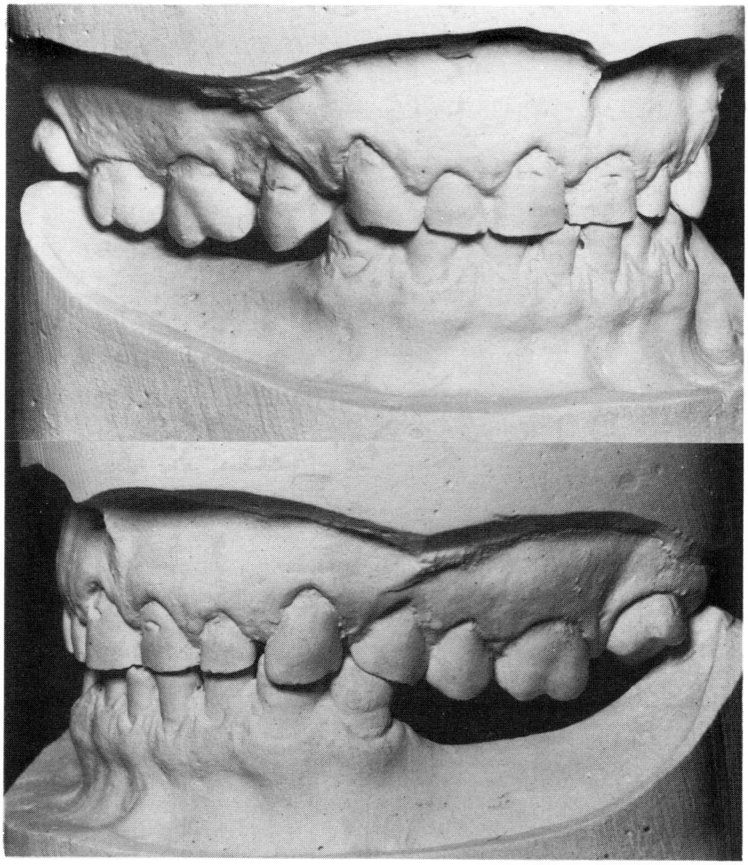

Fig. 1.2. Over-eruption of molars and closure from attrition of anterior teeth leaves insufficient room to place teeth on the opposing partial denture.

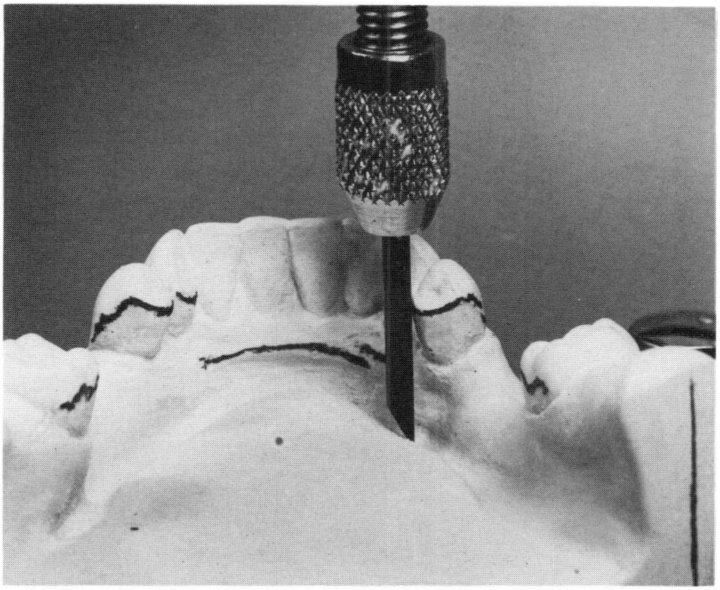

Fig. 1.3. Marked lingual tilting of lower first premolars presents special design problems. Since it is not feasible to place the connectors in such large undercuts, the teeth must be modified or the connectors must cross the occlusolingual surfaces of the premolars.

the mandible. Where possible the crowns of over-erupted teeth should be reduced. Root-filling may be necessary to allow adequate shortening, but if there is exposure of the trifurcation or bifurcation of the roots of the over-erupted tooth, extraction is usually the best course, although Appleton (1980) has advocated the separation of the roots.

Upper and lower third molars that are unopposed often occlude against the opposing mucosa. It is tempting to remove these teeth to solve the occlusal problem, but do not be too hasty about this. Provided there is no interference with the opposing second molars, these teeth might help you to avoid making a free-end saddle denture at some later date. When considering the extraction of a sound but displaced tooth in a partially edentulous patient, the crucial test is to ask yourself whether you would have it extracted from your own mouth in similar circumstances. The answer is usually 'No'. In most cases this is the right answer because the extraction of a molar comprises the loss of approximately 400 square millimetres of periodontal support.

Tilted and Misplaced Teeth

What has been said about extraction of over-erupted teeth also applies to badly tilted and displaced teeth. In patients for whom orthodontic alignment is inappropriate, a tooth may be extracted to avoid complexities in design. A lingually displaced lower premolar that is not in occlusion seems at first an obvious candidate for extraction. The decision to extract should not be taken automatically, but should depend on the proximity of the roots to adjacent teeth and on the tooth's general periodontal condition. In many cases the crown can be modified to avoid the extraction of a tooth that might endanger the adjacent teeth. Always look to the future and imagine whether or not the misplaced tooth would be an advantage or an encumbrance if adjacent teeth were lost.

Lower premolars with marked lingual tilts often make it difficult to connect different parts of dentures (*Fig.* 1.3). The lingual undercuts are such that on insertion a lingual bar has to lie some distance from the soft-tissue surface to pass the in-standing premolars. It is sometimes possible to design the denture so that the lingual bar lies anterior to the in-standing premolars with the remaining connector crossing the lingual part of the occlusal surfaces of the premolars, which are very often out of occlusion (*Fig.* 1.4**A**). A heavy continuous clasp used as a

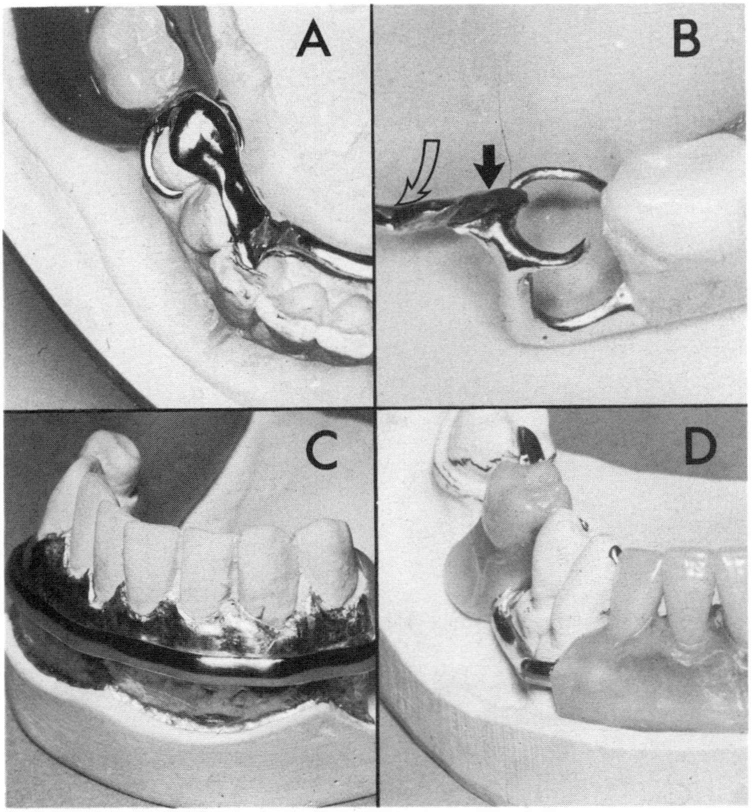

Fig. 1.4. Some solutions for problems arising from lingually tilted lower premolars. **A**, Connector between the lingual bar and the saddle lies on the lingual cusps of the instanding premolars. **B**, A heavy continuous clasp (*open arrow*) used as a primary connector passes through the embrasure (*solid arrow*) and is connected to the saddle with a short buccal bar. **C**, Labial bar on foil-relieved cast. **D**, Buccal bar.

primary connector is a possible alternative in these cases and, if a gap exists anterior to the premolar, the connector can be brought through it to the buccal side, thus avoiding the undercut (*Fig.* 1.4**B**). Another possibility is to fit a labial bar as the primary connector between the saddles (*Fig.* 1.4**C**, **D**). When an anterior tooth is missing in these cases, it can be attached to the labial bar. As a rule such bars are not tolerated well by patients. Connectors are further discussed in Chapter 8.

The undercuts of badly tilted teeth often act as food traps. This is discussed in Chapter 5. Many of these problems can be solved by orthodontic treatment or by careful preparation of teeth and fitting crowns to improve their alignment. This must be done with care to avoid an artificial appearance, as the re-aligned porcelain crowns are seldom of the same size as the rotated teeth and the smaller crowns look artificial. It is usually better to place fixed rather than removable prostheses to avoid problems of relapse after orthodontic correction of misplaced teeth. Canines erupted in the palate can occasionally be brought into the arch by sacrificing a premolar, but in adult patients this may be very difficult, and if it does not succeed the patient is in a worse state than before. Unerupted canines in adult patients can be left, provided they are covered with sufficient bone and do not show any pathology. If removal is contemplated, it should be done without the loss of any other tooth in the arch. It is acceptable to extract a canine tooth that has erupted in the palate of a patient with an arch in which all the teeth are in mesiodistal contact. When lower first molars have been lost and there is marked

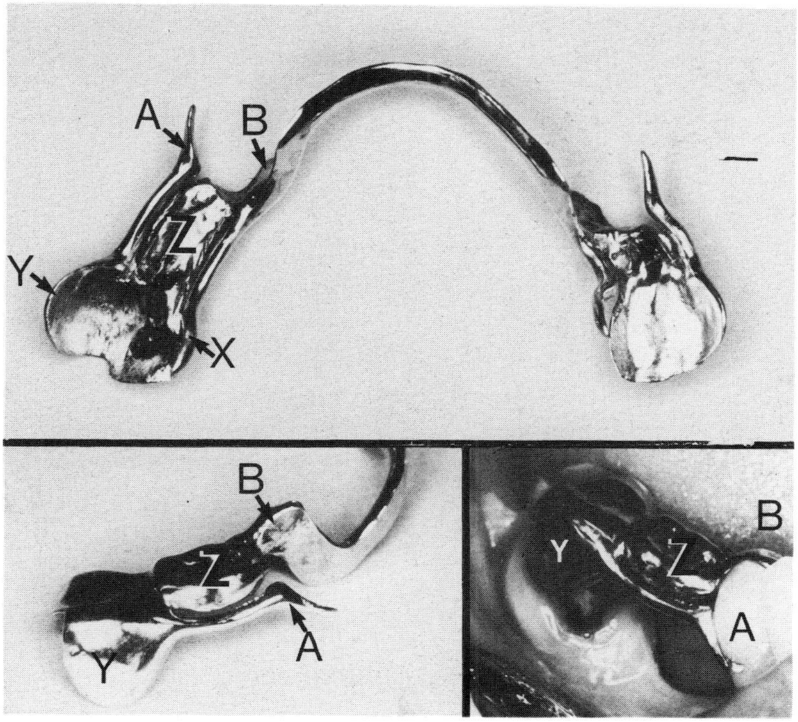

Fig. 1.5. *Upper,* Undersurface of a metal denture to replace mandibular first molars where the abutment teeth are tilted towards each other. *Lower,* Buccal views of right saddle outside and inside the mouth. The clasp 'A' is reciprocated by the lingual plate 'B' and the clasp 'X' by the buccal plate 'Y'. The pontic 'Z' spans the gap in the arch and ensures that the gingival margins are self-cleansing.

forward tilting of the second molars and backward drift of the second premolars, the pontic and clasp design shown in *Fig.* 1.5 is most suitable for a removable partial denture. This design avoids the mesial and distal food traps that a more conventional denture produces, but we recommend fixed restorations in such cases. If a tooth-borne appliance is necessary, we think that the fixed partial denture provides the best restoration regardless of the tilting of the abutment tooth. The technical problems produced by such tilting can easily be solved by the use of various prefabricated attachments (Matsuo and Shimegi, 1981).

Deep anterior overbites often leave very little room for placing removable partial dentures. It is usually unwise to try to increase the vertical dimensions in these cases and a fixed bridge may be the best prosthesis to use. Sometimes removable partial dentures can be constructed with very thin (0·35 mm) cobalt-chromium alloy without interfering with the occlusion, provided the connectors are carefully positioned. In the case illustrated in *Fig.* 1.6 there is just enough room to attach the upper left central incisor to the palatal connector, but the cingulum rest seats had to be located very carefully to avoid occlusal interference.

The space left in the dental arch after extraction of a tooth becomes smaller and orthodontic treatment may be required to restore it, but this approach is fraught with difficulties unless fixed partial dentures are made, as the gaps tend to close up if a removable prosthesis is left out for any length of time. In the case illustrated in *Fig.* 1.7 a mucosa-borne acrylic partial denture had been worn for some time and the tissue destruction from this damaging appliance is obvious. The soft tissue destruction might have been avoided by making a fixed or removable tooth-borne appliance.

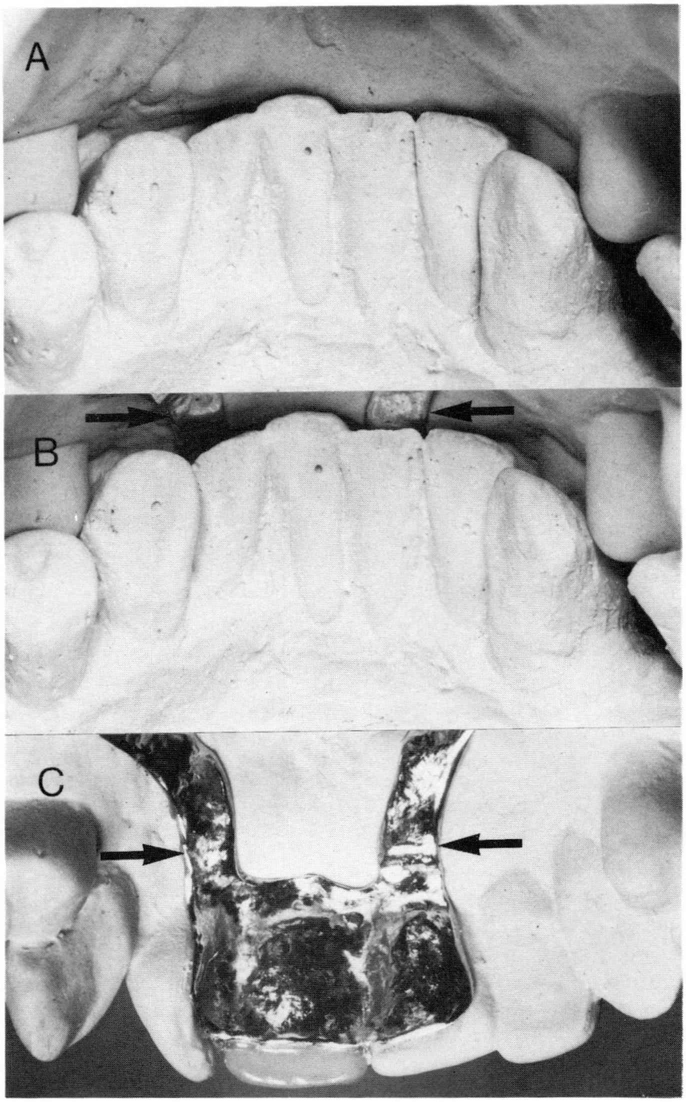

Fig. 1.6. **A**, A deep overbite leaves little room for a removable partial denture. **B**, By careful placement of the connector it is possible to avoid occlusal interferences. **C**, The thin (0·35 mm) cast denture replaces a missing upper left central incisor.

Occlusion

We have considered some gross discrepancies of occlusion that may be found on examination of patients who require partial dentures. However, before designing partial dentures we must be aware of the much smaller discrepancies that can cause patients' discomfort. These discrepancies of occlusion may be as little as 0·1 mm. While most patients will adapt to an amount as small as this, the process of adaptation often gives rise to other occlusal changes and a vicious circle is set up. Small faults in occlusion (less than 0·3 mm) are often difficult to diagnose and locate without the use of a stereostethoscope and thin articulating papers, tapes and shimstock (*Table* 1.1). Should you be in any doubt about the effect of a discrepancy of this order, take a piece of tin foil about 0·3 mm thick and place it between

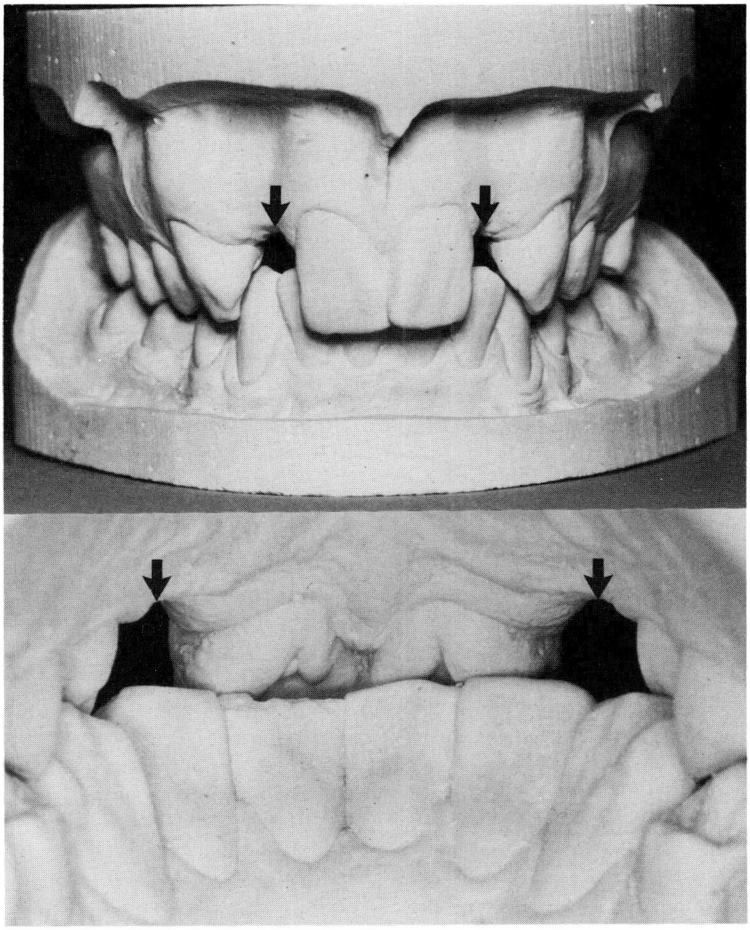

Fig. 1.7. The gaps caused by the loss of the lateral incisors have been reduced by the canine teeth drifting. Much tissue destruction (*arrows*) from an ill-fitting mucosa-borne partial denture can be seen.

Table 1.1 **Thickness of some articulating papers and tapes**

Thickness	*Type*	*Manufacturer*
0·020 mm	Accu film	Parkell, Farmingdale, NY 11735, USA
0·025 mm	Mylar tape (shimstock)	Artus Corporation, Englewood, NY 07631, USA
0·042 mm	Detex red	Associated Dental Products, Purton, Wilts, England
0·060 mm	Detex blue	Associated Dental Products, Purton, Wilts, England
0·062 mm	Ash extra thin	Amalgamated Dental Trade Distributors Ltd, London, England
0·102 mm	Silk dental tape	Denar Corporation, Anaheim, CA 92805, USA
0·160 mm	Cottrell's thin	Cottrell & Co., London, England

the teeth on one side of your mouth. You will find that this feels like a huge interference that would be intolerable if produced by a partial denture. Yet, while partial dentures are being made occlusal discrepancies of between 0·1 mm and 0·5 mm can occur and the utmost care is necessary at all stages to reduce these occlusal errors to the minimum.

Before discussing the details of occlusion the following facts about natural teeth should be recognized:

1. Teeth move with every heart beat.
2. Teeth are intruded into the alveolus with every occlusion and after their initial recovery return rather slowly to their former position.
3. A change in tooth form that changes the forces on the tooth causes a change in its position.
4. Occlusion modifies muscle activity and muscle activity modifies occlusion.

The occlusal surface of a dental arch should not be thought of as an occlusal table because the movements of the teeth make it more like a piano keyboard than a table top. An impression of a dental arch records tooth position at a moment in time and an impression of the opposing arch records a tooth position at a different time. A wax or paste registration of the occlusion provides a third sample of tooth position that is different from either of the samples already taken. It is not surprising that the occlusion of partial dentures is frequently a cause of difficulty. It is therefore necessary to 'put occlusion on a time base' so that the influence of one occlusion upon another can be assessed and so that a stable occlusion can be developed in each patient before construction of partial dentures is started. The gnathosonic techniques for establishing a stable occlusion are described by Watt (1981) and the biomechanics of occlusal splints are discussed by Ash and Ramfjord (1982).

In addition to the variability of tooth position we must also reconsider some of our concepts of jaw relationships. Ideas like the 'terminal hinge axis' and the position of 'centric relation' are dental concepts that we may use to help us to mount casts on an articulator. However, we must remember that these dental concepts have little anatomical or physiological reality and the positions vary according to the muscle activity. In order to establish a comfortable occlusion of the teeth, we should not dictate a forced relationship of the patient's jaws that we feel is correct because *we* can reproduce it, as it is unlikely we will get the correct functional position for the patient. Instead, with the patient we should seek the appropriate position, so that when it is found both are satisfied that it is the correct position. This 'correct' position is the position of maximum intercuspation of the teeth at the termination of the path of closure produced by optimum muscle activity.

We can say the following things about this position of maximum intercuspation:

1. There is stable tooth contact all round the dental arch in this position.
2. Teeth do not slide over each other in order to reach this position and when the jaws are opened from this position there is no sliding of teeth out of occlusion and therefore no separation noise.
3. When the teeth are snapped together in this position, the sound they produce is a single impact noise of short duration that is reproducible on successive contacts.
4. This position must be established in the patient's mouth and checked gnathosonically and clinically for stability. The patient 'feels the difference' when the position is established and is aware of its stability. Only after its establishment should casts be made and mounted in the intercuspal position on the articulator.
5. If so many teeth are missing that a stable intercuspal position cannot be found, then temporary appliances should be made in the retruded contact position and fitted and adjusted to establish the intercuspal position before permanent restorations are made (Ash and Ramfjord, 1982; Ramfjord and Ash, 1983).

Functional Malocclusion

When there has been considerable tooth loss, there is usually some postural adaptation of the mandible to accommodate the loss. If the tooth loss is on one side only, a unilateral chewing habit will be present, possibly with a reduced joint space on the side of tooth loss

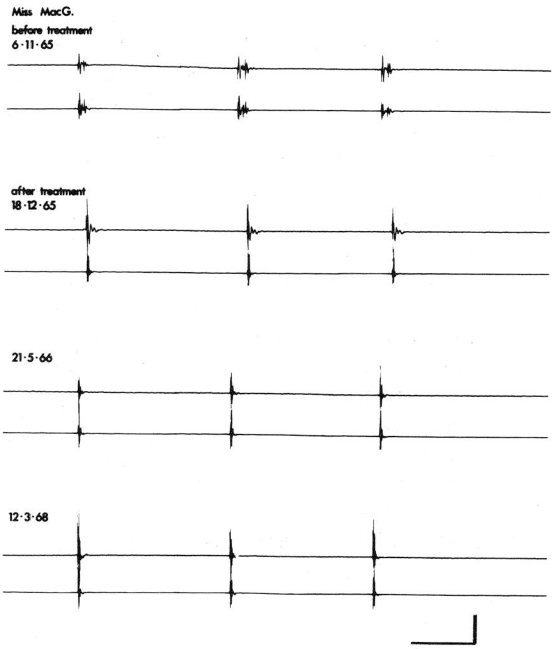

Fig. 1.8. Oscillographic records of the sounds of occlusion of the teeth before and after the occlusion was stabilized. *Upper two records:* The prolonged double peaked sounds of the unstable occlusion before correction. *Other six records:* After correction the single impact sounds of short duration indicate that the occlusion remained stable during the following period of 2 years and 8 months. (*Scale:* 200 ms, 40 mV.)

and asymmetrical muscle activity. If the patient has pain in the muscles or noises in the joints, active steps should be taken to correct these before the partial denture is constructed. These steps might include the construction of a temporary bite plate to stabilize the occlusion and relax the muscles. Correction of the occlusion is possible only after muscle relaxation (Watt, 1981). It is fundamental to the success of partial dentures that the occlusion should be stabilized before the dentures are constructed (*Figs.* 1.8, 3.6, 3.7, 3.8). It is very unwise to make partial dentures for a patient with an unstable occlusion as the denture increases the unfavourable forces on the remaining teeth and makes damage to their periodontium more likely. The method of stabilizing occlusion is described in Appendix II.

Apart from the stabilization of the occlusion, a thorough clinical and radiographic investigation of the remaining teeth and of the saddle areas should be carried out to locate the presence of any buried roots and other pathology and to indicate the amount of supporting bone round the abutment teeth.

Chapter 2

Morphological changes following tooth loss

When a tooth is extracted the contour of the tissues changes quickly. Within 2 weeks a millimetre of buccal contour is commonly lost and a greater loss of height of the residual ridge takes place (Watt, 1960). Immediately after the tooth has been extracted the gingival margins collapse towards the tooth socket (*Fig.* 2.1).

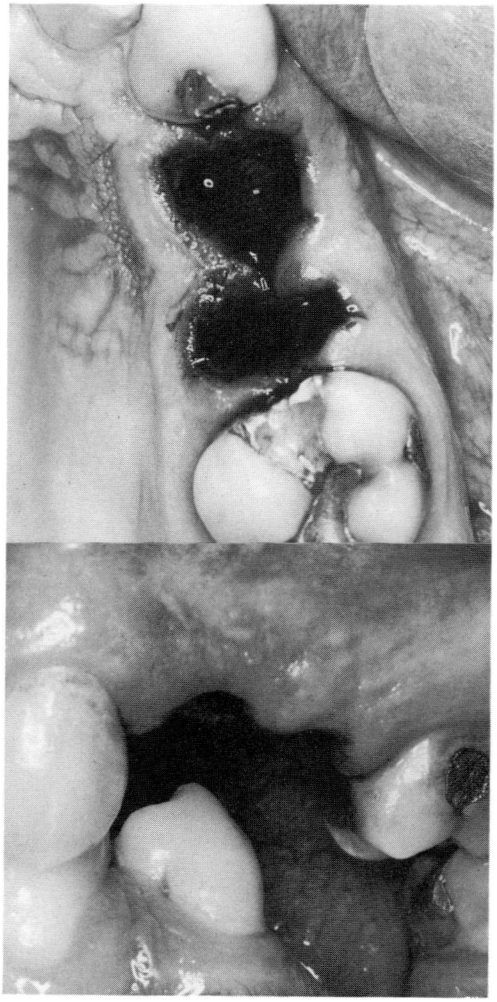

Fig. 2.1. After teeth have been extracted the gingival margins collapse towards the tooth sockets and cause marked loss of contour, which must be restored by the prosthesis. Occlusal and buccal views 15 min after extraction of left upper premolars.

Collapse of Gingival Margins

In a study of morphological changes following extraction of maxillary teeth (Watt, 1960), observations showed that in every case the gingival margins collapsed towards the sockets when teeth were extracted. This collapse was encouraged by pressure of the operator's fingers at the time of extraction and had the effect of reducing the buccolingual diameter of the extraction wounds. The amount of collapse and the effect on measurements of postextraction changes varied considerably between extractions. In the majority of cases the collapse of the lingual gingival margin was reflected by a dip in the graph of lingual vertical change shortly after extraction; thereafter the change proceeded more slowly (*Fig.* 2.2, *Table* 2.1). The collapse of the buccal gingival margins produced similar dips in the graphs of buccal change in cases where the collapse was sufficiently extensive to involve the buccal measurements (*Fig.* 2.2, *Table* 2.2). It seemed reasonable to assume that differences in the amount of the free gingivae accounted for some of the variations in the gingival collapse. Different degrees of trauma during extractions were also likely to have contributed to the variations observed.

The gingival collapse eventually results in

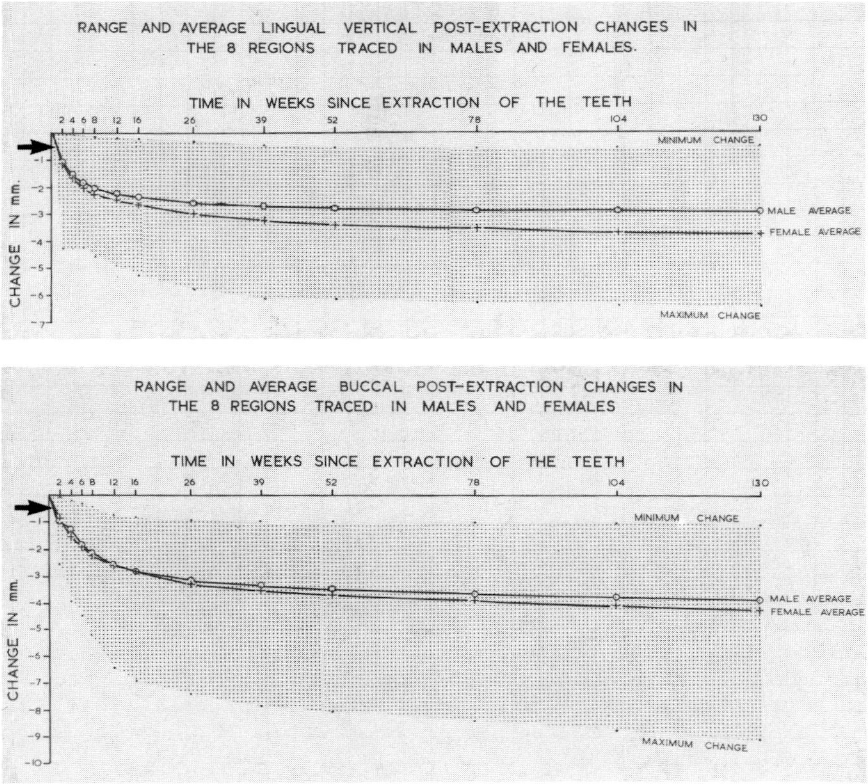

Fig. 2.2. Graphs of range and average tissue loss following extraction of maxillary teeth. *Upper,* Lingual vertical loss. *Lower,* Buccal horizontal loss. The arrows indicate the sudden collapse of gingival margins followed by the slower loss caused by bone resorption. There were wide variations among the 25 patients in the sample, as can be seen by the stippled areas, which represent the range of tissue loss. The differences between males and females were not significant. The changes in millimetres are shown in *Tables* 2.1 and 2.2 (Watt, 1960).

Table 2.1 **Average lingual vertical changes in 8 regions traced in males and females and range of lingual vertical changes in a sample of 25 subjects**

	Lingual vertical changes		*Range of changes in the whole sample*	
Weeks since extractions	Males (mm)	Females (mm)	Minimum (mm)	Maximum (mm)
2	1·06	1·13	0·00	4·25
4	1·54	1·62	0·06	4·25
6	1·82	2·02	0·09	4·25
8	2·02	2·22	0·12	4·55
12	2·26	2·48	0·18	4·91
16	2·34	2·66	0·22	5·25
26	2·60	3·00	0·33	5·78
39	2·72	3·24	0·49	6·12
52	2·81	3·40	0·55	6·19
78	2·91	3·58	0·60	6·34
104	2·96	3·77	0·60	6·45
130	3·03	3·86	0·60	6·54

Table 2.2 **Average buccal changes in 8 regions traced in males and females and range of buccal changes in a sample of 25 subjects.**

Weeks since extractions	*Buccal changes* Males (mm)	Females (mm)	*Range of changes in the whole sample* Minimum (mm)	Maximum (mm)
2	0·87	0·96	0·07	2·50
4	1·52	1·23	0·21	3·89
6	1·90	1·82	0·33	4·45
8	2·21	2·12	0·42	5·20
12	2·57	2·55	0·75	6·40
16	2·82	2·82	0·84	6·88
26	3·13	3·26	0·91	7·35
39	3·31	3·50	0·94	7·82
52	3·46	3·69	0·97	8·02
78	3·62	3·89	1·00	8·40
104	3·75	4·08	1·05	8·75
130	3·86	4·26	1·10	9·10

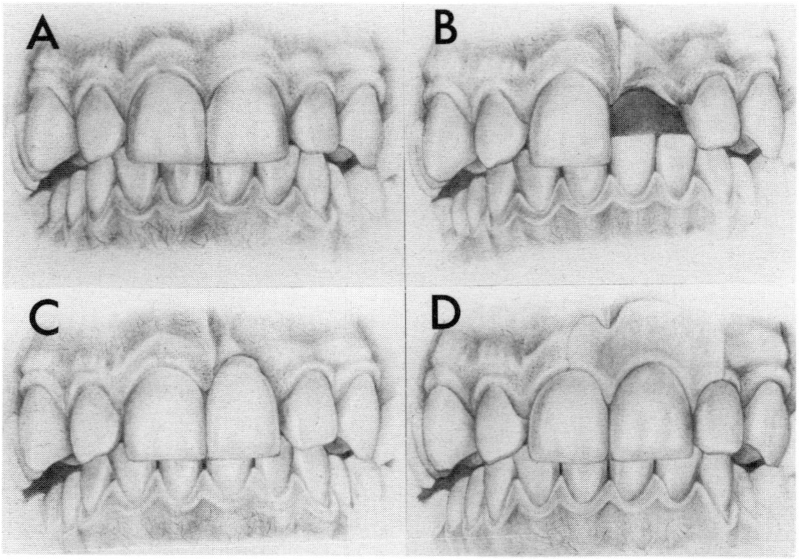

Fig. 2.3. When a tooth is extracted the interdental papillae between it and adjacent teeth are lost and should be replaced by the partial prosthesis. **A,** Before extraction. **B,** Post-extraction changes. **C,** 'Gum-fitted' replacement does not restore all the lost tissue. **D,** Soft tissue loss restored with labial flange.

the loss of the interdental papillae between the extracted tooth and the remaining teeth on each side of the gap (*Fig.* 2.3).

Bone Loss

The morphological changes described are also accompanied by bone loss on the side of the abutment tooth nearest the gap. Thus, any tooth next to a gap is less satisfactory as an abutment than a tooth within an intact portion of the dental arch (*Fig.* 2.4). This is further discussed in Chapter 4.

When making partial dentures to replace anterior teeth, all the lost tissues should be replaced in order to restore the patient's appearance. *Fig.* 2.5 shows a patient who has lost the upper right lateral incisor and canine as well as the upper left canine. The papillae between the two central incisors can be clearly seen, but there is no papilla on the distal side of the upper right central incisor. To make a

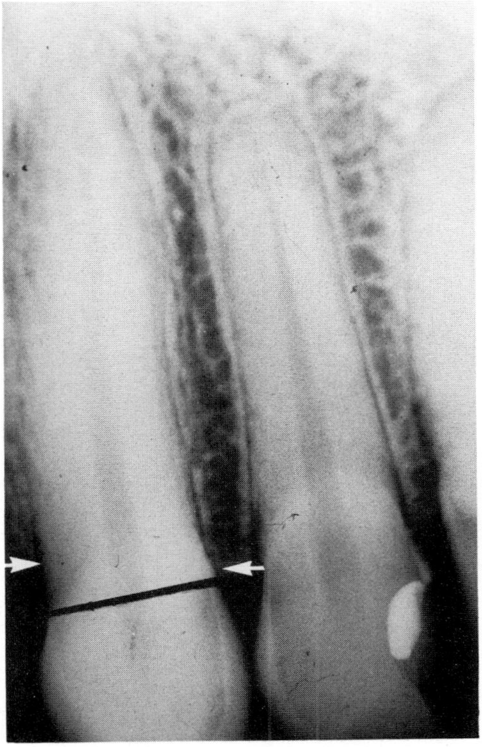

Fig. 2.4. Upper left canine after extraction of the left premolars shows a marked difference between the mesial and distal levels of the alveolar bone (*arrows*). The black line has been drawn between the mesial and distal parts of the amelocemental junction.

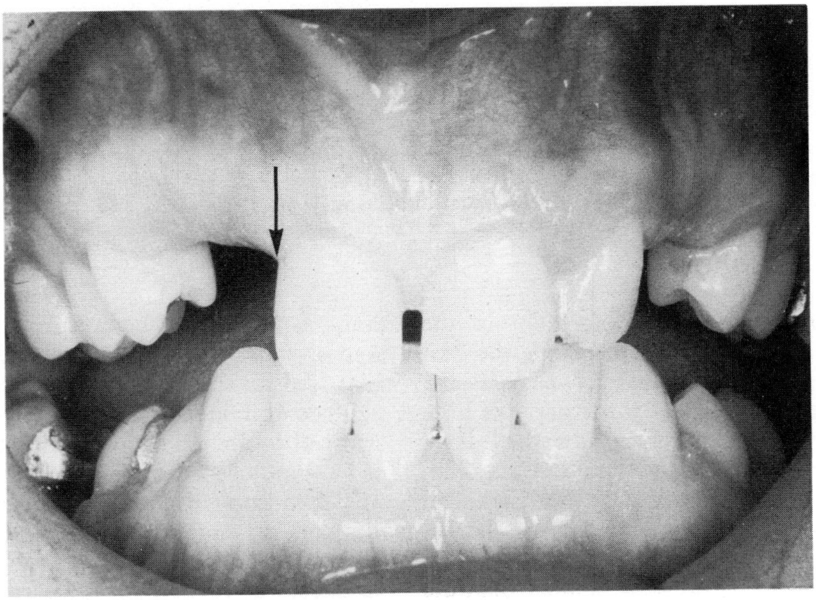

Fig. 2.5. The loss of the right lateral incisor and canine has caused the loss of the interdental papilla distal to the right central incisor (*arrow*). Note the marked difference in gingival contour between the mesial and distal borders of the right central.

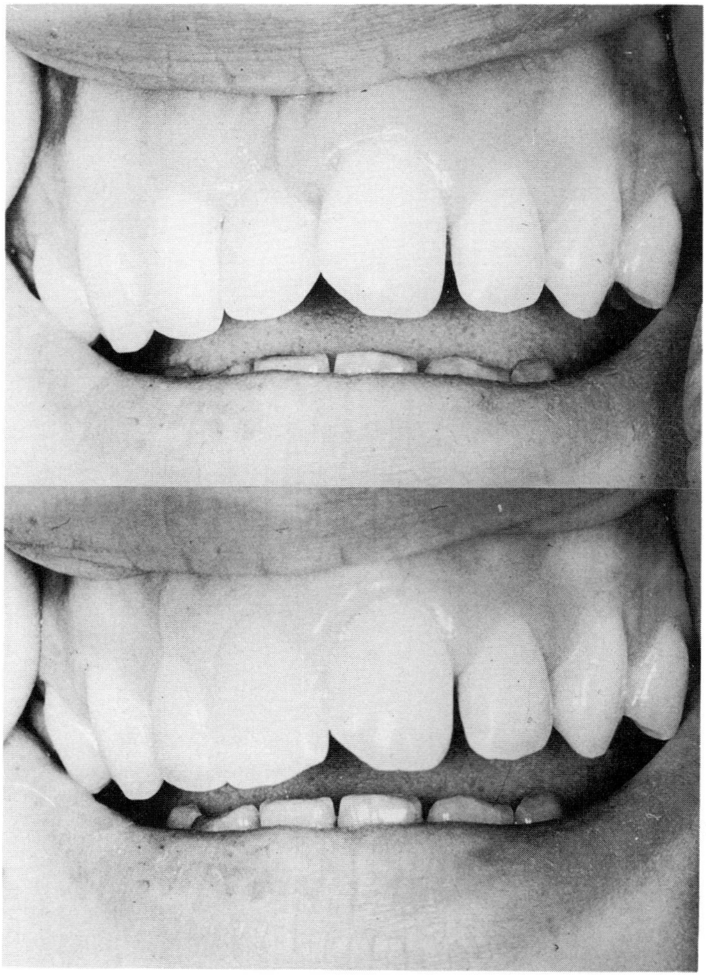

Fig. 2.6. *Upper,* Replacement of right central incisor by gum-fitted tooth that is too small because there is insufficient space in the position where it fits the gum. In addition the prosthesis fails to restore the lost soft tissue contour. *Lower,* A more satisfactory prosthesis. This has a flange that replaces the lost gingival contour. The flange also makes it possible to use an artificial tooth of the correct size, positioned more labially where there is space for it. In addition the flange provides retention for the anterior part of the denture. Thus clasps can be placed out of sight on the posterior teeth.

partial denture virtually undetectable in the mouth it is necessary to replace all the lost tissues—not only the teeth, but also the interdental papillae and that part of the alveolar process that has been absorbed since the teeth were extracted. To position the teeth correctly it is usually necessary to make an acrylic flange. 'Gum-fitted' teeth must be set further lingually because of resorption of the ridge. In this position they are smaller than the natural teeth. If placed in the correct position in the arch they must of necessity be longer than their natural counterparts in order to contact the mucosa. This point is illustrated in *Figs.* 2.3 and 2.6, in which you see the upper right central incisor replaced by a gum-fitted artificial tooth. There was loss of buccal bone at the time of extraction and because the tooth was gum-fitted it was set further back; since the gap had narrowed, a tooth narrower than its natural counterpart was fitted. This produced a very poor appearance.

For good appearance it is essential that the artificial tooth should be of the same size and shape as the tooth it is replacing. In this patient, by fitting a small acrylic flange to replace the lost tissues, the right central incisor was placed in its proper position, where there was sufficient space for a tooth of the correct size.

The type of flange used for a restoration of this kind is made of a mottled acrylic with a little clear acrylic added. The fine edges of the flange are finished opposite the middle of the gingival margins of the two abutment teeth. These edges are thinned to a knife-edge on the attached mucosa. This makes the flange virtually undetectable in the mouth. The pink mucosa shines through the thin margins of the flange and makes it difficult to see where the denture stops and the patient starts. A similar case is shown in *Fig.* 2.7 where the upper right lateral incisor was replaced by a

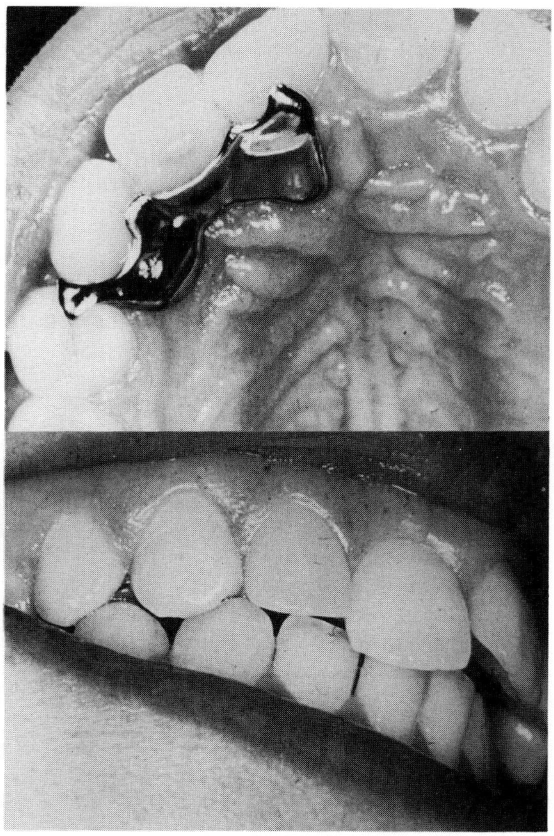

Fig. 2.7. Lost right lateral incisor replaced by sectional denture with contoured flange (*see* Chapter 12).

sectional denture. Stippling of the labial flange of the denture made it difficult to detect.

If possible the flanges of partial dentures should replace only the lost tissues. The lower diagram in *Fig.* 2.8 shows a horizontal cross-section of a flange replacing soft tissue lost after the extraction of an upper right central incisor. Note that the remaining central incisor

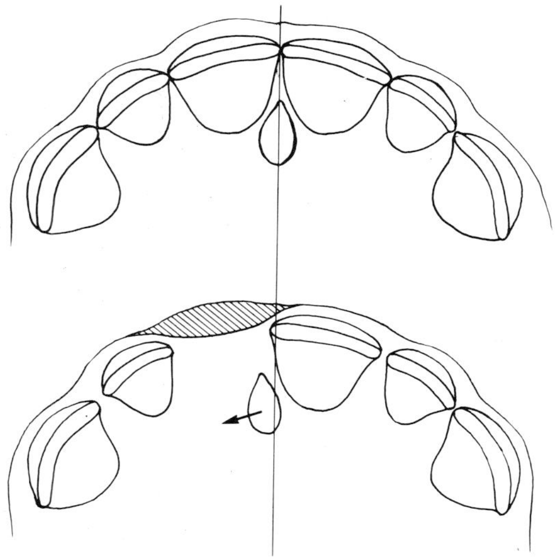

Fig. 2.8. *Upper,* Pre-extraction. *Lower,* Soft tissue and bone loss following the extraction of the central incisor. Note changes in the position of the adjacent teeth and of the incisive papilla. Hatched area represents cross-section of denture flange required to replace lost tissue.

and the incisive papilla deviate towards the side of tooth loss. When a denture has been fitted soon after extraction of a central incisor, the scar tissue in the socket drags the papilla towards the side of tooth loss and the papilla may become inflamed by trauma from the denture. The general loss of buccal contour following extraction of teeth is illustrated in *Fig.* 2.9, which shows horizontal tracings through the maxillary alveolar process of a partially edentulous patient. The buccal contour of the alveolar process was reasonably smooth before any of the teeth were lost and the stippled areas of the diagram represent horizontal sections of the buccal flanges of a partial denture replacing the teeth that had been extracted.

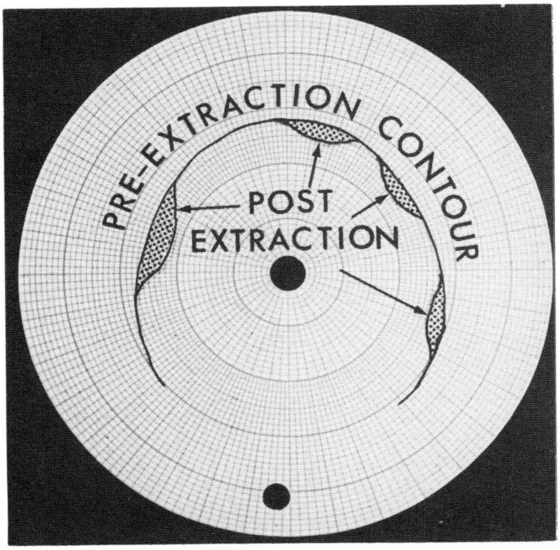

Fig. 2.9. Horizontal tracing through the maxillary alveolar process approximately midway between the mucogingival line and the gingival margin of a partially edentulous patient. The stippled areas represent the tissue loss that should be replaced by the partial denture. (Polar graph scale in mm.)

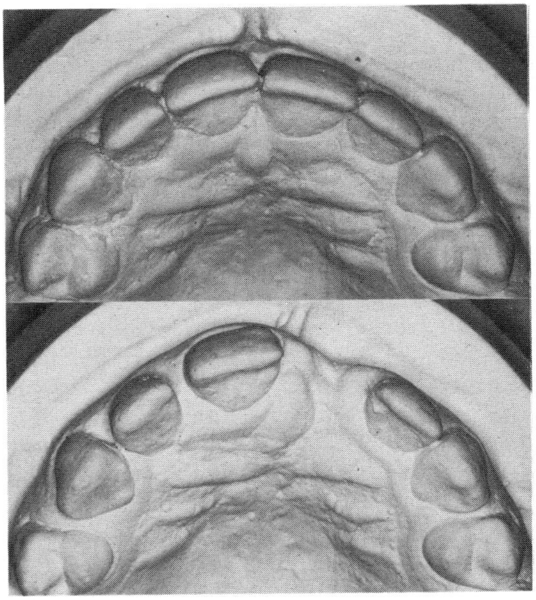

Fig. 2.10. Loss of the left central incisor caused drifting of the right anterior teeth and deviation of the incisive papilla towards the gap. Note the increased spaces between the right anterior teeth.

A common complaint of partially edentulous patients is that food sticks round the partial denture after eating. This can be reduced by correctly designing the flanges with fine margins on the attached gingivae. As far as possible the flanges should be 'streamlined' to reproduce the former alveolar contour.

After extraction the adjacent teeth frequently drift towards the gap. *Figs.* 2.8 and 2.10 illustrate this. In *Fig.* 2.10 the loss of the upper left central incisor has caused the right central incisor to drift towards the space and increased the interdental spaces between all three anterior teeth on the right side. A temporary denture that carries finger springs may be made to reposition the drifted teeth. This type of treatment is necessary if a fixed bridge is going to be fitted, but if removable partial dentures are made the teeth sometimes drift back and create problems if the dentures are left out for any length of time. Even leaving the denture out overnight can lead to uncomfortable wedging when it is replaced the following morning. This repeated trauma may damage the periodontium.

Streamlined Partial Dentures

We can make a great contribution to the comfort of our patients by designing 'streamlined' partial dentures. In effect this means that as far as possible the partial denture should replace only the lost parts and have as few 'extra-anatomical' parts as possible. One of the problems of wearing partial dentures is the amount of food that is left sticking to them after a meal. Many partial denture wearers have to take the denture out as soon as possible after eating in order to remove the unwanted debris. Streamlined partial dentures minimize this difficulty, but other factors in the design of partial dentures sometimes make streamlining impossible.

Saddles

The borders of saddles that lie on the attached mucosa should be knife-edged. In the sulcus the borders should be rounded but only to the extent necessary to replace the lost tissues. *Fig.* 2.11 shows a common error in design of a saddle margin compared with the streamlined

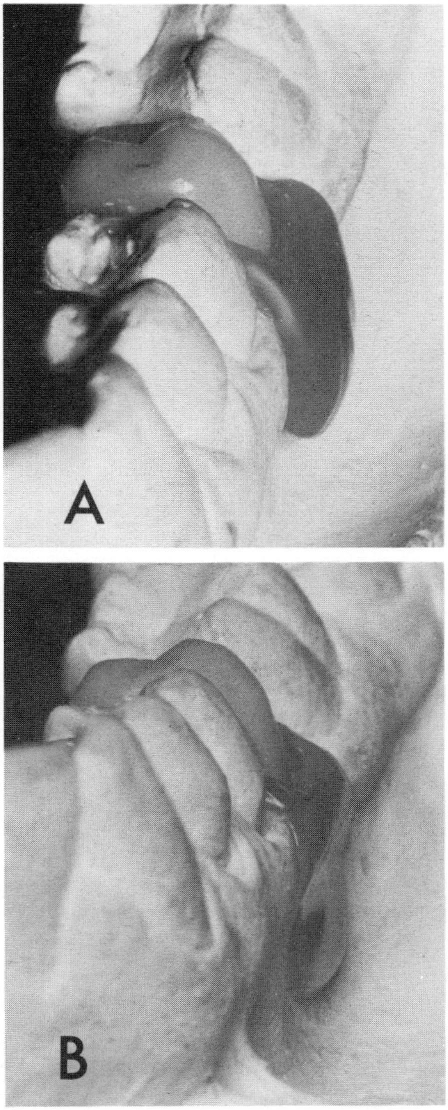

Fig. 2.11. **A,** Common error in design of saddle margins. **B,** Streamlined designs are less likely to trap food.

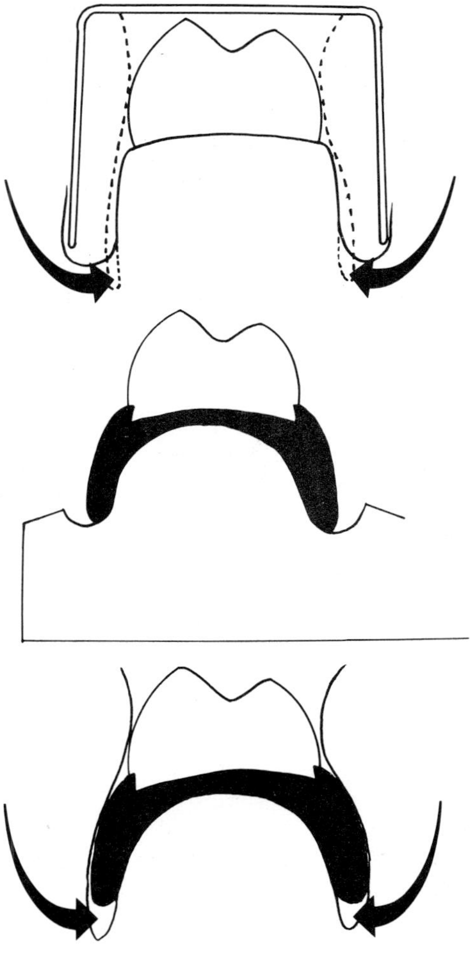

Fig. 2.12. *Upper,* Tray made with 2·5 mm spacer pushes cheek outwards and the tongue inwards and therefore distorts and reduces depth of buccal and lingual sulci. Dotted lines show true positions of cheek and tongue. *Middle,* The denture flanges are usually waxed to arbitrary thickness which is almost invariably less than the width of the distorted sulci, but is frequently greater than the amount of tissue lost. *Lower,* When the denture is placed in the mouth the cheek almost returns to its former position. Thus the sulcus deepens and a space (*arrowed*) appears below the margin of the denture flange. Food is trapped in this space when the denture is worn.

design that we recommend. You can see that the streamlined design replaces only the lost tissues and presents a smooth contour between the intact alveolar process and the denture, thus preventing the lodgement of food.

Streamlined margins can be formed on the cast by laying a wax knife parallel to the contour of the unabsorbed ridge and shaping the wax to the same contour. The margins in the sulcus present more of a problem as partial denture impression trays invariably distort the sulcus by stretching the reflected mucosa and drawing it away from the underlying bone (*Fig.* 2.12). When the denture is fitted the cheeks and tongue tend to fall back against the buccal and lingual sides of the ridge and leave gaps below the denture margins that were formed on a cast made from the over-extended

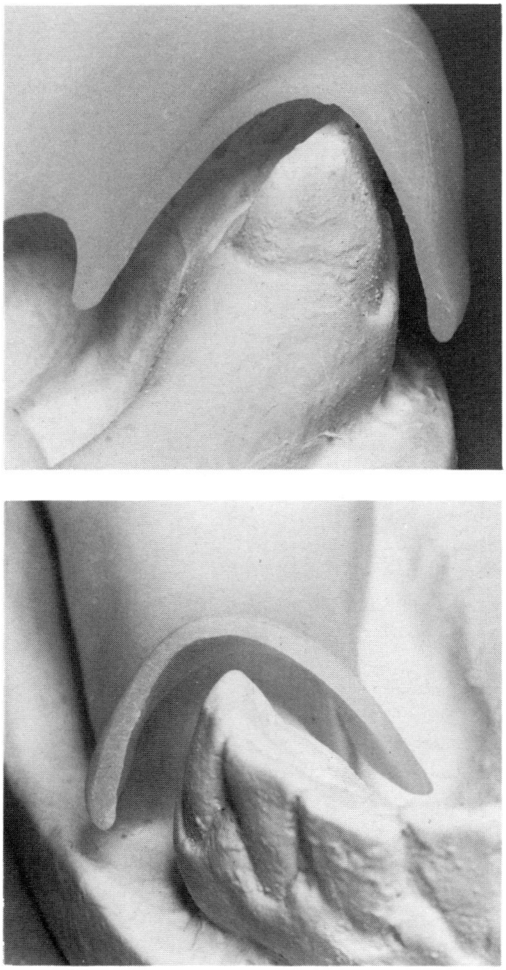

Fig. 2.13. *Upper,* Even an individual tray will produce sulcus distortion as sufficient room for impression material must be left between the tray and the teeth. *Lower,* The distortion is most evident in the section between the dentulous and edentulous parts of the tray.

impression. These gaps are a common cause of food trapping under the margins of partial dentures. Even individual trays produce sulcus distortion (*Fig.* 2.13), as sufficient room for the impression material must be left between the tray and the teeth. However, excessive distortion can be avoided by designing individual trays with closely fitting saddles and carefully adjusted margins, so that they do not stretch the mucosa. Impressions of the saddles are taken with impression paste, which is then trimmed back from the abutment teeth. When

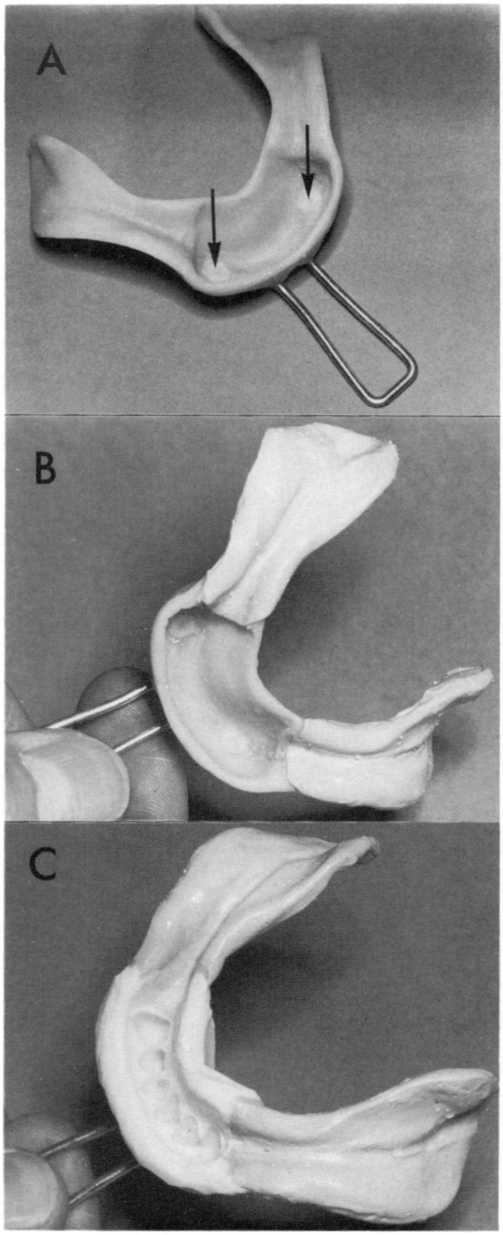

Fig. 2.14. **A,** Special impression tray for free-end saddle lower denture. The tray fits closely over the saddle area (0·5 mm spacer), but has a 2 mm spacer in the area of the teeth. Arrows indicate locating stops, which are removed after the saddle impressions are complete. **B,** Zinc-oxide–eugenol impression paste records the saddle areas. **C,** The impression is completed with alginate in the region of the teeth, while the saddle areas are compressed with finger pressure.

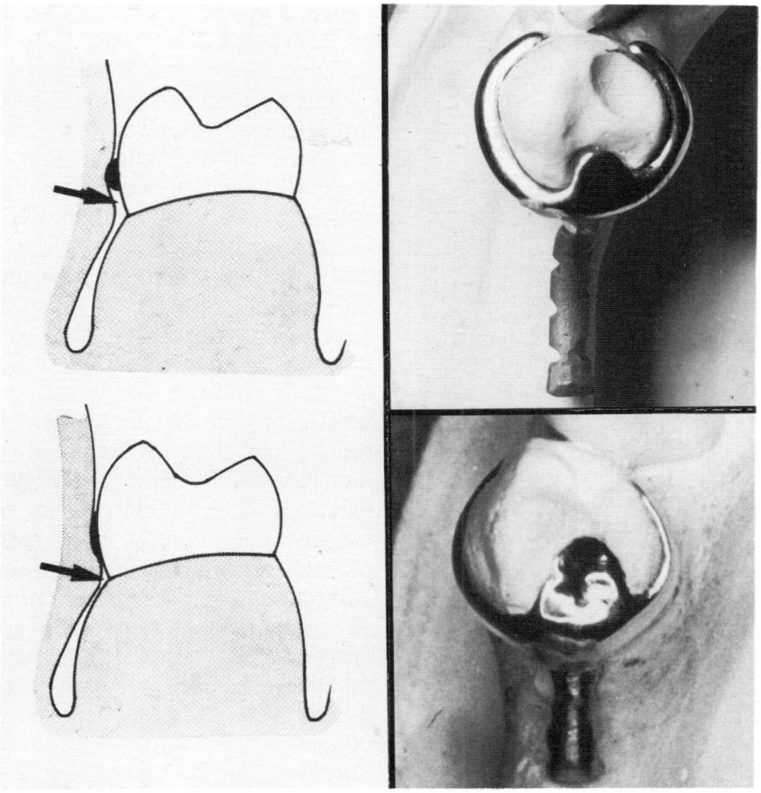

Fig. 2.15. Designs of clasps. *Upper,* A bulky clasp of half-round cross-section is likely to be uncomfortable and to trap food between cheek and tooth (*arrow*). *Lower,* A broader, flatter clasp is more comfortable.

the saddle contours are correct, the remainder of the impression is taken with alginate impression material while finger pressure is applied over the saddles. This technique improves the denture form and the comfort of the patient (*Fig.* 2.14).

A modification of the above method gives still more accuracy. The tray is constructed in much the same way, but the buccal flange is removed round all standing teeth, except for those to be used as abutments. Impression paste is used as before in the saddle areas, but a rubber impression material is used instead of alginate for taking the impression of the teeth. In this way the tray can be made with less space round the teeth and consequently there is less distortion of the sulcus. With this method it is essential to retain the occlusal stops on the tray to avoid distortion of the rubber impression material as it polymerises.

Retainers

Not only the saddles present food traps, but also the clasps. By their very nature external retainers are 'extra-anatomical' and distort the denture space. Buccal arms of clasps press into the cheek that enfolds them and trap the food around the clasp arms. Clasp arms are usually designed to taper in breadth and thickness towards their tips so that the stresses are distributed as evenly as possible throughout their length. We suggest that the narrow tapering clasp arms should be replaced by broader arms that taper more in breadth than in thickness. Although this design does not distribute stress so evenly throughout the structure, it is much more comfortable for the patient. An example of such a clasp is shown in *Fig.* 2.15.

Preparation of abutment teeth and provision

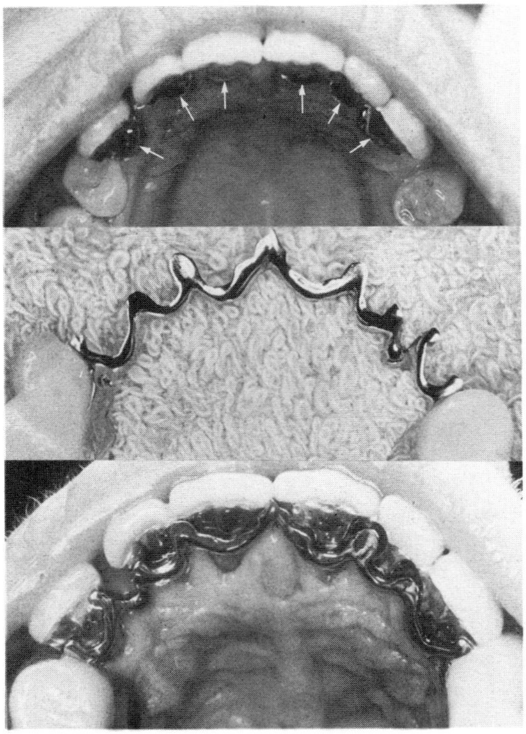

Fig. 2.16. *Upper,* Milled grooves in anterior restorations (*arrows*) to accommodate continuous clasp. *Middle,* Continuous clasp connector. *Lower,* Denture in mouth.

of slots and grooves in the abutment pieces to accommodate clasps and connectors can help to streamline the partial denture (*Fig.* 2.16). Complex partial dentures that have some fixed parts (such as abutment pieces) and some removable parts can be made to follow the principles of streamlining more easily than simple partial dentures with external retainers. Intra-coronal attachments (*see* Chapter 7) used in complex partial dentures help to streamline these appliances (*Fig.* 2.17). In complex dentures guide planes can be arranged so that there are no undercut spaces, whereas the simple denture has food traps in every area where undercuts have been blocked out to allow the insertion of the denture.

Connectors

Connectors on the lingual and palatal surfaces are additions to the anatomical contours and to some patients they are unacceptable encumbrances that interfere with the tongue so badly that the dentures cannot be tolerated (*Fig.* 2.18). Connectors, clasp arms and other parts of partial dentures that are added to the normal anatomical contours on the lingual side are less well tolerated than 'extra-anatomical' additions on the buccal side. Thick narrow bars or clasps are worse than thin flat bars and clasps. Thus, when designing a reciprocal arm to counter-balance a buccal clasp arm, it is better for the comfort of the patient to extend the lingual plate on to the tooth rather than have a clasp arm on the lingual side. For instance, a lingual bar plus a continuous clasp is often difficult for a patient to tolerate, whereas a thin flat lingual plate is much more easily accepted, although it may be more damaging to the gingival margins. As might be expected, bars or clasps near the edge of the tongue cause more interference than those placed elsewhere. For instance, a sturdy continuous clasp used as a primary connector is less easily tolerated than a sublingual bar (*Fig.* 2.19). Patients find bars crossing the palate near the postdam region are more comfortable than anterior or middle palatal connectors. Anterior connectors are least well tolerated of all parts of a partial upper denture. Farrell (1969, 1971) showed that the anterior part of the palate should not be covered in any way if it is possible to design the denture to avoid it. Bars that cross the anterior part of the palate should be positioned in the grooves between the rugae.

Peripheral Length

A general principle of sound denture design is to keep it simple. Since simplicity in design is often associated with the peripheral length of a denture, it is reasonable to suggest that the shorter the periphery of a denture, the more easily it is tolerated. Complicated dentures of 'skeleton' design often have unnecessary connectors and unduly long peripheries. Examples of these are shown in *Fig.* 2.20. These dentures may be difficult for the patient to tolerate. Palatal bars running parallel to the gingival margins, and 4 or 5 mm away from them in the premolar region, lie in positions that are constantly being tapped and rubbed by the tongue, as the direct palatograph in *Fig.* 2.21 shows. Where a single tooth is standing on its own, it is not worth making the connector

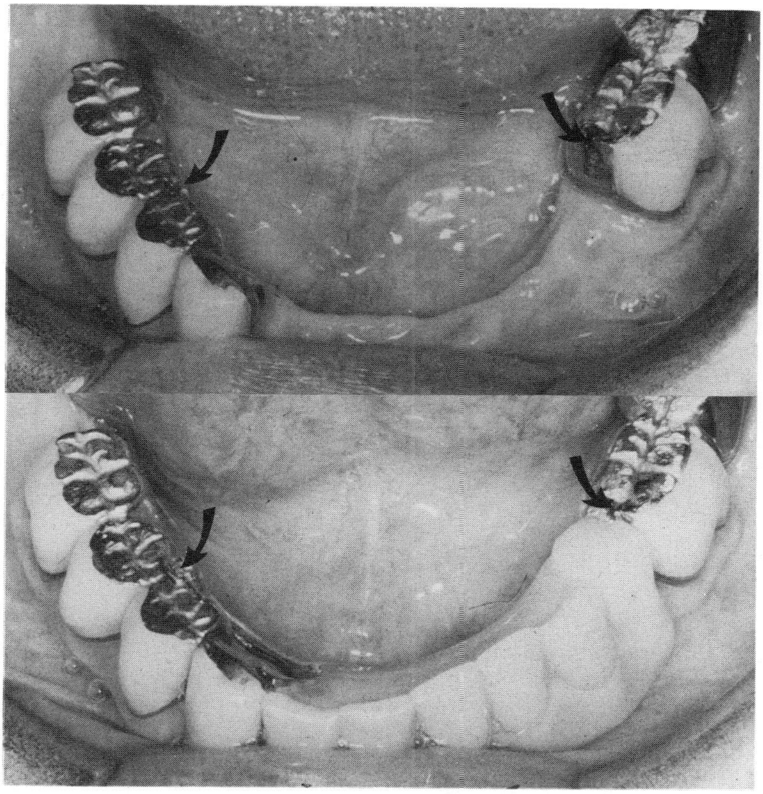

Fig. 2.17. Intracoronal attachments (*arrows*) help to streamline this mandibular partial denture.

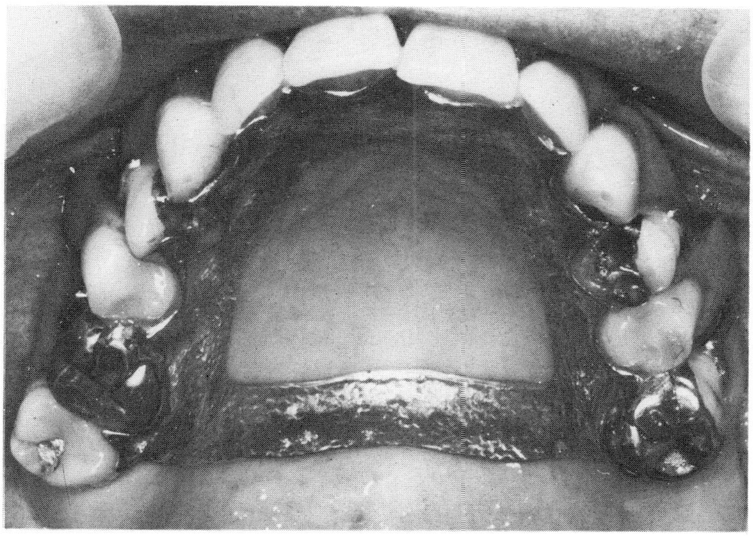

Fig. 2.18. Thick major connectors crossing the palate obstruct the tongue and are unacceptable encumbrances for some patients.

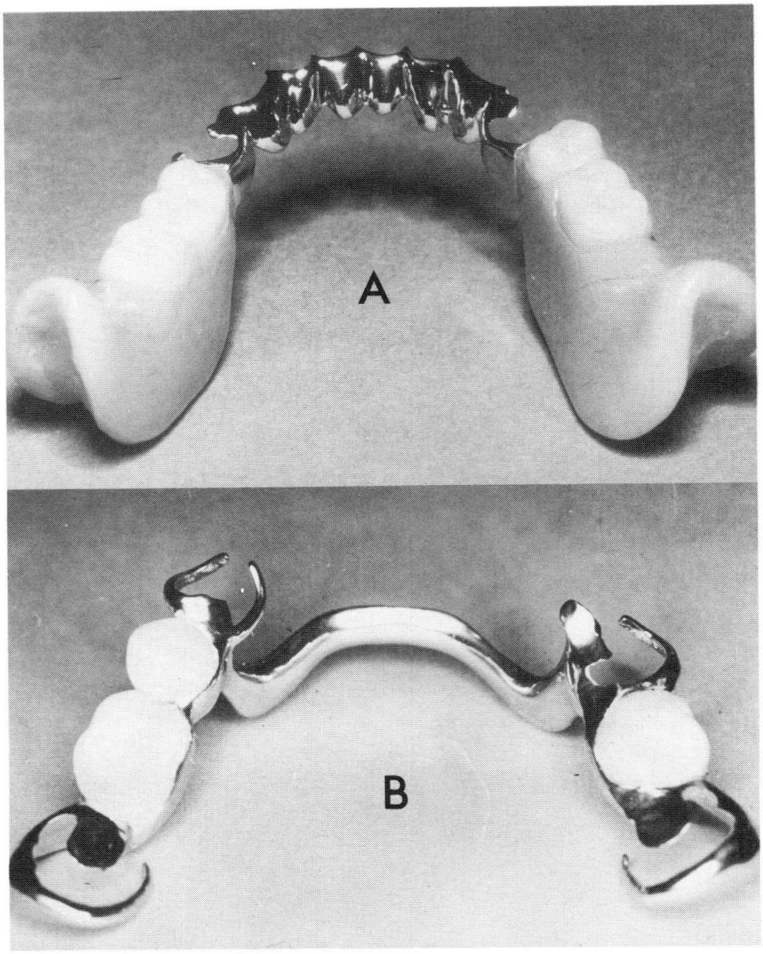

Fig. 2.19. Bars or clasps near the edge of the tongue cause more interference than when placed elsewhere. For instance, a sturdy continuous clasp **(A)** used as a primary connector is less easily tolerated than a sublingual bar **(B)**.

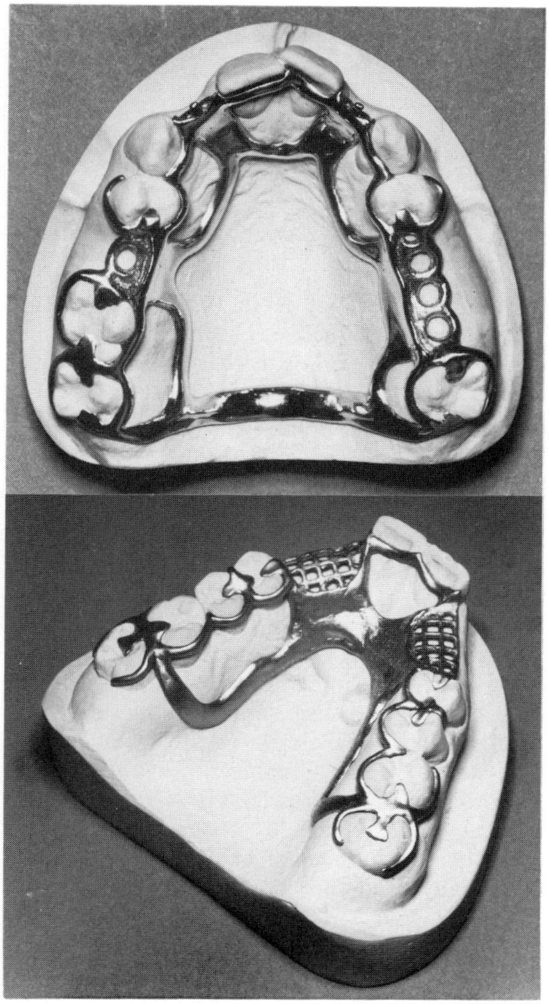

Fig. 2.20. Examples of dentures with unnecessarily complicated designs which might be difficult for patients to tolerate.

avoid the gingival margin as this leaves an uncomfortable food trap that irritates the

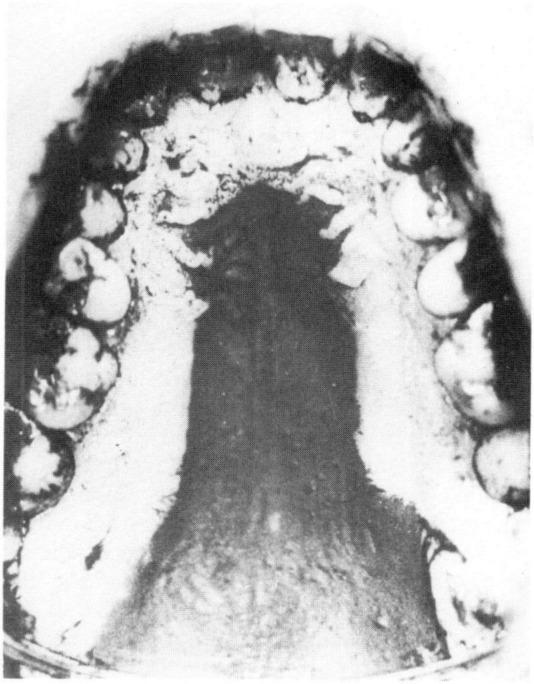

Fig. 2.21. Direct palatograph following the pronunciation of the word 'tea'. Where possible the edges of connectors should not be placed in the lateral areas that are wiped clean by tongue contact.

tongue. In such cases the design can be simplified by carrying a lingual plate connector over the gingival margins. Details of individual clasp and connector designs are given in Chapters 6 and 8.

An important guiding principle in designing is that as far as possible all partial dentures should be streamlined; that is, they should lie within the normal anatomical contours of the mouth.

Chapter 3

The supporting tissues

Support Deficit

At this point it is appropriate to consider the structures that support partial dentures. When a natural tooth is lost the total area of its periodontium is also lost and the area of mucosa that remains to support the load on an artificial replacement is less than the periodontal area of the lost tooth. There is therefore a deficit in the support available for all partial dentures. An indication of the size of this deficit is given by the ratio of the support area of the residual mucosa in the gap to the periodontal area of the extracted tooth or teeth. For example, a lower first molar has a mucosal/periodontal ratio of approximately 1 : 4. This means that the area of the periodontium of the molar is about four times that of the mucosal support area left in the gap after the extraction of the tooth (*Fig.* 3.1).

Several authors have measured the periodontal areas of teeth (*Table* 3.1). Ante (1926) produced figures, but gave no details of either the number of teeth measured or the method of measurement. Watt et al. (1958) measured the periodontal areas of five teeth of each type by coating the roots with a plastic film that was removed and measured (*Fig.* 3.2). Their results were later confirmed by Jepsen (1963) (*Table* 3.1). A paper by Crabb and Wilson (1974) described a method of measuring periodontal areas of canine teeth.

In a statement by Johnston et al. (1971), designated as 'Ante's Law', it was proposed that the root surface area of the abutment teeth should equal or be greater than that of the teeth being replaced with pontics. According to Kantorowicz (1979) this is good clinical advice and a convenient way of assessing the number of abutments is to count how many teeth are to be replaced and add

Table 3.1 **Average measurements of root surface areas in mm²**

Type of tooth	*Ante (1926)*	*Watt et al. (1958)*	*Jepsen (1963)*
Upper			
Central incisor	139·0	204·5	204·0
Lateral incisor	112·0	177·3	179·0
Canine	204·0	266·5	273·0
1st premolar	149·0	219·7	234·0
2nd premolar	140·0	216·7	220·0
1st molar	335·0	454·8	433·0
2nd molar	272·0	416·9	431·0
3rd molar	197·0	305·3	—
Lower			
Central incisor	103·0	162·2	154·0
Lateral incisor	124·0	174·8	168·0
Canine	159·0	272·2	268·0
1st premolar	130·0	196·9	180·0
2nd premolar	135·0	204·3	207·0
1st molar	352·0	450·3	431·0
2nd molar	282·0	399·7	426·0
3rd molar	190·0	372·9	—

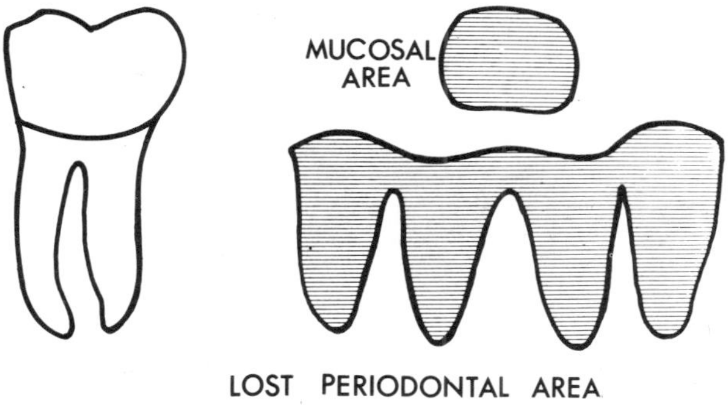

Fig. 3.1. Periodontal area of extracted first lower molar compared with the area of mucosa left in the gap. The support deficit is the ratio between these areas and is 4 : 1 = 75%.

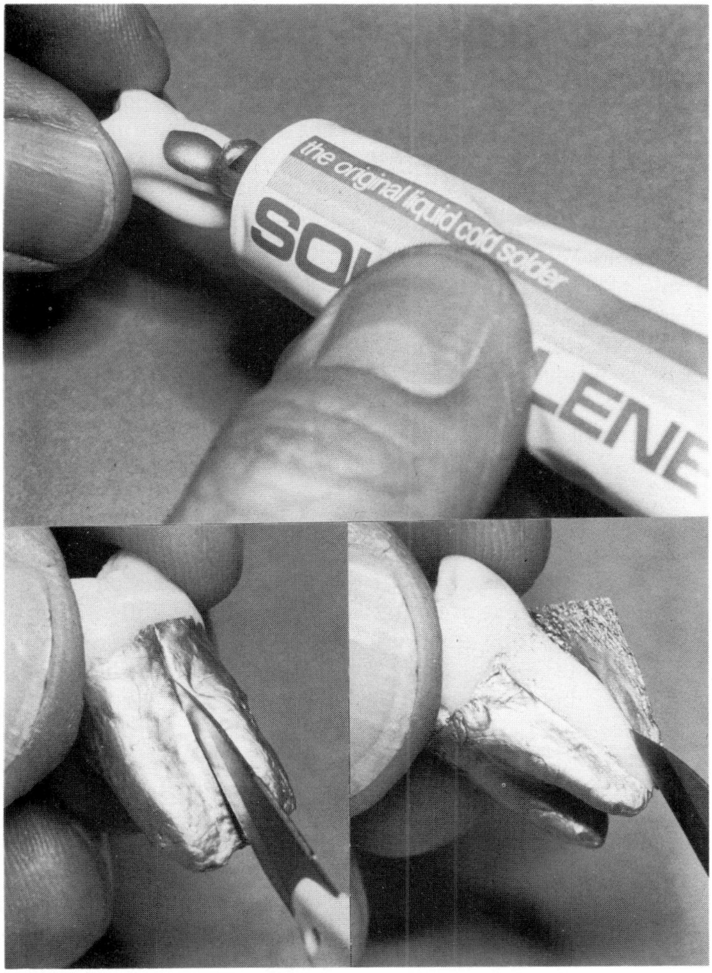

Fig. 3.2. A method of measuring the periodontal area by coating the root of a tooth with plastic film, then removing the film and measuring its area.

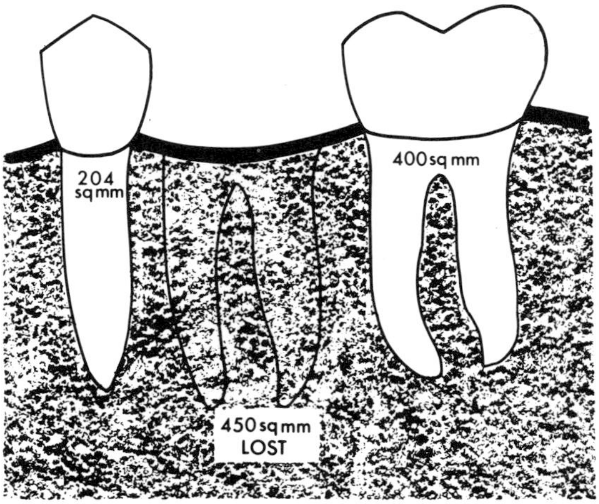

Fig. 3.3. The ratio between the *R*emaining and *L*ost tooth support (R/L ratio), as measured by periodontal surface areas, gives a quantitative assessment of the support available for partial dentures. In this case the remaining tooth support is 204 + 400 sq mm = 604 sq mm and the lost support is 450 sq mm. The R/L ratio is 604/450 = 1·3. The area of mucosa in the gap was 97 sq mm, 21·6% of the lost periodontal area.

one to the total. We would not dispute this as it is a safe general rule. The 'R/L ratio' is the ratio of the periodontal area of the *R*emaining teeth to the periodontal area of the *L*ost teeth (*Fig.* 3.3). While it is desirable to have an R/L ratio of at least 1·0, R/L ratios of 0·75 are acceptable in some instances. *Table* 3.2 shows that the R/L ratios of most one-tooth and two-tooth gaps exceed 1·0 (Ante's requirement), but two-molar gaps have an R/L ratio of only 0·6. These ratios are based on the assumption that the teeth immediately next to the gap are the only ones used as abutments, but of course if two molars were missing in one quadrant both premolars could be used as anterior abutments and that would improve the R/L ratio to about 0·85. In free-end saddles, where there is only one abutment tooth, the R/L ratios are very low.

The Effect of Periodontal Disease

Periodontal disease may reduce the amount of periodontal area quite spectacularly. For instance, a 2 mm reduction of the alveolar margin all round a maxillary first premolar reduces the periodontal area by about 15 per cent. The R/L ratio should be modified accordingly where periodontal disease is present. It is therefore essential that an appropriate measurement of periodontal disease should be made before partial dentures are constructed. Various periodontal indices are available for this (Miller, 1938; Russell, 1956; Laster et al., 1975; Lindhe and Nyman 1975; Hibberd, 1981).

Nature of Tooth Support

Teeth are not objects embedded firmly in inanimate bone, but are vital structures that move with every heart beat (Parfitt, 1960, 1961, Manderson, Wills and Picton, 1979). They are connected to the bone through the periodontal membrane, which not only transmits the heart beat to the teeth, but also enables the teeth to move into their sockets when vertical forces are applied and to move sideways when horizontal forces are applied. The mathematics of tooth movement has been extensively studied (Synge, 1933; Bien, 1966; Mühlemann, 1967; Körber, 1971; Wills, 1974; Wills, Picton and Davies, 1976). Some of these are classic mathematical studies (Synge, 1933; Thompson, 1933; Hay, 1939), while others are related to studies of animal and human teeth. It is the latter that interest us most.

First, displacement and force are related by a power function:

$$\text{Intrusion} = K(\text{force})^M$$

(where K and M are positive constants).

The actual intrusion varies according to the amount and direction of the applied force. The tooth does not fully return to its rest position until 1 or 2 minutes after the release of loading (Parfitt, 1960), but after 10 seconds it has recovered most of its position, although it is still partly intruded (*Fig.* 3.4). The simple factor that characterizes the intrusion of teeth is not true for the recovery phase from maximum displacement. This phase has been compared to that of a Voigt element (Voigt, 1928).

During chewing the recorded loads on pressure transducers tend to become larger towards the end of mastication, starting at 2 kg of force and ending at 6 kg of force when carrot is being chewed (Anderson, 1956a, b).

Table 3.2 **R/L ratios for different gaps in the dental arch**

Extracted teeth	*Lost tooth support (sq mm)*	*Abutment teeth*	*Remaining tooth support (sq mm)*	*R/L ratio*
⌊1	205	1⌋⌊2	382	1·9
⌈1	162	1⌉⌈2	337	2·1
⌊2	177	⌊13	472	2·7
⌈2	175	⌈13	434	2·5
⌊3	267	⌊24	397	1·5
⌈3	272	⌈24	372	1·4
⌊4	220	⌊35	484	2·2
⌈4	197	⌈35	476	2·4
⌊5	217	⌊46	675	3·1
⌈5	204	⌈46	647	3·2
⌊6	455	⌊57	634	1·4
⌈6	450	⌈57	604	1·3
⌊7	417	⌊68	760	1·8
⌈7	400	⌈68	823	2·0
⌊12	382	1⌋⌊3	472	1·2
⌈12	337	1⌉⌈3	434	1·3
⌊45	437	⌊36	722	1·6
⌈45	401	⌈36	722	1·8
⌊56	672	⌊47	637	0·9
⌈56	654	⌈47	597	0·9
⌊67	872	⌊58	522	0·6
⌈67	850	⌈58	532	0·6
21⌋⌊12	764	3⌋⌊3	534	0·7
21⌉⌈12	674	3⌉⌈3	544	0·8
⌊456	892	⌊37	684	0·8
⌈456	851	⌈37	672	0·8
⌊567	1089	⌊48	525	0·5
⌈567	1054	⌈48	570	0·5
⌊678	1177	⌊5	217	0·2
⌈678	1178	⌈5	204	0·2
⌊5678	1394	⌊4	220	0·2
⌈5678	1382	⌈4	197	0·1
⌊45678	1614	⌊3	267	0·2
⌈45678	1679	⌈3	272	0·2

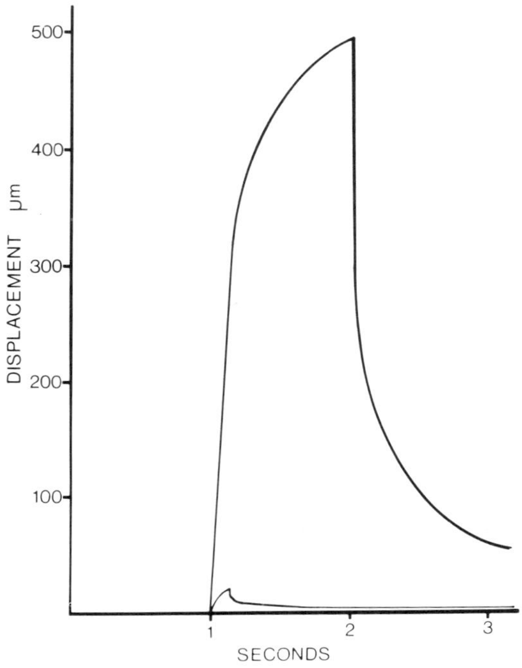

Fig. 3.4. The displacement of a tooth (*lower graph*) and of mucosa (*upper graph*) in response to an axial load of 4 Newtons applied at a rate of 4 N/sec. It can be seen that the mucosal displacement is very much more than the tooth displacement. Note that on removal of the load recovery is not completed in the time indicated. (*After* Manderson, Wills and Picton, 1979, pp. 98–101.)

The delayed creep compliance of teeth decreases with increasing force and time. This reduction of creep as the supporting structures become more and more stressed is consistent with a progressive transfer of load to the more rigid structures around the teeth, but this is not always applicable for loading intervals of less than 0·5 sec (Wills and Manderson, 1977). The only component of the linear Voigt element found to change consistently is the spring constant added to account for the instantaneous recoil. For recovery from 250 g force, this spring accounts for 50–60 per cent of the displacement, while for recovery from 40 g force this proportion is reduced to 30–40 per cent. The relationship between force F, displacement S and time t is:

$$S = at^nF^m$$

(where t and F do not equal zero and where a, m and n are positive constants).

This was first propounded by Nutting (1921). Skin also shows a power relation between force and stretching under tension (Gibson et al., 1965; Ridge and Wright, 1965; Kenedi and Cowden, 1976). The tooth support tissues also follow this law.

In practical terms there is less intrusion of teeth caused by suddenly applied forces than by slowly applied forces and once intruded teeth take some time to recover their former positions.

Periodontal Responses to Loads

The periodontal response to forces on the teeth has been investigated by a number of clinicians and their results are important when designing partial dentures for mouths already mutilated by the loss of a number of teeth. Gottlieb and Orban (1931) studied tissue changes in experimental traumatic occlusion and Waerhaug (1955) investigated the effect of occlusal stress in a sample of dogs and concluded that the supporting structures seemed to be well suited to prevent permanent damage caused by occlusal overloading. However, under unfavourable conditions undue occlusal stress can increase the depth of clinical pockets below the amelocemental junction. Wentz et al. (1958) studied the effects of buccolingual jiggling occlusal trauma in a sample of Macacus monkeys. The periodontal space widened to more than three times the original width, but the periodontal fibres were histologically normal and functionally arranged. The teeth were hypermobile, but neither gingivitis nor periodontitis was evident.

Ramfjord and Kohler (1959) pointed out that the alveolar crest fibres maintain the alveolar crest bone and are the most persistent fibres in preventing any downgrowth of epithelium and pocket formation in relation to traumatic changes. From their study, which involved adults from 16 to 68 years, the following conclusions were made:

1. The most stable periodontal structures with regard to changes in occlusal stress appear to be Sharpey's fibres entering the cementum and the periodontal fibres coronally to the margin of the alveolar crest.

2. Most of the adaptation of periodontal

fibres to change in functional demand takes place at the surface of the alveolar bone and the middle zone of the periodontal membrane.

3. Disuse atrophy of functionally-orientated periodontal fibres in adults is a slow process.

4. Loss of posterior teeth may lead to traumatic occlusion of anterior teeth with such sequelae as resorption of the surface of the root (extending into dentine) and resorption of the alveolar bone with perforation of the labial wall of the alveolar process.

5. Remodelling of the alveolar process in response to changes in functional occlusal stress occurred in all subjects of the study.

In a later paper Ramfjord (1974) discussed other periodontal aspects of restorative dentistry. Glickman (1963) believed that trauma from occlusion did not cause inflammation or periodontal pockets in periodontitis, but when trauma was combined with inflammation it caused destruction of the supporting tissues.

Lindhe and Nyman (1977) reviewed the literature on the significance of occlusal trauma in the aetiology of periodontal disease and commented on their own experiences with Beagle dogs. They concluded that the forces produced by occlusal trauma were unable to induce progressive destruction of the periodontal tissues when the supporting tissues were markedly reduced but not infected by plaque. Jiggling occlusal trauma did not cause further destruction of the attachment once the plaque-induced disease had been cured. These results indicate that, when large-span bridges are placed on teeth with markedly reduced but not inflamed periodontal tissues, the mobility of the isolated abutment teeth is not a problem. It is critical, however, that the fixed prosthesis as a whole shows no increasing mobility or migration with time. The bridge can be stable in spite of a minimal amount of supporting tissue and in spite of hypermobility of isolated abutment teeth, especially when the prosthesis has a cross-arch design. It should be understood that the term 'stability' as used by Lindhe and Nyman (1977) does not necessarily imply no mobility, but merely that the mobility of the bridge does not increase with time.

In further investigations Nyman et al. (1978) demonstrated that repetitive mechanical injury, resulting in a progressive increase of tooth mobility, produced an enhanced rate of destruction of the supporting apparatus in dogs that already had periodontal tissue breakdown. This observation should be compared with the results produced by Svanberg and Lindhe (1973) and Lindhe and Svanberg (1974). They studied the effect of jiggling forces on premolars of dogs that had either a normal periodontium or an ongoing experimentally-induced periodontitis. In dogs with normal periodontium, jiggling forces induced one phase of increasing tooth mobility which had a duration of around 60 days, and was followed by a phase during which the tooth mobility was increased, but no longer increasing. During this latter phase, the periodontal tissues became adapted to the altered functional demands; the periodontal membrane was wider than normal, but contained a normal number of blood vessels. The vessels did not display signs of altered permeability, the bone surface of the periodontal ligament presented only a few osteoclasts, and there was no loss of connective tissue attachment. When the same experiment was repeated in dogs with experimental periodontitis, similar jiggling forces produced an extended phase of progressive (i.e. increasing) tooth mobility. During the entire period of jiggling the periodontal tissues were unable to adjust to the abnormal occlusal load. Hence, throughout 6 months of observation the gradually increasing tooth mobility was accompanied by an increase in size of the periodontal membrane space. In addition, the periodontal tissues contained an increased number of osteoclasts and an increased number of vessels that displayed signs of altered permeability. In these dogs trauma from occlusion was accompanied by an increased rate of attachment loss and downgrowth of pocket epithelium.

Galler et al. (1979) found no evidence that splinting of teeth benefits the periodontium following osseous surgery and that the only justifications for splinting were patient comfort, replacement of missing teeth or post-orthodontic retention.

Polson (1980) reviewed the investigations

on squirrel monkeys and Beagle dogs and noted that mesiodistal jiggling displacing forces result in morphological alterations in the periodontal membrane and alveolar bone. These changes, however, do not initiate the loss of connective-tissue attachment, which is a characteristic of marginal periodontitis. Elimination of trauma, in the presence of existing marginal inflammation, does not reduce tooth mobility or increase bone volume. He concluded that resolution of marginal inflammation is of prime importance in the management of periodontal disease.

In orthodontic treatment the duration of the application of force is important since a light force over a period of time may overcome the natural resiliency of the periodontal membrane and act like a heavier force over a shorter time. In other words, a small force over a period of time can cause changes in tooth position. A tooth in normal occlusion with opposing teeth can be moved into a traumatic relationship by such a force (Weinstein et al., 1963).

The direction of the force applied to a tooth causes different responses in the periodontium and this determines the amount of resulting damage (Moyers and Bauer, 1950). For example, Clayton (1966) has shown that an axial force of 90 lb on a tooth displaces it no more than a transverse force of 5 lb—eighteen times less than the axial force. Changes in the periodontium caused by increased force on the teeth are reversible in the healthy periodontium, although tooth mobility is increased (Stuteville, 1937; Bhaskar and Orban, 1955), while in an unhealthy periodontium, force can be destructive to the supporting tissues (Glickman and Smulow 1962).

Picton and Moss (1973) have demonstrated experimentally the importance of the trans-septal fibres in maintaining tooth position in adult monkeys. The contraction of the trans-septal fibres, together with the shape and continuity of contact areas between teeth, maintain the correct relationship of teeth (Moss and Picton, 1974).

Lilja et al. (1981) presented a method that correlated the compression of the periodontium with orthodontic forces and evaluated the histological changes. When orthodontic forces are applied to teeth, there is immediately a small tooth movement, which is restricted to periodontal membrane alterations. Then there is a period when no tooth movement takes place and the tissues show signs of damage. After this rapid tooth movement occurs because of bone resorption (King and Fischlschweiger, 1982).

Adaptive Responses

Provided it is within physiological limits, a constant force applied to a tooth causes remodelling of the bone around the tooth. There is intermittent resorption and repair (active bone resorption where there is pressure and deposition of bone where there is tension) (Goldman and Gianelly, 1972), and thus the tooth moves into a position that reduces the applied force. Equal intermittent forces applied to a tooth from opposite directions result in an increase in width of its periodontium. This adaptive change causes an increased mobility of the tooth so that the forces can be sustained without damage to the underlying bone and periodontal structures. When the intermittent forces are removed from such a tooth, the periodontium generally returns to its normal thickness and the mobility of the tooth reduces to within normal limits (Mühlemann, 1967). Intermittent forces on a tooth that come from different directions are seldom balanced, usually being greater in one direction than in another. When a thin wrought clasp arm is opposite a rigid clasp arm, unequal forces are exerted on the abutment tooth and as a result the adaptive response of the periodontium is unequal (Catena, 1972). In the cervical third of the root it thickens more on the side opposite the rigid arm, so that the difference in the flexibility of the two components of the clasp is balanced by the difference in the compressibility of the adapted periodontium owing to rotation of the tooth. Near the apex the thickening takes place on the same side as the rigid arm (*Fig.* 3.5). This may account for a partial denture becoming more comfortable after some weeks. It may also account for the changes in tooth position that can occur if the partial denture is left out of the mouth for any length of time. The periodontium tends to recover its normal thickness in relation to the forces of natural teeth upon it, having been

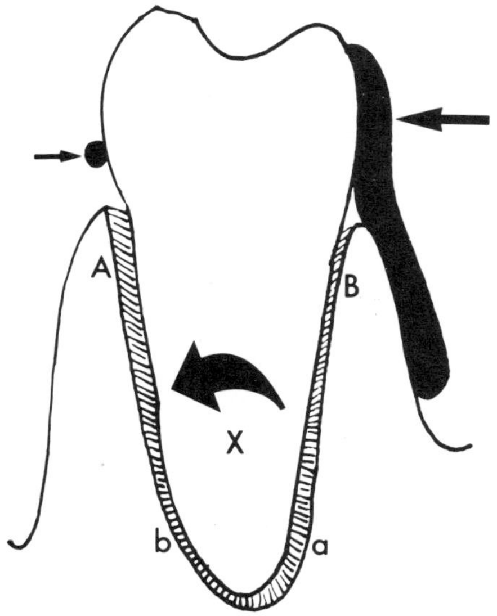

Fig. 3.5. The theoretical effects on the periodontium of a rigid plate exerting large forces on one side of a tooth opposed by a flexible clasp arm transmitting smaller forces on the opposite side. The buccal periodontal width (A) increases opposite the rigid lingual arm, while the lingual periodontium (B) opposite the flexible arm is less affected. Since the tooth rotates in the direction of the curved arrow around a fulcrum (X), compensating changes are also found at 'a' and 'b'. Thus thickening at 'A' and 'a' provides cushioning for the larger forces from the rigid plate, while the flexible arm absorbs some of the energy, and 'cushioning' at 'B' and 'b' is not required. Thus, the forces on the tooth are equalized.

relieved from the abnormal forces produced by the partial denture. This highlights the complexity of designing partial dentures and the need to take into account all the responses that can occur in the mouth.

The general principle to be followed is that the appliance should require the least possible adaptation by the tissues, since any adaptive response can be considered to use up the 'adaptive potential'. Hence the mouth is less able to cope with additional trauma or changes in occlusal forces. Before a partial denture is made the occlusion should be stabilized and the final impressions should be postponed until the periodontium has recovered sufficiently to ensure that the teeth remain in stable positions. *Fig.* 3.6 shows the gnathosonic record of a patient before and after the occlusion has been stabilized. Note that once stabilized the occlusion remains stable (*Fig.* 3.7) (Watt, 1981). It is unwise to make a partial denture for a patient unless the occlusion has first been stabilized in the mouth, because premature contacts of teeth call forth postural adaptive responses (*Fig.* 3.8) and the whole masticatory activity is upset by this. Such abnormal activity puts excessive stresses on the partial denture and hence on the abutment teeth. Stabilization of the occlusion ensures that minimum adaptation is required by the periodontium. In patients

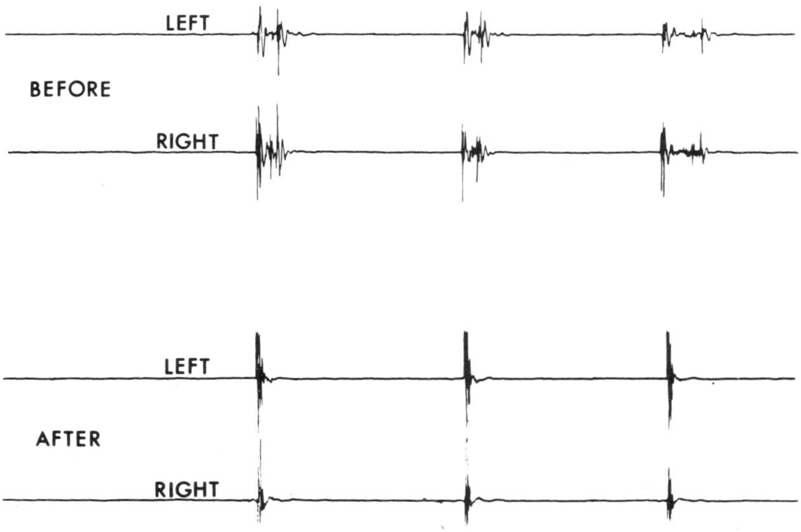

Fig. 3.6. Gnathosonic records of a patient before (*upper*) and after (*lower*) stabilization of occlusion.

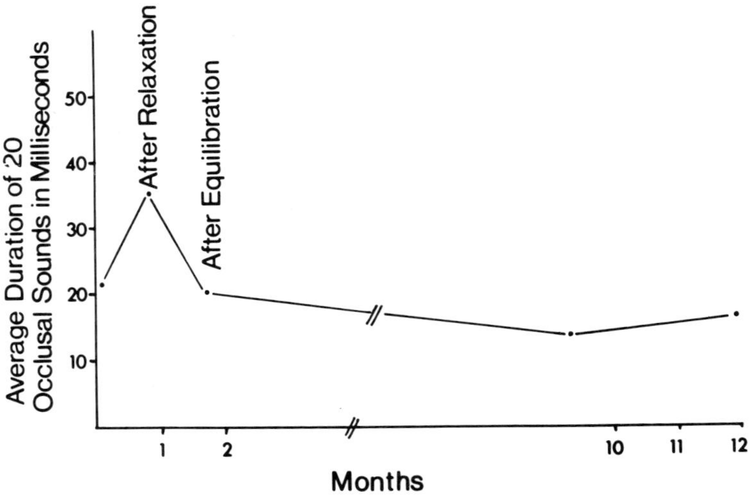

Fig. 3.7. The average duration of the sounds of 20 snapping contacts of teeth provides a measure of the stability of the occlusion. This graph shows that after relaxation of the hypertonic muscles the average duration of occlusal sounds increased. This indicated an unstable occlusion. After the premature contacts were located and removed, the occlusion became stable, as indicated by a low average sound duration, and remained so over the course of 12 months.

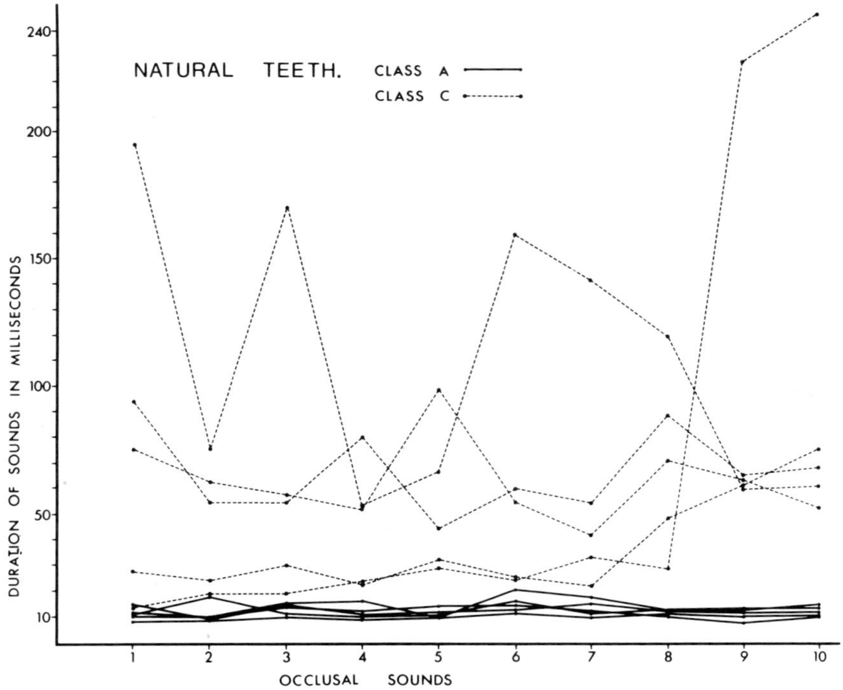

Fig. 3.8. The durations of 10 successive occlusal sounds in each of 5 patients with Class C unstable occlusions (dotted lines) and in 5 patients with Class A stable occlusions (continuous lines) (Watt, 1981, p. 57).

with a stable occlusion the natural teeth remain in position when the dentures are removed, but when the occlusion is unstable the teeth move and a new periodontal trauma occurs each morning as the denture is forced into place. This indicates either a fault in the denture or a failure to stabilize the occlusion of the natural teeth and when the denture is newly fitted the patient may have considerable difficulty accommodating to it.

The periodontium is never called upon to make the full adaptive response required to accommodate to a patient's malocclusion. This is because the patient's first response to a malocclusion is postural, whereby high cusps are avoided by altering the position of the mandible. If this postural adaptation is completely successful and can be maintained without muscle pain, the periodontium may be required to adapt very little or not at all. However, considerable periodontal adaptation may be necessary if an occlusal dilemma develops (Watt, 1981), whereby postural adaptation to avoid one high contact produces another traumatic contact of the teeth. Such dilemmas produce jiggling forces that may harm the periodontium.

The adaptation could be expressed as:

$$A = P + p + j$$

(where A is total adaptation, P the postural component, p the periodontal component and j the joint component).

The greater the amount of postural adaptation, the less periodontal adaptation is required. The joint remodelling component of adaptation is likely to require a longer time and its contribution, while recognized, is not considered to be large. In effect, the periodontal component $(p) = A - P$. The fundamental point is that the adaptation required by the periodontium is a comparatively small part of the total adaptation to a malocclusion, and only becomes significant in dilemma situations.

Nature of Mucosal Support

Far less is known about the deformation characteristics of oral mucosa than about periodontal membrane and the supporting structures of teeth. However, if a load is sustained for a long period, the mucosa may be compressed to 45 per cent of its original thickness, the distortion and recovery being viscoelastic in nature (Picton and Wills, 1978).

When mucosa is under load its displacement obeys a power law in much the same way as periodontal membrane, but according to Wills and Manderson (1977) the mucosa appears to take rather longer to recover its original position than the teeth, so that in tooth-and-mucosa-borne dentures over time a change will take place in the relationship between the mucosal surface and the tooth surface. In other words, the mucosa of a saddle will remain depressed long after the natural teeth have returned to their resting position. The amount of displacement of mucosa can be up to twenty times that of teeth (Manderson et al., 1979) and if the area of contact of the saddle is small there is greater intrusion into the mucosa than with large saddles (Picton and Wills, 1978). These findings should be seen in relation to the thickness of mucosa of the alveolar ridge crests of a sample of edentulous human subjects (Kydd et al., 1971):

In the mandible,	anterior mucosal thickness	$= 1{\cdot}9 \pm 0{\cdot}6$ mm
	premolar region	$= 2{\cdot}3 \pm 0{\cdot}5$ mm
In the maxilla,	premolar region	$= 1{\cdot}2 \pm 0{\cdot}5$ mm
	molar region	$= 4{\cdot}2 \pm 0{\cdot}7$ mm

Kydd and Daly (1982) reported on the effect of load on the mucosa of dogs. They confirmed that the behaviour was viscoelastic. On release of load there was an instantaneous elastic recovery followed by a delayed elastic recovery that lasted up to 2 hours. The system was highly non-linear since doubling the load only increased the change in thickness by an additional 5 per cent. Initially there was a greater degree of deformation in the epithelial layer than in the submucosa, but both layers reached maximum deformation in 15 minutes under a 20-gramme load.

The recovery of mucosa after removal of load is not a simple elastic one, the rate partly depending on the return of extracellular fluids to the area. Recovery is faster when the loading rate (cyclic loading) is high, since in that case the fluid has less chance of being displaced from the tissues. In older patients (68–70 years) a longer period is needed for the recovery of displaced mucosa than in a younger group of patients (21–27 years).

The various features of mucosal behaviour under load must be taken into account when designing partial dentures that derive part of the support from teeth and part from mucosa. In later chapters we consider the implications in greater depth.

Chapter 4

Use of support

We have discussed the structures that provide support for partial dentures and now we will consider the loads to which the dentures are subjected. Dentures should be designed to ensure an efficient distribution of load over the available support. We shall first consider the vertical loads and the support given to these loads by the teeth and mucosa (Watt et al., 1958) and then discuss the more complex lateral loads to which partial dentures are subjected.

Support of Partial Dentures in Relation to Vertical Loads

The greatest loads to which teeth are subjected are applied along their long axes approximately at right angles to the occlusal plane. We can divide these loads into two groups: masticatory loads and clenched loads.

Masticatory Loads

Masticatory loads are applied to a denture and its supporting tissues during mastication. The loads vary with the muscle activity, type of food and the occlusal surface area of the teeth.

Several workers have studied masticatory loads. Bearn (1973) used a hydraulic system to measure chewing forces between artificial teeth and denture bases. He found that the greater the area of the contacting teeth, the greater the force that could be applied. He used three sizes of occlusal surface and found that forces ranged from 0·4 to 2·5 kg when different foods were being chewed. Lundgren et al. (1975) measured chewing forces on long-span bridges and found that the mean was 4·8 kg. De Boever et al. (1978) found that the occlusal forces exerted on partial dentures during normal function were relatively low and seldom exceeded 4·5 kg. Gibbs et al. (1981) used a sound transmission system to measure chewing and swallowing forces on natural teeth. The mean forces were 26·7 and 30·2 kg respectively. The variations in the forces were rather large, the standard deviations being 20·7 for chewing and 25·0 for swallowing forces. Farrell (1956) found that in masticatory performance the number of natural teeth in the mouth seems to be relatively unimportant because of the adaptive capacity of the stomatognathic system. Substantial evidence on the effect of loss of teeth on masticatory performance in man is lacking, but there is some evidence that partial dentures can significantly improve chewing performance (Watson, 1977). Agerberg and Carlsson (1973, 1981) studied functional disorders of the masticatory system in a sample of adults and concluded that impaired mobility of the mandible was most common where a number of teeth had been lost.

Clenched Loads

The clenched load is the load applied to the denture and its supporting tissues when the teeth are clenched. It may be thought of as the vertical component of bruxism loads and may be damaging to the supporting structures (Leof, 1944; Miller and Firestone, 1947). Since 1861 data have been published on biting force (*Table* 4.1). This force is equivalent to the clenched load, although it may be slightly less since a certain amount of jaw separation is necessary to allow for the insertion of the bite-load gauge between the teeth. It can be seen that there is a large variation in clenched loads, and it seems that the results depend on the individual who measures the loads and on the equipment used.

Atkinson and Ralph (1973) used a gnathodynamometer with strain gauges to

Table 4.1 **Clenched loads (in kilograms)**

Authors	Natural Teeth						Dentures	
	Incisors	*Canines*	*Premolars*	*Molars*	*Single (unspec.)*	*Total*	*Complete*	*Partial*
Burras (1861)						225		
Dennis (1893)	7–12·5		11·3–18	14·5–21·5	7–21·5	113·4	1·1–4·5	
Black (1895)				77·6*	16–159 max		9·0–13·5	18–36 (upper)
Reschofsky (1906)							20–25	
Eckermann (1911)	20–40			40–80	20–80			
Dietz (1920)	30		50	100				
Morelli (1920)	15							
Schulze (1921)	20							
Haber (1926)	15–25 $\overline{x}$ 58 max	22–36 $\overline{x}$ 86 max	26–40 $\overline{x}$ 110 max	36–72 $\overline{x}$ 120 max	15–120	224(f) $\overline{x}$ 352(m) $\overline{x}$		
Howell and Manly (1948)				90 max				
Watt et al. (1958)					21·7 $\overline{x}$			7·4 $\overline{x}$ (mucosa-borne) 11·2 $\overline{x}$ (tooth-borne)
Atkinson and Ralph (1973)	19·6(m) 13·5(f)			29·3(m) 21·3(f)				
Garner and Kotwal (1973)	11·3							
Lundgren et al. (1975)					16·1			
Helkimo et al. (1977)	18·0(m) 11·0(f)			39·0(m) 22·0(f)				

m = male
f = female
$\overline{x}$ = mean

* $\overline{x}$ clenched load, 1000 young adults

measure the biting force of a control group of dental students. The results were as follows:

Incisor biting force:	males	19·6 kg
	females	13·5 kg
Molar biting force:	males	29·3 kg
	females	21·3 kg

In a study that used a strain gauge gnathodynamometer to measure incisal biting forces of a group of young males and females, Garner and Kotwal (1973) reported a mean biting force of 11·3 kg. Like Worner and Anderson (1944), they found that males bit harder than females and that biting forces increased with age up to adolescence. Lundgren et al. (1975) used bite-forks with strain-gauge transducers to measure chewing and clenching forces on long-span fixed bridges. They found the mean clenched force was 16·1 kg. Pacer and Bowman (1975) believed that the clenched force was related to the following factors: psychological condition and age of the patient, the individual level of pain tolerance, the measuring methods and the periodontal structures. Linderholm and Wennström (1970) could not relate biting force to the height and weight of their subjects and found similar values for men and women in a study of 58 males and 14 females (age range 18–31 years). The biting force of 125 Skolt Lapps (aged 15–65) was measured with a bite-fork between the first molars and between the incisors (Helkimo et al., 1977). In the males the maximal biting force in the molar region was 39 kg and in the incisor region 18 kg. The values for the females were 22 kg in the molar region and 11 kg in the incisor region. The biting force decreased with increasing age, especially in females. Most of this reduction with increasing age was probably due to the age-dependent deterioration of the dentition. In both sexes the biting force was notably less among the denture-wearers than among those with teeth. There was a close relationship between the biting force and the number of natural teeth; the greater the number of natural teeth, the greater the biting force. In our own studies (Watt et al., 1958) we found some correlation between the periodontal disease score and the biting load; the higher the periodontal disease score, the lower was the biting load (*Fig.* 4.1).

We used measurement of biting load to assess the designs of tooth-borne dentures and

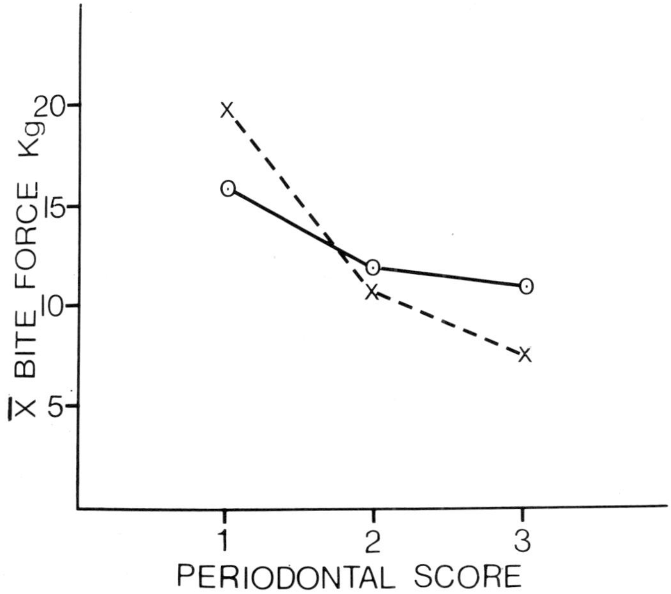

Fig. 4.1. Relationship between biting force and periodontal disease score. The biting force was measured between the upper and lower central incisors (continuous line) and between the upper and lower lateral incisors (interrupted line). The periodontal disease score is indicated as mild (1), moderate (2) or severe (3).

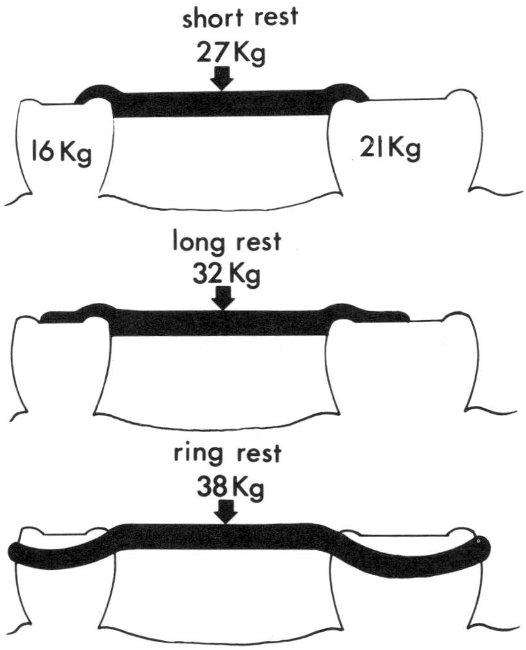

Fig. 4.2. Average maximum biting loads on experimental tooth-borne saddles with different types of occlusal rests (five estimations of each load were averaged). *Upper,* The average maximum load on the natural premolar tooth was 16 kg and on the molar tooth 21 kg, so theoretically the patient should have been able to bite with a 37 kg load on the experimental saddle, but where short occlusal rests were used he could only exert 27 kg. *Middle,* Where long occlusal rests were used, he could exert a force of 32 kg (still below the theoretical 37 kg load). *Lower,* Where ring rests surrounding the tooth above the survey line were used, the theoretical load was exceeded by 1 kg. (*After* Geddes, 1958.)

mucosa-borne dentures. The mean of 215 measurements of biting loads on natural teeth was 21·7 kg, whereas it was only 11·2 kg when 16 measurements were taken of biting loads on short bounded tooth-borne saddles with conventional occlusal rests. As this figure was much lower than expected, we investigated why the average maximum biting load on tooth-borne dentures was only about 50 per cent of the biting load of natural teeth. We were puzzled by this, because theoretically it should be the same. This was investigated by Geddes (1958), who made a variety of cobalt-chromium castings with different types of occlusal rests; he found that the biting load on tooth-borne saddles was closely related to the kind of occlusal rest used. *Fig.* 4.2 shows some results of his experiments. On average the natural teeth could accept loads of 16 and 21 kg, so that theoretically a load on the saddle fairly distributed between these two natural teeth should accept a 37 kg load. With narrow rests (both short and long) the 37 kg load was not reached, but where ring rests were used the theoretical load was exceeded by 1 kg. This suggested that these rests directed the load to the periodontium in the most favourable manner.

The most likely reasons for the reduced biting load on tooth-borne saddles with conventional occlusal rests are:

1. The rests do not transmit the load down the long axes of the teeth.
2. The relatively small area of the rest exerts crushing and shearing forces on enamel and dentine to which the patient is sensitive.

The compressive strength of dentine is approximately 297 MN/m^2 (Waters, 1980) and the surface areas of conventional occlusal rests vary from about 2 sq mm to 7 sq mm (mean 4·5 sq mm), so that it is quite possible that stresses approaching the compressive strength of dentine can be exerted through the rests, especially if they do not fit well and contact at only a few points (*Fig.* 4.3). The hardness of metal rests exaggerates this effect. We found that the use of a bite-load gauge with unpadded metal ends invariably resulted in a lower bite-load being registered than when the ends of the gauge were padded.

Many clinical and laboratory methods have been used to examine the effects of loading partial dentures. These have been reviewed by MacGregor et al. (1983).

Distribution of Clenched and Masticatory Loads

We must now ask ourselves how clenched and masticatory loads can best be distributed to the remaining teeth. Measurements were made from radiographs of teeth adjacent to a gap in the dental arch (Watt et al., 1958). The measurements were made from the amelo-cemental junction to the crest of the residual alveolar ridge, and from the amelocemental junction to the top of the interdental table between the abutment tooth and its neighbour.

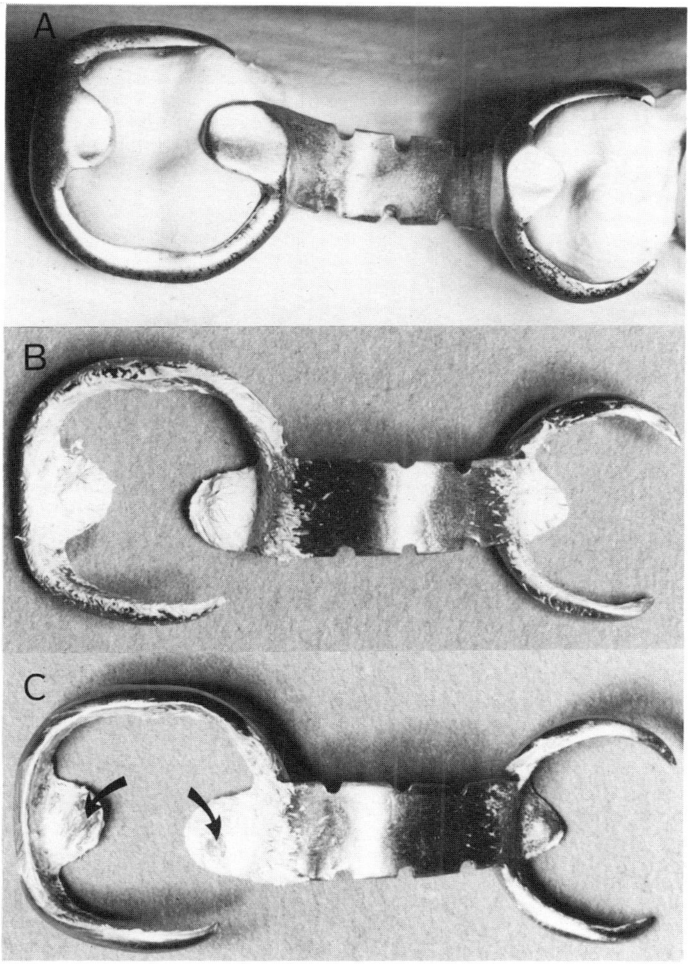

Fig. 4.3. **A**, Occlusal rests of experimental appliance apparently fit the cast well. **B**, Disclosing pressure paste applied to the fitting surfaces of the rests. **C**, After loading in the mouth it is apparent that the premolar rest fits better than the molar rests, which contact at only two small areas (*arrows*). Thus, stresses approaching the crushing strength of dentine might be generated at these points.

In 36 patients the mean difference between these two measurements was 3·1 mm. This indicates that there is a considerable loss of bone on the side of the abutment tooth nearest the gap, with a corresponding loss of the periodontal membrane (*see Fig.* 2.4). Thus, in the dental arch the teeth adjacent to a gap are perhaps the least suitable teeth to accept the loads applied to tooth-borne dentures. A review of 61 cobalt-chromium partial dentures showed that there was fremitus or mobility in many of the teeth carrying occlusal rests if they were adjacent to saddles. When possible, it is best to place occlusal rests for tooth-borne dentures on teeth within the intact portions of the dental arch. As pointed out by Chick (1953), when applied to premolars but not molars, this arrangement has the additional advantage of relatively decreasing the load on the premolar by increasing the distance from the point of application of the load to the rest (*Fig.* 4.4). We have already shown that the periodontium of a premolar is approximately half the area of the periodontium of a molar and that the maximum biting load on the experimental saddles increased as the point of

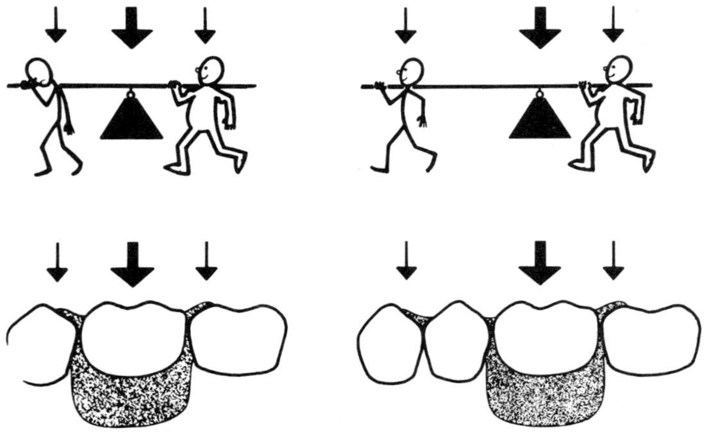

Fig. 4.4. The periodontal area of the premolar is approximately half that of the molar. By placing an occlusal rest on the first instead of the second premolar, the point of application of the load is further from the weaker tooth and hence is reduced. In addition the first premolar, lying within an intact part of the dental arch, is likely to have more periodontal and bony support than the tooth adjacent to the saddle.

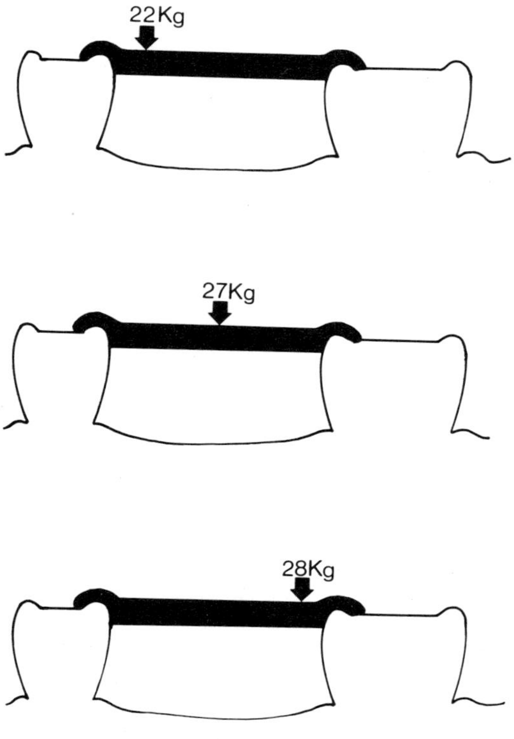

Fig. 4.5. Maximum loads that the patient can exert on a tooth-borne saddle. As the load is placed nearer the major abutment, the amount accepted increases. In this case the maximum load accepted by the premolar was 16 kg and the molar 27 kg. (cf. upper diagram, *Fig.* 4.2).

application of the load was placed nearer the molar (*Fig.* 4.5) (Watt et al., 1958).

In Chapter 3 we discussed the R/L ratio (the ratio of the periodontal area of the remaining teeth to the periodontal area of the lost teeth) and suggested limits for tooth-borne dentures. These limits should be kept in mind when selecting abutment teeth. However, in many separate calculations of biting loads we were impressed by the fact that, regardless of the type of tooth, the average area of periodontium that supported a 1 kg load was 13 sq mm, with a narrow range of 10·2–15·5 sq mm. This figure is useful when calculating loads and support for partial dentures. It is usually necessary to prepare seats on natural teeth for the occlusal rests of removable partial dentures. This is further discussed in Appendix II.

Our conclusions about occlusal rests on tooth-borne dentures are as follows:

1. Occlusal rests should fit closely (*Fig.* 4.3).

2. Occlusal rests should cover an area of tooth substance large enough to avoid stresses that are nearly as great as the crushing strength of dentine.

3. The load on removable tooth-borne saddles is distributed to abutment teeth best by ring rests.

4. Occlusal rests should be placed on teeth within the intact portions of the dental arch whenever possible.

Support of Partial Dentures in Relation to Lateral Loads

The conditions required for the support of lateral loads (bracing) are quite different from those required for the support of vertical loads. We have seen that there are significant differences in the amount of vertical load that can be sustained by a tooth if the load is applied in the long axis of the tooth or to one side of the occlusal surface. Axial loads induce much smaller tooth movements than horizontal thrusts (Mühlemann, 1967). Clayton (1966) has shown that a 90 lb axial load would result in no more displacement than a transverse load of 5 lb—that is, one-eighteenth of the vertical force, when applied laterally, can produce the same displacement of a tooth. We must keep this fact in mind when designing the support against lateral loads.

Let us consider a theoretical case in which the abutment teeth for a partial denture have conical roots of circular cross-section. The point of application of a horizontal load makes little difference to the total area of periodontium loaded, although it decides the translations and rotations of the teeth and the parts of the periodontium that are loaded (Pryputniewicz and Burstone, 1979). *Fig.* 4.6 illustrates this point. You can see that when the bracing element extends halfway round the teeth, lateral loads towards the buccal side are borne by the cervical part of the buccal periodontium in compression and by the cervical part of the lingual periodontium in tension. Shearing forces operate on mesial and distal periodontium. If the bracing element is short, a force applied on the lingual side loads the mesiobuccal surface of the cervical part of the periodontium in compression and the distolingual part of the cervical part of the periodontium in tension. The less the bracing elements encroach on the lingual surface, the more like a wedge does the saddle become when thrust towards the buccal side, and the more mesial and distal are the forces on the teeth. Also, the narrower the wedge, the greater is the buccal movement of the saddle and the greater are the mesial and distal forces on the teeth. In the limiting case, if no bracing was present all the support would come from the lingual and buccal surfaces of the mucosa of the saddle areas. Thus, the proportion of lateral load delivered to the periodontium depends on the extent of the bracing round the teeth (*Fig.* 4.6). The limiting case at the other end of the argument occurs when the bracing is extended to the transverse diameter of the tooth, in which case the mucosa is compressed

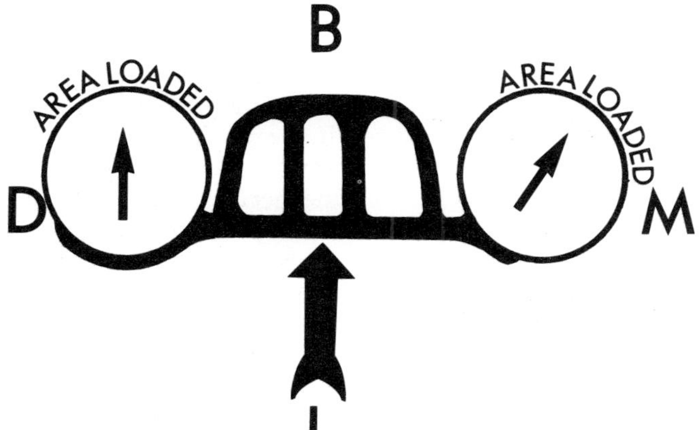

Fig. 4.6. Simplified diagram of the distribution of compressive load at the alveolar margin when a force is applied on the lingual side of a partial denture saddle between two conically rooted teeth. The teeth are shown in horizontal cross-section. Note that the areas loaded are of the same size but in different positions depending on the length of the bracing arms. (B, buccal; L, lingual; M, mesial; D, distal.)

to the same degree as the periodontium is compressed and consequently accepts only a very small part of the lateral load as it is much more compressible than the periodontium (Manderson et al., 1979).

Just as the reduction in occlusal surface area of the teeth on mucosa-borne saddles reduces the masticatory load on the mucosa, so the provision of a generated occlusal surface in bilateral free-end saddle dentures reduces the lateral thrusts on the denture and the lateral loads on the remaining abutment teeth. The lateral thrusts on occlusion of partial dentures are probably the most damaging ones to the abutment teeth.

The most useful method of generating the occlusal surface is by lateral sliding movements against a record block bearing a displaceable wax or an abradable surface. A reverse of this surface is then made in artificial stone and against that the artificial teeth are set on the saddle of the partial denture. It is important to maintain the vertical dimension with supporting cusps or a central bearing point during the procedure. Many dentists feel that the technique of generating an occlusal surface is time-consuming and difficult, but it need not be so; provided the dental technician understands what is required, this technique gives the patient the most comfortable type of partial denture occlusion. It is particularly useful in patients with bilateral free-end saddles opposed by natural teeth, since it gets rid of the occlusal interferences that may accompany the conventional setting of this type of denture.

Wrought flexible clasps placed at the ends of long mucosa-borne saddles permit the lateral thrusts on the saddles to be mainly absorbed by the mucosa. Rigid clasp arms on single teeth at the ends of such saddles transmit the lateral thrusts to the teeth and may cause the patient discomfort. A mucosa-borne or tooth-and-mucosa-borne partial denture that is rigidly attached to its abutment teeth makes the patient more conscious of the teeth being tugged and stressed during eating than does a denture that is disjoined from the abutment teeth, or flexibly attached to them. Forces transmitted to the teeth (and hence sensations to the patient) vary indirectly with the flexibility of the connectors.

In dentures with free-end saddles the amount of movement permitted by the connector between the retainer and the denture is important to the patient. The more rigid the connector, the more uncomfortable is the denture, and the more likely it is that the abutment teeth will be traumatised. A possible exception is the swing-lock denture, which uses multiple abutments. Flexible connectors generally make the dentures more comfortable and less likely to traumatise the teeth. The connector should be designed so that the masticatory forces are transmitted to the abutment teeth in the direction in which the teeth are best able to sustain them. If the connectors are too flexible, the mucosa takes too large a proportion of the masticatory load and may be damaged by it, but if the connectors are too rigid, the tooth may be traumatised, since the R/L ratio is extremely unfavourable for single abutment teeth at the ends of free-end saddles. Many so-called stress-broken designs do not transmit masticatory loads down the long axis of abutment teeth and rock round a fulcrum axis through the occlusal rests in much the same way as rigid designs do (*see* Chapter 8). A rigid transverse hinge, such as a dimple hinge (Watt, 1972), distributes the load over the widest area of mucosa in bilateral free-end saddles. As the hinge lies within the tooth-borne element, it has the advantage that it distributes the load evenly over the remaining teeth. MacGregor (1958) has shown that the amount of vertical load transmitted to the abutment tooth is directly proportional to the length and stiffness of the connector (*Fig.* 4.7). If the connector is quite rigid, the abutment tooth takes 100 per cent of a load applied near the occlusal rest and takes 50 per cent of a load applied at the midpoint of the saddle, the other 50 per cent being supported by the mucosa at the distal end of the free-end saddle (*see Fig.* 8.14). On the other hand, a load applied near the free end of the saddle is limited by the ability of the mucosa to accept it. However, where load is distributed between the teeth and the mucosa, the periodontal afferents appear to take precedence in the brain. Provided the periodontal membrane is not overloaded, severe and even traumatic pressures can fall on the mucosa without the

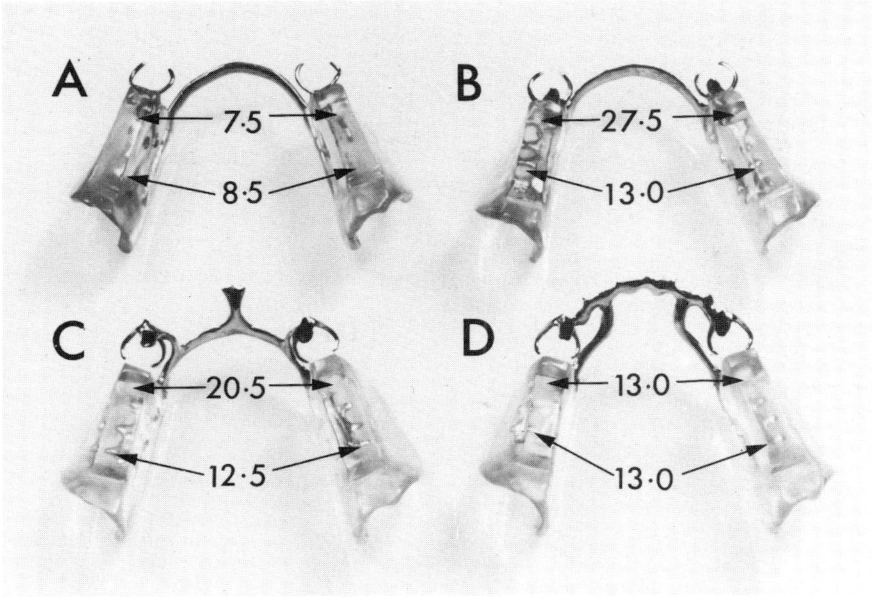

Fig. 4.7. Experimental appliances for assessing the influence of retainers and minor connectors on the mucosal loads of bilateral free-end saddles. Each number is the mean of 8 measurements of maximum biting loads (kg) on the anterior and posterior ends of free-end saddles. **A**, Mucosa-borne with wrought clasps and no rests. **B**, Tooth-and-mucosa-borne with rigid direct connection between saddles and cast occlusal rests. **C**, Tooth-and-mucosa-borne with connectors of medium length between saddles and rests. **D**, Tooth-and-mucosa-borne with long flexible connectors between saddles and rests.

Note that the maximum loads sustained on the anterior and posterior ends of the saddles are related to the rigidity of the connectors and the position of the rests. **A**, On the mucosa-borne saddles there is little difference between the anterior and posterior average loads that could be supported. **B**, With a rigid minor connector, the anterior load is greater than the posterior. **D**, Where the minor connector has some flexibility, the distribution of load is similar to the mucosa-borne denture; this finding is also partly due to the position of the occlusal rest.

patient being aware of them. This is clearly seen in entirely mucosa-borne dentures that prop the natural teeth apart. In a very short time the denture is forced into the mucosa until the natural teeth contact. We believe that this is because the occlusal loading on the periodontium is minimal while the denture that 'props the bite' is present, so that the thrust of elevator muscles is maximum until the teeth can contact. The periodontal afferents then limit the occlusal thrust to what the periodontium can accept. Severe damage to the mucosa can occur if a mucosa-borne denture that props the natural teeth apart is worn for any length of time. Mucosa-borne dentures replacing anterior teeth invariably damage the mucosa (*Fig.* 4.8).

An acrylic denture can be made tooth-borne by cutting rest seats in the marginal ridges of the abutment teeth and extending the acrylic on to these. Additional retention can be obtained by extending arms distal to the last molars (*Fig.* 4.9). When cutting rest seats for such a denture the cavo wall should be made parallel to the labial undercut of the tooth to improve retention.

Realities of 'Gum-stripping'

Acrylic mucosa-borne dentures that cover the gingival margins and have neither clasps or rests are often called 'gum-strippers'. They are probably the commonest type of partial denture made throughout the world today. Some dentists salve their consciences by relieving such dentures at the gingival margins in the mistaken belief that this will prevent damage to the margins, but the gingival tissues

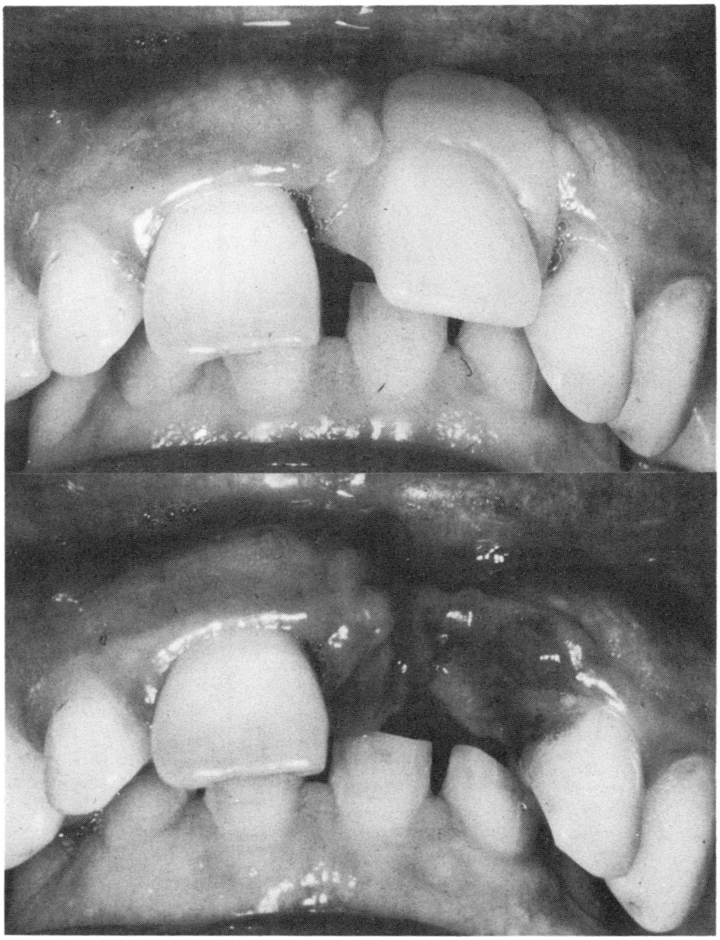

Fig. 4.8. Mucosa-supported acrylic partial upper denture that caused severe damage to the saddle area.

often proliferate into the relieved areas (Hobkirk and Strahan, 1979). Although these dentures are simple in construction, their movements in function are by no means simple. We have all had the experience of finding patients who have worn such 'damaging' appliances for many years without apparently harming their mouths too badly, while others who have worn them for a comparatively short time have suffered severe damage to the gingival margins of the abutment teeth and the mucosa (Koivumaa, 1956; Koivumaa et al., 1960; Bergman et al., 1977). (*See also* Appendix I.)

The Effect of the Form of Saddle Areas on Movement of Free-end Saddles

In order to understand these apparent contradictions, it is necessary to remember that the mucosa-borne partial denture tends to rotate round a soft-tissue fulcrum in much the same way as a raft on water (*Fig.* 4.10). While it is easy to predict such movements on a flat surface of mucosa, it is much more difficult to predict movement on a complex surface like the partially edentulous mouth. We shall start with a simple diagram (*Fig.* 4.11A) of a flat mandibular free-end saddle area covered by evenly compressible mucosa.

Application of a load at the distal part of the denture saddle causes rotation round a fulcrum between the point of application of the load and the gingival margins of the abutment teeth. This makes the denture rise from the gingival margins (*Fig.* 4.11B), removing pressure from them rather than loading them as the term 'gum-stripping' might suggest. Using the same model, a load applied near the anterior end of the saddle undoubtedly puts pressure on the gingival margins of the abutment teeth (*Fig.* 4.11C) and causes 'gum-stripping'. Let us now modify the model (*Fig.* 4.11D) and make it a little closer to reality by introducing an anteroposterior curve rising posteriorly on the saddle area. In this model application of load on the posterior part of the saddle makes the denture move forward down the slope of the residual alveolar ridge and brings pressure to bear not only on the gingival margin distal to the abutment tooth, but also on the lingual attached gingivae of the anterior teeth. If the curve is as shown in *Fig.* 4.11E with its most dependent part about the midpoint of the saddle, a backward movement takes place when the occlusal load is applied at the anterior end of the saddle and damage to the gingivae is thus avoided. If the patient loads the posterior end of the saddle, forward pressure on the gingival margins occurs (*Fig.* 4.11F) and if he loads the middle of the saddle above the most dependent part, no anteroposterior movement takes place and the saddle moves vertically as far as the compressibility of the mucosa allows (*Fig.* 4.11G).

When a curved rigid body is depressed into a closely fitting, evenly compressible curved surface by a load opposite its most dependent

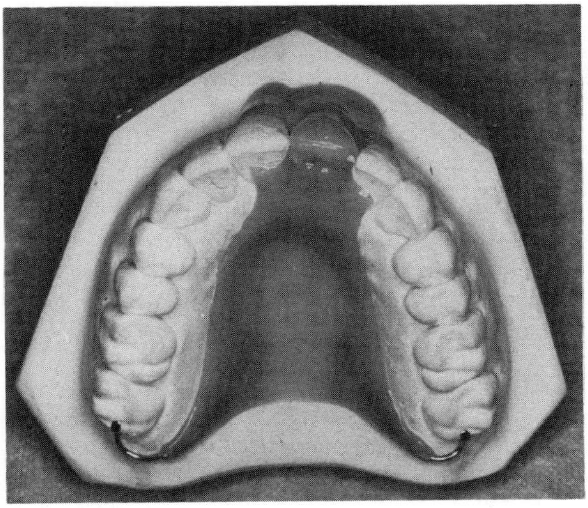

Fig. 4.9. A tooth-borne 'spoon' denture. Note the extension of the acrylic base into the rest seats on the marginal ridges of the central and lateral incisors. Wrought wires engaging the distal surfaces of the last molars improves the retention of this appliance by preventing forward movement that would disengage the labial flange from the labial undercuts.

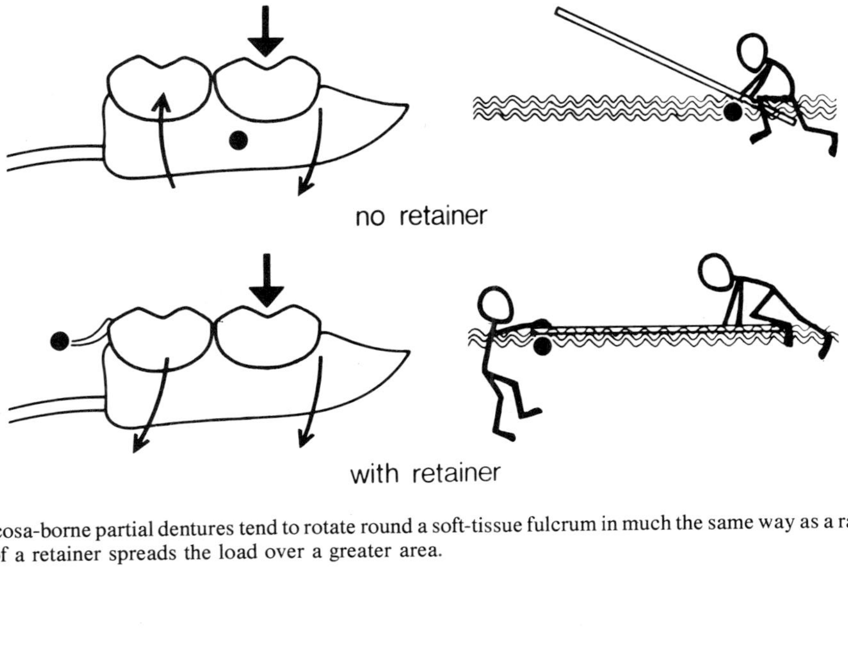

Fig. 4.10. Mucosa-borne partial dentures tend to rotate round a soft-tissue fulcrum in much the same way as a raft in water, but the presence of a retainer spreads the load over a greater area.

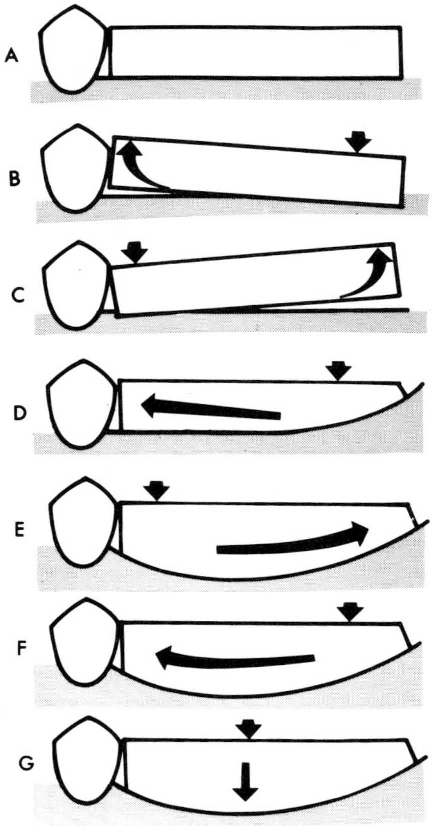

Fig. 4.11. Theoretical model of movements of free-end saddle on evenly compressible mucosa. The movements depend on the shape of the saddle area and the point of application of load. **A**, No load; **B**, **C**, **D**, **E**, **F**, **G**, Short arrows indicate point of application of load; long arrows indicate displacement of denture. (*See text.*)

part, the degree of compression opposite the load is greater than the compression at the ends and the difference is related to the steepness of the curvature. This explains why patients wearing free-end saddle dentures complain of pain under the most dependent parts of the saddles. Relief with thin foil (0·06 mm) over the centre of the saddle areas prevents this complaint. In the limiting case, where the ends of the curve turn through 90° to become parallel to each other, no compression of the surface occurs at the ends and an increasing degree of compression occurs towards the midline.

Thus, when designing dentures for bilateral free-end saddles, care must be taken to identify the type of saddle before the denture is designed. If the saddle area is relatively flat, the danger of damage is less than if the saddle area slopes upwards at its distal end, but even in these cases damage can be minimized by placing teeth only above the flat part of the ridge. If the saddle has its most dependent part at its midpoint, it is best to concentrate the occlusal load by placing the teeth on the part of the saddle above the most dependent part of the ridge (*Fig.* 4.12). In this way damage can be minimized with these simple acrylic dentures.

Effect of Compressibility of Mucosa on Movement of Free-end Saddles

The difference in compressibility of the anterior and posterior ends of the saddle area determines whether or not there will be pressure on the gingival margins of the anterior teeth when a load is applied to the middle of the saddle. If the anterior end of the saddle area is more compressible than the posterior end, the acrylic denture rotates towards the anterior teeth when the load is applied and 'gum-stripping' may take place. If the anterior end of the saddle area is less compressible than the posterior mucosa, the denture rotates away from the anterior teeth and damage is less likely to occur.

The compressibility of the mucosa can be measured with the instrument shown in *Fig.* 4.13, which comprises a spring-loaded plunger that delivers a thrust of 100 g to 1 sq mm of mucosa. The clear plastic disc at the end of the instrument is placed against the mucosa and the amount of protrusion of the plunger beyond the disc serves as a measure of mucosal compressibility at the point and is recorded in millimetres on the dial of the instrument. *Fig.* 4.14 shows a typical result of measurement of mucosal compressibility on a free-end saddle area. These figures are only indications of immediate compressibility and, as Wills and Manderson (1977) have shown, when mucosa is compressed it takes some time to recover (*Fig.* 3.4) and may stay in its distorted form for a considerable length of time. *Fig.* 4.15 also illustrates this and shows superimposed profile tracings of casts made from different impression materials. At the top

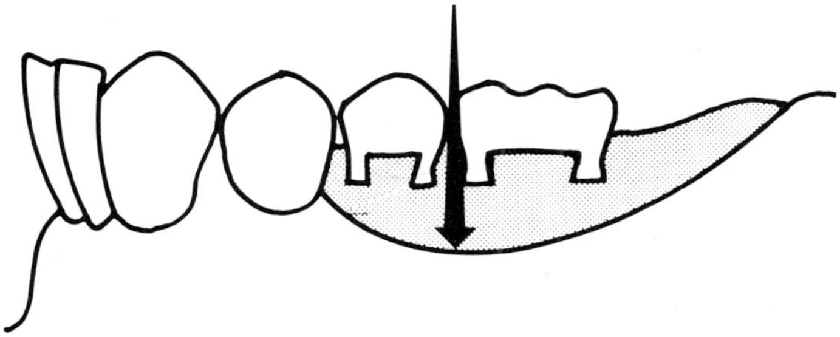

Fig. 4.12. The most dependent part is at the middle of this free-end saddle area. Teeth should be positioned so that the load falls on this part of the saddle area. The second molar is omitted to ensure that the main load (*arrow*) is accepted by the most dependent part of the saddle area.

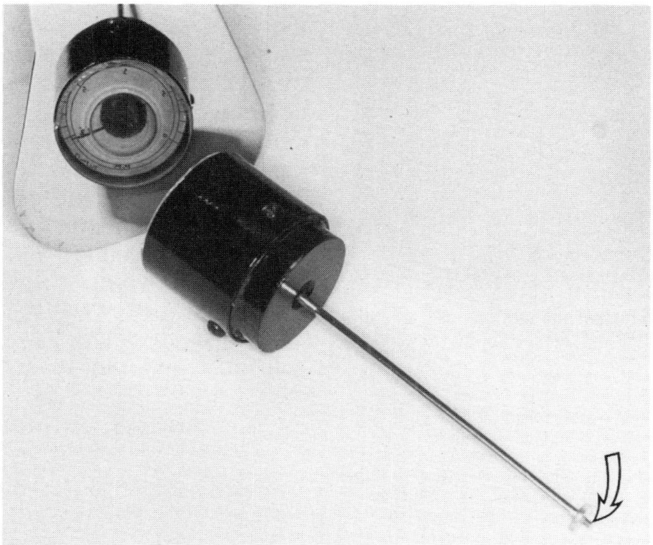

Fig. 4.13. Mucosa-compressibility gauge. The protrusion of the spring-loaded plunger (*arrow*) beyond the clear plastic disc, which is held against the mucosa, indicates the amount of compression in millimetres on the gauge (shown reflected in mirror).

a tracing of a cast from an alginate impression has been superimposed on a tracing of a cast from a compression impression of the saddles made with impression compound. Differences of up to 2 mm in the level of the mucosa in the free-end saddles can be seen. The dark line on the middle tracing represents the profile of a cast from an alginate impression that was made the following week, the patient having worn during that week a partial lower denture made on a cast from the compression impression. It can be seen that the mucosal level of the alginate impression now corresponds to that of the previous compression impression. The lower trace represents the profile tracing of another alginate impression made 30 minutes later. Some recovery of mucosa can be seen. The rather large differences in position of the free-end saddles obviously took place and this indicates the importance of making provision in partial denture designs for movement of the free-end saddles towards the tissues to avoid trauma to the teeth.

When a patient chews on a bilateral lower free-end saddle denture, the working side may sink into the tissues 1 mm or more and there is a tendency for the opposite side to rise from the tissues since the fulcrum round which the denture tilts is provided by the occlusal rests

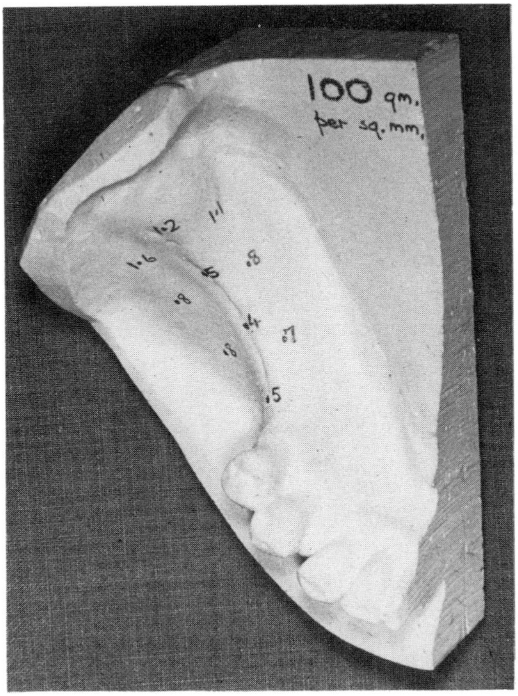

Fig. 4.14. The compressibility of the mucosa of a free-end saddle area measured in points of a millimetre with the gauge shown in *Fig.* 4.13.

nearest the saddle on the working side. The implications of the torsional forces involved in this and the means of avoiding them are further discussed in Chapters 8, 9 and 10.

The loading of a saddle on the right side of a mucosa-borne upper denture makes the denture rotate round the vault of the palate and brings down the left side of the denture. Similarly, if the left side is loaded, the right side tends to come away from the tissues and the palatal gingivae are sucked. Thus, it is very common to see proliferative gingivitis in patients who wear mucosa-borne acrylic partial upper dentures covering gingival margins. Other factors, such as neglected hygiene and direct trauma from food, may also contribute to the gingivitis. Further mucosal damage is done by the movement of these dentures in the vault of the palate. If the patient has had some papillary hyperplasia of the palate before the impression is taken, the surface of the denture will be rough and will fit into the grooves between the papillae, producing a sucking action every time the denture moves (Watt and MacGregor, 1976).

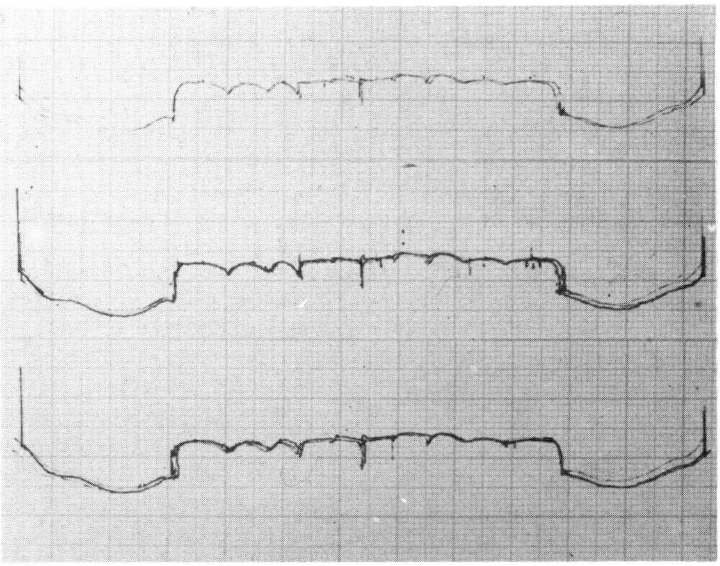

Fig. 4.15. Superimposed profile tracings of mandibular casts of a patient with bilateral free-end saddle areas. *Top, upper trace*—cast from alginate impression; *lower trace*—cast from compression impression. *Middle,* Dark line superimposed on previous tracings is a tracing of cast from alginate impression taken immediately after the patient had removed a denture that had been worn for one week. The denture was made on a cast from the compression impression. *Bottom lower,* Dark line tracing of a cast from an alginate impression half-an-hour after removal of the denture shows some recovery of the mucosa.

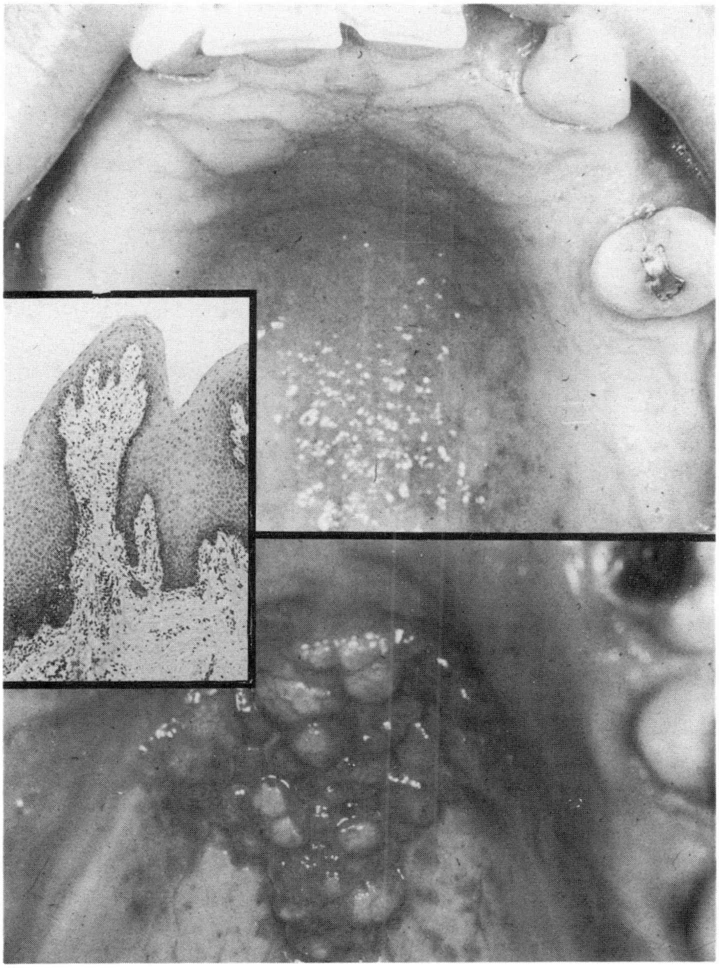

Fig. 4.16. Papillary hyperplasia of the palate caused by movement of mucosa-borne dentures. *Upper,* Early stage. *Lower,* More advanced stage. *Insert:* Histological section of papilla.

This causes an increase in the size of the papillae, which become further traumatised by movement of the denture (*Fig.* 4.16).

Relationship between Support and Retention

Indirect Support

The retainer on one side of a direct supporting element (occlusal rest) can provide indirect support for part of the denture on the opposite side of the supporting element (*Fig.* 4.17). The amount of support that can be obtained from this cantilever system is relatively small, since pressure on the indirectly supported saddle causes an extracting force on the tooth with the retainer. This can be uncomfortable for the patient and may damage the periodontium.

Indirect Retention

Similarly, a supporting element on one side of a direct retainer can provide indirect retention for part of the denture on the opposite side of the retainer (*Fig.* 4.17).

Retainer's Contribution to Support of a Mucosa-borne Denture

As already mentioned, a mucosa-borne denture is supported like a raft on water (*see Fig.* 4.10). When loaded, the denture rotates round a soft-tissue fulcrum, the location of

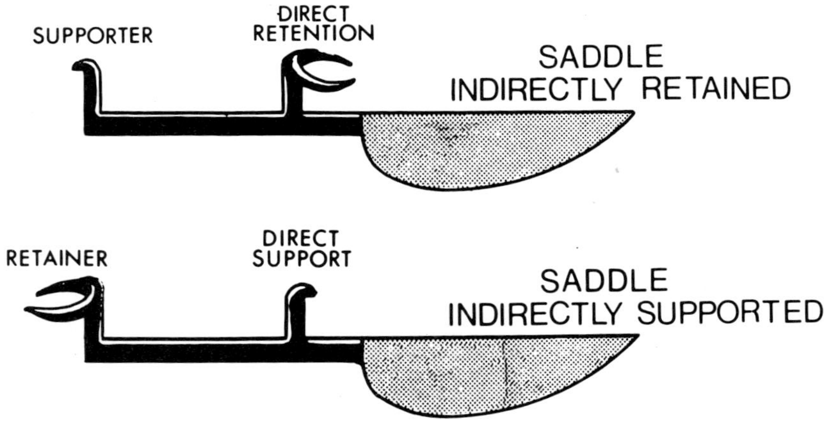

Fig. 4.17. *Upper,* A supporting element provides indirect retention by resisting rotation of the saddle away from the mucosa round the direct retainer. *Lower,* A retaining element provides indirect support by resisting rotation of the saddle towards the mucosa round the direct supporter.

which depends on the point of application of load. On the application of load, if the opposite side of an upper denture is held by a retainer, the area of mucosa compressed is greatly increased, since the position of the fulcrum moves nearer the retainer (*Fig.* 4.18). This is similar to the indirect support described above, except that the fulcrum is not clearly defined but changes according to the compressibility of the mucosa, the effectiveness of the retainer, and the flexibility of the denture base.

The Role of Connectors

The more rigid the connector between the tooth-borne part and the mucosa-borne part of the denture, the greater is the amount of tooth support. The more flexible the connector, the greater is the proportion of mucosal support (*see Fig.* 4.7), but the efficiency of the retainer must always be related to the flexibility of the connector. A stiff retainer with a rigid connector puts more load on the tooth than a stiff retainer with a flexible connector. However, if the connector is rigid and is joined to a mucosa-borne saddle, the retainer is likely to be displaced because the forces of occlusion generated on the saddle are greater than the forces resisted by even the stiffest retainer. Thus, rigid tooth-and-mucosa-borne denture designs rock round the tooth-borne fulcrum axis and the retainers should be designed to allow for this.

Relationship between Support and Occlusion

Muscle Force

We have discussed at some length the amount of support available for dentures in terms of mucosal surface area and periodontal area and we have indicated that deficiency in support might cause breakdown of the supporting tissues through overloading. However, the protective mechanism of the body generally prevents overload and damage. Thus, if the support is deficient, the deficiency will be compensated by a decrease in muscle force on the denture, but if we wish to increase the efficiency of the denture we must also make the best use of the support.

Support from Mucosa and Periodontium

We have already mentioned an exception to the general rule stated in the previous paragraph, an exception that can bring about quite marked resorption of bone under mucosa borne saddles (*see Fig.* 4.8). This occurs when part of the support comes from the mucosa and part from the periodontium. When a mucosa-borne denture props the natural teeth apart, the periodontal afferents do not send warnings to the brain on chewing as the periodontium is not being overloaded, although the mucosa is being traumatised. Yet, because the periodontal afferents appear to take

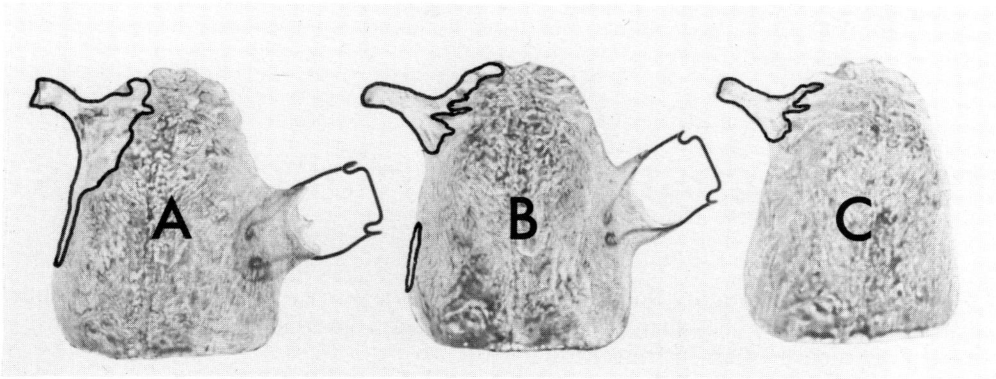

Fig. 4.18. When a 4 kg load was applied to the saddles of base-plates A, B and C, the pressure-indicating paste coating their fitting surfaces was squeezed out and the areas outlined indicate the areas of mucosa that were loaded. The base-plates with clasps (**A** and **B**) show a wider distribution of load, but in the base-plate without clasps (**C**) a smaller area of mucosa is loaded. Base-plate A is made of flexible polythene and shows the widest distribution of the load.

precedence over the mucosal afferents, it is not long before the mucosa is damaged and the denture sinks into the soft tissues far enough to allow the natural teeth to come together. When this occurs, for a short time the support is balanced between the teeth and the mucosa, but as time goes on there is further loss of tissue under the denture and the greater occlusal load is then taken by the remaining natural teeth. There is some evidence (Watt et al., 1958) that if periodontal disease has progressed to a sufficient extent to damage the afferents from these natural teeth, forces in excess of their support capability may be exerted on these teeth to bring about their early loss.

Chapter 5

Surveying casts for partial dentures

Before designing partial dentures the casts of the patient's mouth must be surveyed (*see* Appendix III) by means of an instrument that analyses the casts and draws lines on them that indicate undercut areas in relation to paths of insertion and removal of the dentures. The lines guide the positioning of clasp arms. The surveying instrument can also be used to eliminate unwanted undercuts.

Cast Surveyors

Cast surveyors (*Figs.* 5.1, 5.2) are sometimes called 'clasp surveyors', but as they have other uses the term 'cast surveyor' is more appropriate. In its simplest form the cast surveyor is an instrument that holds a marking rod vertically above a tilting table on which the cast to be surveyed can be mounted and locked in any position of anteroposterior or lateral tilt. The marking rod is usually a piece of graphite, or a pencil lead, and it can be rotated or moved up and down, but must always remain vertical so that the angle it makes to the cast remains constant for any one position of tilt. The marking rod draws survey lines on the cast that indicate the greatest horizontal width of the object being surveyed. More complicated cast surveyors have attachments that hold milling and drilling instruments (*Fig.* 5.2).

Survey Line

The survey line (*Fig.* 5.3) is a line drawn round the greatest girth of a tooth in relation to the common path of displacement or to the path of insertion and removal of the denture. Those parts of the teeth on the gingival side of the survey lines are in undercuts in relation to the path in which the cast is being surveyed, while the parts of the teeth on the occlusal side of the survey lines do not lie in undercuts in relation to that path.

Paths of Displacement

Paths of displacement are all possible paths along which all or part of the denture may be displaced during function.

Common Path of Displacement

The common path of displacement is the path along which a denture is most likely to be displaced during function. This path is at right angles to the occlusal surfaces of the teeth, since sticky food tends to dislodge the denture along this path when the jaws are opened. In the first instance the cast is therefore surveyed with a marking rod parallel to this common path of displacement.

Path of Insertion and Removal

The path of insertion and removal is the path along which the denture is inserted into the mouth and removed from the mouth. This path must be decided before the denture is designed. The table of the surveyor is adjusted so that the marking rod is parallel to this path. A second survey line is then drawn round the teeth and mucosal surfaces of the cast in relation to this path. The colour of the marking rod should be different from that used to make the survey lines in relation to the common path of displacement.

Undercut

The BSI Glossary of Terms Relating to Dentistry (1983) defines an undercut as 'that area of a tooth or soft tissue surface which is beyond the survey line when viewed from a

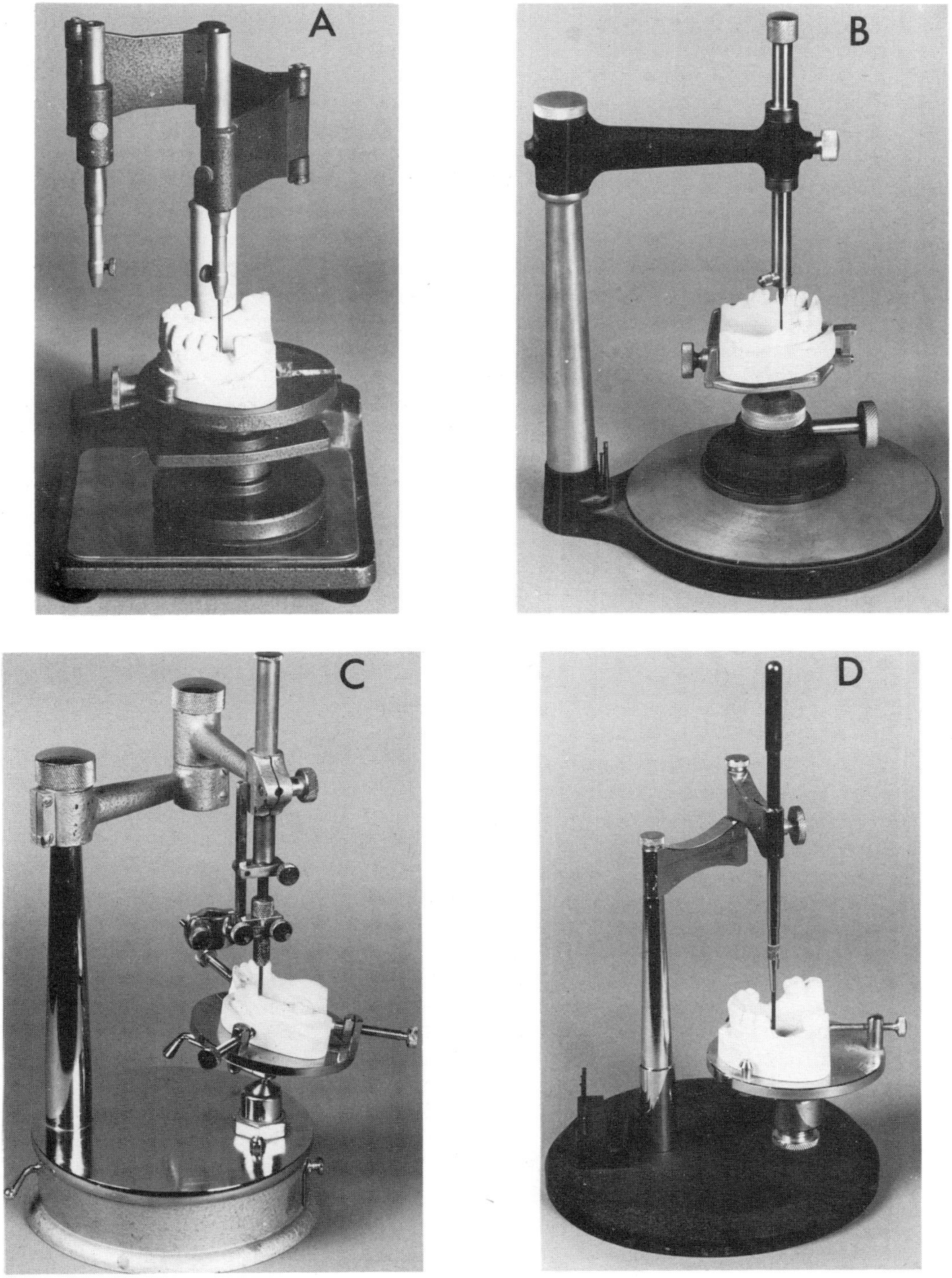

Fig. 5.1. Various types of cast surveyors (simple parallelometers). A, Krupp model K3 (Krupp, Essen, West Germany). B, Ney fixed arm (J M Ney Co., Bloomfield, Conn., USA). C, Nesor model D (Nesor Products Ltd, London, England). D, Anthogyr model 1670 (Anthogyr, Sallanches, France).

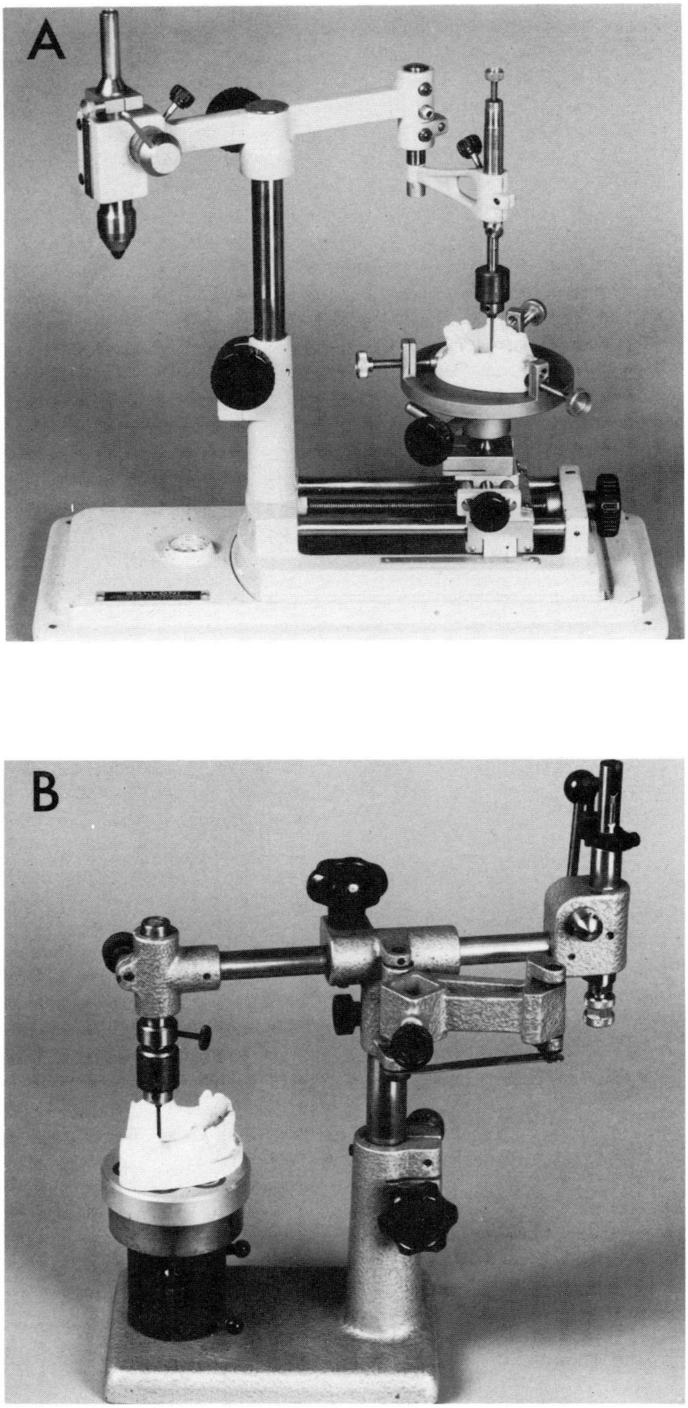

Fig. 5.2. Advanced parallelometers with milling facilities. **A,** Galloni isoparallelometer model 1020 (Galloni ASEG, South Colombano, Italy). **B,** Bachmann parallelometer (Cendres et Metaux, Biel-Bienne, Switzerland).

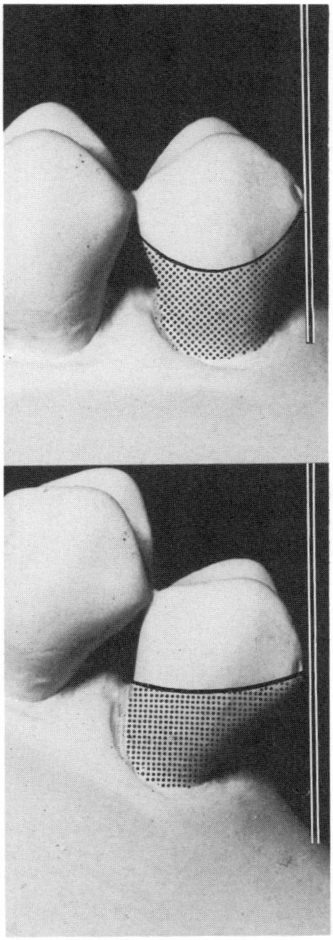

Fig. 5.3. Survey lines, showing how the tilt of the tooth alters the line and consequently the undercut area (*shaded*).

particular direction' (*Fig.* 5.3). Undercuts may be divided into true or false undercuts. True undercuts are those in relation to the common path of displacement and provide resistance to removal of the denture along this path. False undercuts are undercuts produced by tilting the cast. They provide resistance to removal of the denture along the path in which the survey has been made, but not in the common path of displacement. When the path of insertion and removal of the denture has been chosen, the tips of the clasp arms should lie in undercuts in relation to both the path of removal and insertion of the denture and to the common path of displacement.

Guiding Surfaces

Guiding surfaces of teeth (*Fig.* 5.4) guide removable partial dentures towards their final position in the mouth. It is advantageous if the guiding surfaces are parallel to each other, but this is seldom possible as the surfaces of the teeth are curved. Guiding surfaces decrease the number of paths along which the denture may be displaced. The choice of the path of insertion and removal of the denture is influenced by the guiding surfaces that are located on a cast of the mouth by the analysing rod of the surveyor (*Fig.* 5.4).

Objects of Surveying

The object of surveying is to ensure that no rigid portions of a partial denture lie in undercuts in relation to the path of insertion and removal of the denture, although they may lie in undercuts relative to the numerous possible paths of displacement. The flexible ends of clasp arms must lie in undercuts in relation to all possible paths of insertion, removal or displacement, since they are responsible for the retention of the denture (*Fig.* 5.5). As mentioned above, the most likely path of displacement is at right angles to the occlusal plane of the teeth. One must therefore ensure that the tips of the clasp arms and, if possible, the denture base itself, resist displacement along this path. However, a patient must be able to insert and remove the denture easily and the springiness of the clasp arms must provide the only resistance to insertion and removal along the single path of insertion and removal (*Fig.* 5.6).

The objects of surveying may be summarized as follows:

1. To mark the most bulbous parts of the teeth and soft tissues.
2. To identify undercut areas on teeth and alveolar ridges of a cast relative to any given path of insertion, removal or displacement of partial dentures.
3. To locate tooth surfaces that may help to guide partial dentures to their exact position in the mouth.
4. To find the undercuts that can be used for retention and to measure the amount of horizontal undercut on the teeth selected for clasping.

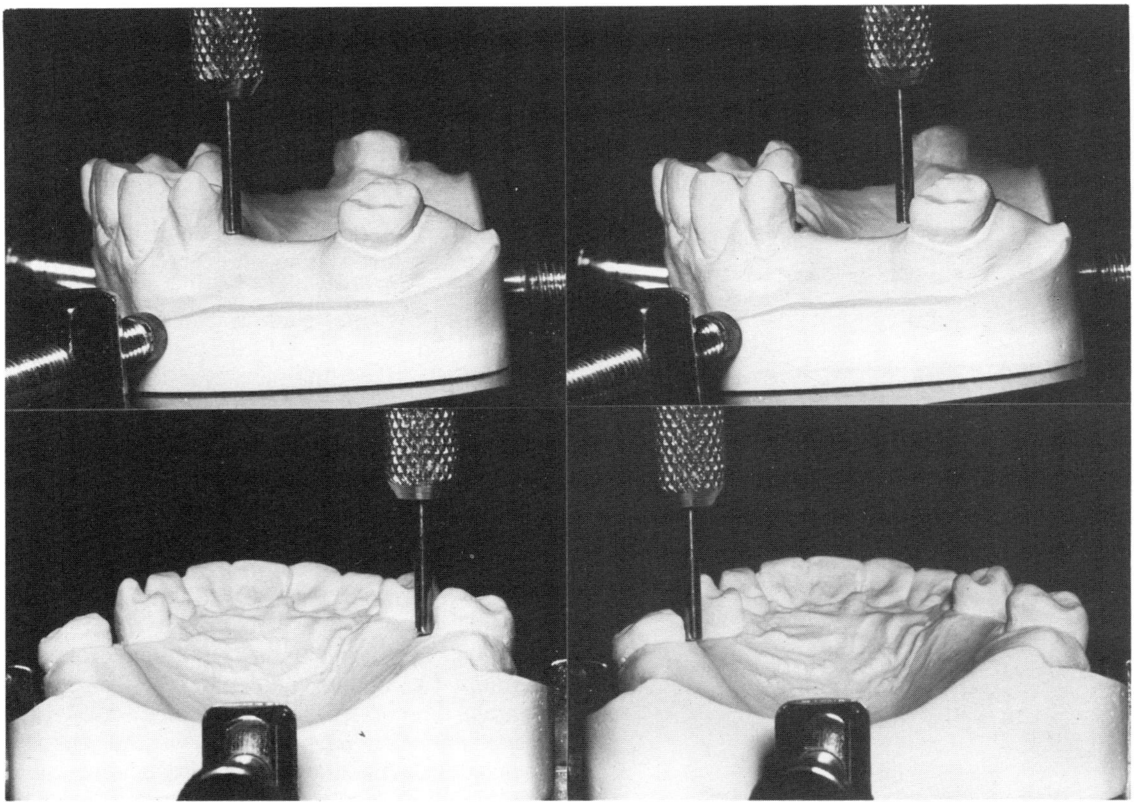

Fig. 5.4. The analysing rod on the surveyor is used to locate guiding surfaces on the teeth prior to the selection of a path of insertion and removal of a partial denture. As far as possible the guiding surfaces should be parallel to each other. (*See* text: Choosing the path of insertion and removal.)

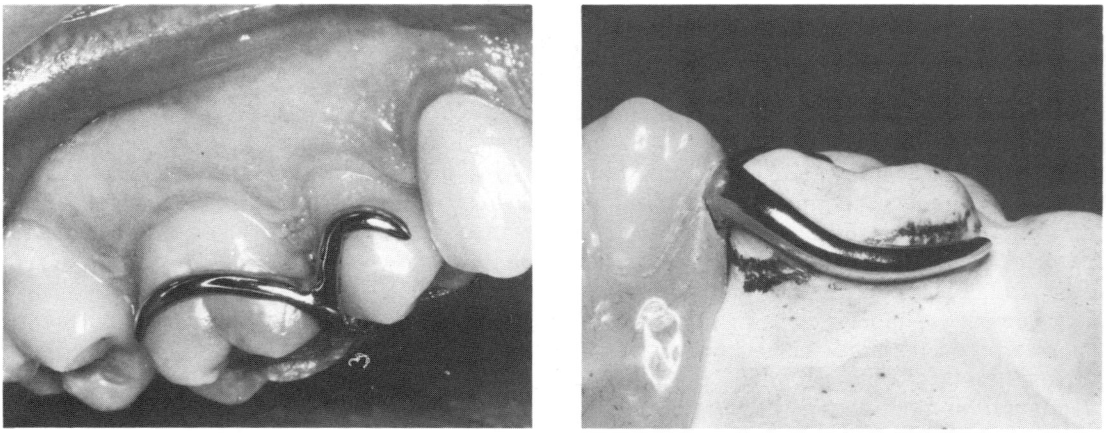

Fig. 5.5. The flexible ends of clasp arms lie in undercuts and provide retention for partial dentures.

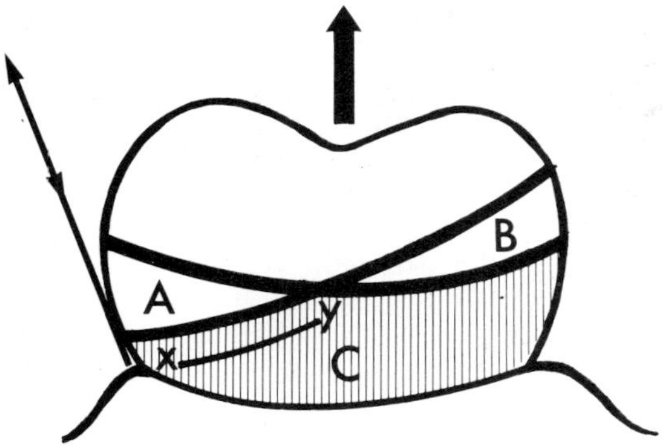

Fig. 5.6. The area A + C is undercut in respect to the common path of displacement (*thick arrow*), but 'A' is not undercut in respect to the path of insertion and removal (*thin arrow*). 'B' is undercut in respect to this path, but as it is not undercut in respect to the common path of displacement it cannot be used for retention. 'C' is undercut in respect to both the common path of displacement and the path of insertion and removal, and if the clasp tip lies on the line X–Y it will be in a specified undercut (say 0·25 mm) in respect to the path of insertion and removal, but the nearer it is to 'X' the more resistant it will be to displacement of the denture at right angles to the occlusal surface of the teeth.

5. To aid the design and exact location of the clasp arms.
6. To block out unwanted undercuts on the cast.
7. To help to define where the margins of the denture base should lie in relation to the survey lines on the natural teeth, and thus ensure that no gaps are left between the teeth and the denture base.
8. To assist the planning of fixed partial denture work before preparation of the teeth.
9. To aid the location and parallelism of precision attachments.
10. To mill parallel surfaces, or surfaces at specified angles, on abutment pieces and bars, and to drill parallel holes.

Method of Surveying

1. Lock the cast on the tilting table of the surveyor so that the occlusal plane of the teeth is parallel to the base of the surveyor and is therefore at right angles to the graphite marking rod (*Fig.* 5.7).

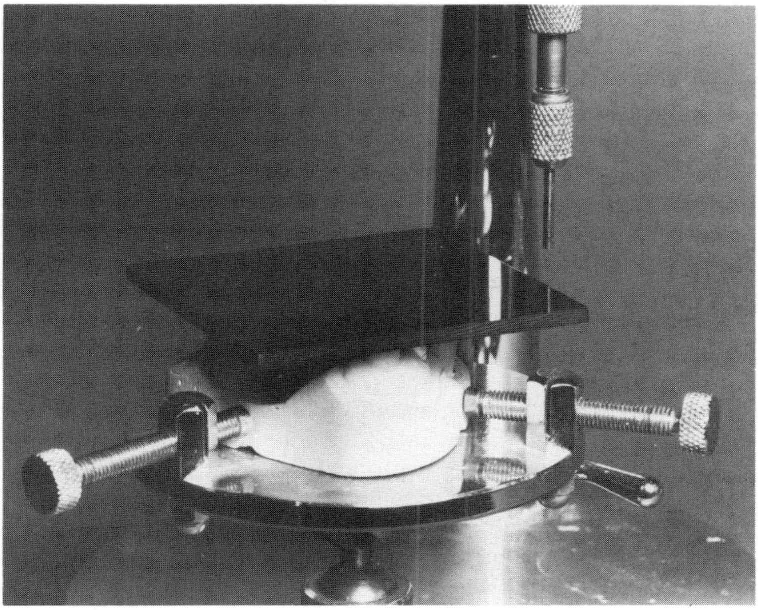

Fig. 5.7. The cast locked on the tilting table of the surveyor is positioned so that the occlusal plane of the teeth is parallel to the base of the surveyor. In this case a Perspex slab laid on the teeth defines the 'occlusal plane' of the cast.

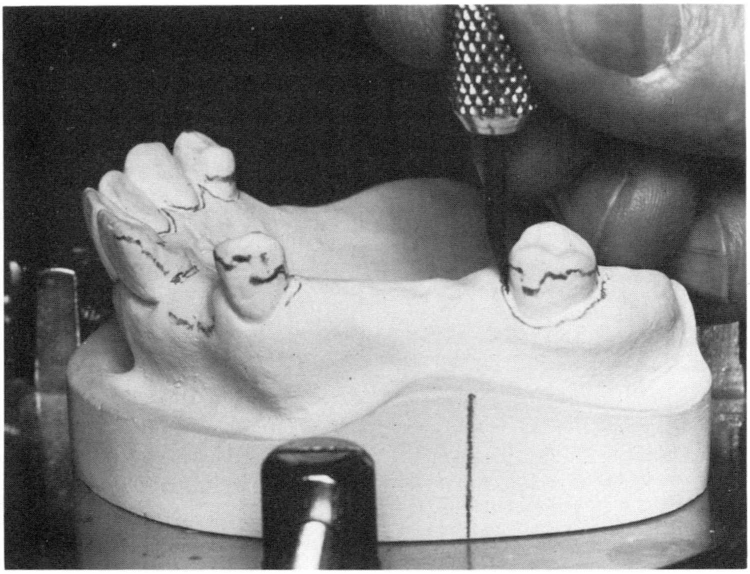

Fig. 5.8. The side of the marking rod is used to mark the widest parts of each tooth in turn in respect to the common path of displacement as represented by the long axis of the rod. The tip of the rod marks the horizontal extent of the undercut on the cast.

2. Examine the graphite marking rod and make sure that it is not worn and has a straight, vertical edge.

3. With the table locked in position, bring the side of the marking rod into contact with each tooth in turn and move it around the tooth with the tip of the rod touching the cast. In this way the side of the rod touches only the widest parts of the teeth in relation to the common path of displacement and the tip of the rod outlines the horizontal extent of the 'undercut' area relative to that path (*Fig.* 5.8). The survey line represents the greatest girth of the teeth in respect to the common path of displacement. It indicates those parts of the teeth that *can* be used for retention; those parts of the teeth on the occlusal side of the line *cannot* be used. The survey line on the tooth may be broken where a hollow on the tooth lies between horizontal ridges on the tooth surface (*Fig.* 5.9). Where there are vertical grooves on the tooth, graphite rods trimmed to a knife-edge produce better survey lines than rods of circular cross-section (*Fig.* 5.10).

4. When the teeth and the soft-tissue undercuts have been surveyed in relation to the common path of displacement, replace the graphite with the analysing rod and decide the path of insertion and removal of the denture (*Fig.* 5.11). The factors influencing this decision are discussed in detail later, but if no teeth are tilted the path of insertion and removal should generally be at right angles to the occlusal plane and no further surveying is necessary. Misplaced teeth or teeth lying at awkward angles usually indicate that a different path of insertion of the denture should be chosen.

5. When the path of insertion and removal of the denture has been chosen, the cast should be surveyed in relation to that path, using a marking edge of a different colour to outline the undercut areas (*Fig.* 5.12). A number of these areas may lie above the survey line in relation to the common path of displacement. They are useless for retention of the denture since they do not provide undercuts in the path along which it is commonly displaced. Thus clasp arm tips should be positioned in the area of the undercut below both survey lines, preferably at the appropriate degree of undercut in relation to the path of insertion and removal (say 0·25 mm in the case of a cobalt-chromium clasp arm), but in a much deeper undercut in

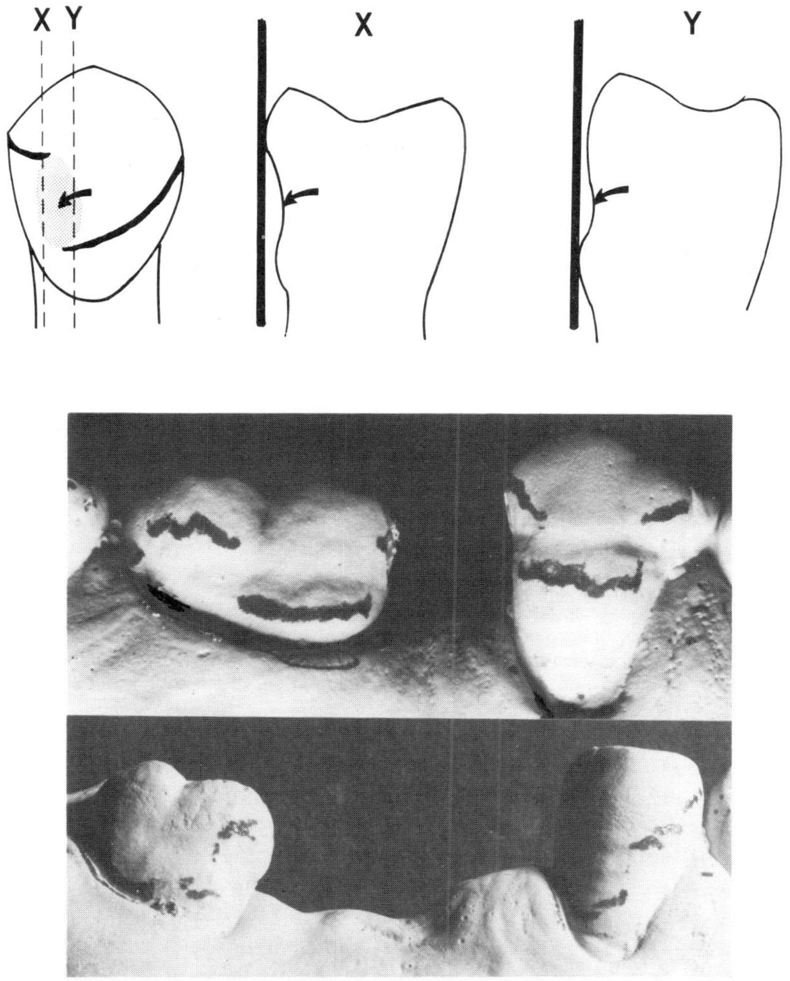

Fig. 5.9. The survey lines on the teeth may be broken by hollows on the surface of the natural teeth. *Upper left,* stippled area indicates hollow; interrupted lines show positions of sections 'X' and 'Y'. Diagrams 'X' and 'Y' show how the surveying lead contacts above and below the hollow (*arrowed*) and causes interruption of the survey line.

relation to the common path of displacement (*see Fig.* 5.6). In this way the clasp gives a denture adequate retention when the patient tries to remove it, and the denture is much more resistant to displacement when sticky food is chewed. Undercut gauges are used to decide the exact positions of the clasp arm tips (*see* Appendix III).

Choosing the Path of Insertion and Removal

The choice of the most suitable path for insertion and removal of the denture depends upon the answers to two questions:

What are the positions and angles of the guiding surfaces?

Is a labial flange required?

What are the Positions and Angles of the Guiding Surfaces?

Loosen the screw that locks the tilting table of the surveyor so that the table can be tilted easily but will stay in the position of tilt in which it is placed. Look at the saddle areas on the right side of the cast and place the

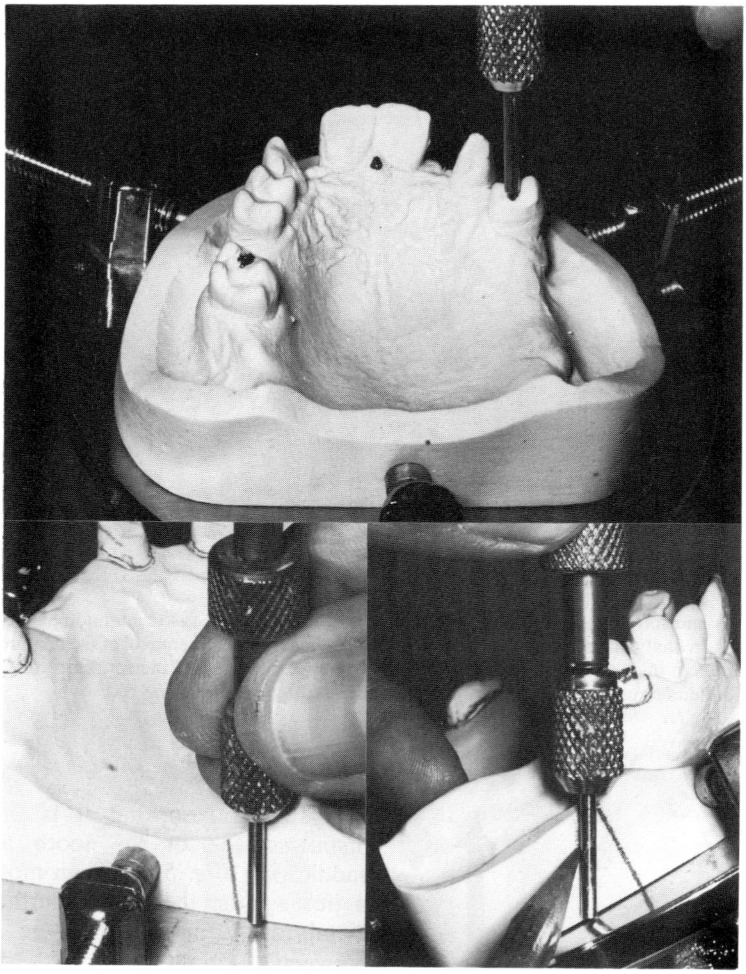

Fig. 5.13. Two methods of marking the cast so that it can be relocated on the surveyor. *Upper,* With the marking rod locked, three widely separated marks are placed on the cast in the same horizontal plane. *Lower,* The analysing rod is used to mark the anteroposterior tilt on the side of the cast; a similar mark on the back of the cast indicates the lateral tilt (*see also Fig.* 5.14).

alternatively, make marks at three widely separated points in the same horizontal plane (*Fig.* 5.13). A triangular location plate and mandrel can also be used to relocate a cast on the surveyor (*Fig.* 5.14). This method is particularly applicable to fixed prostheses as damage to the palate of the cast in these cases does not usually matter.

It may be that during the foregoing analysis of the cast you find some of the surfaces are parallel and some divergent or convergent. You must make up your mind whether or not you will grind the surfaces of the teeth or modify them with fillings or crowns to provide a larger number of parallel guiding surfaces (Holt, 1981).

Regardless of the type of retainer used, its effectiveness depends on the number of paths along which it must provide retention. Where there are numerous possible paths along which the denture can be displaced, it is less easy to make an effective retainer, but if the denture can only be displaced along a single path, the demands placed upon retainers are less

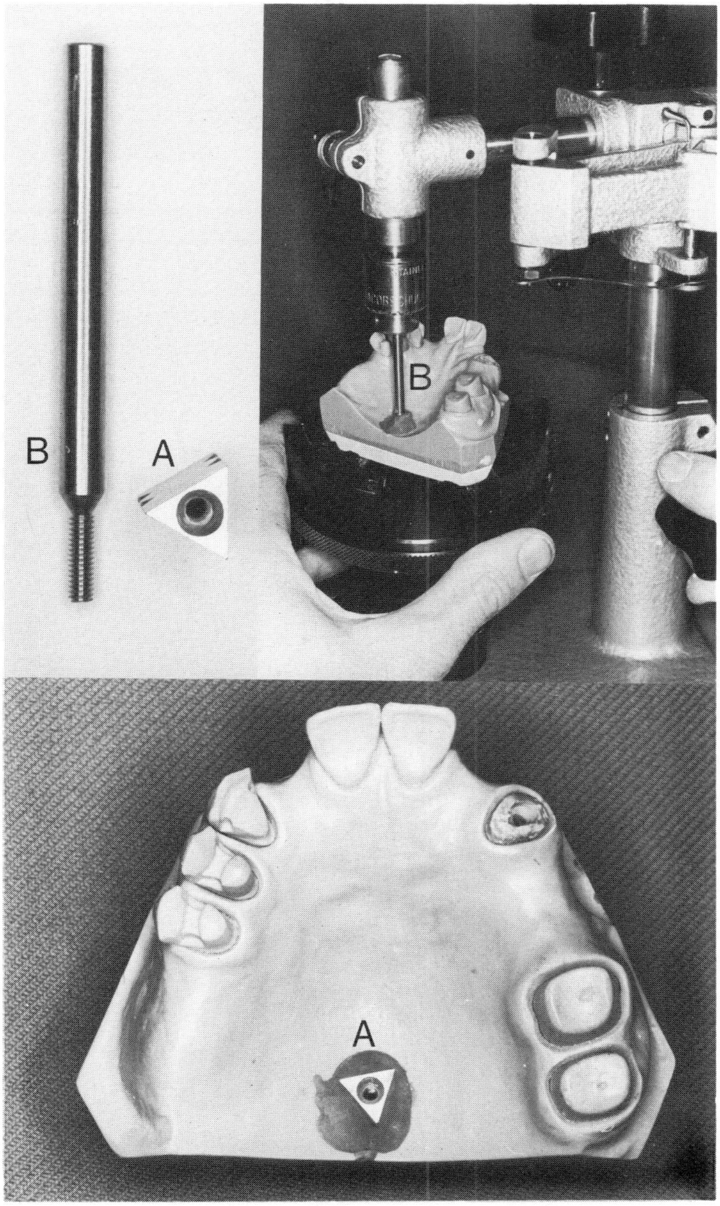

Fig. 5.14. A third method of relocation of a cast on the surveyor is by using a triangular location plate (A) screwed to a mandrel (B) which is held in the chuck of the surveyor. The location plate is then lowered into a hole in the palate of the cast and attached to it with artificial stone or cold-curing resin. When the resin is set the mandrel is unscrewed and can be used at any time to relocate the cast accurately on the surveyor for milling or other purposes.

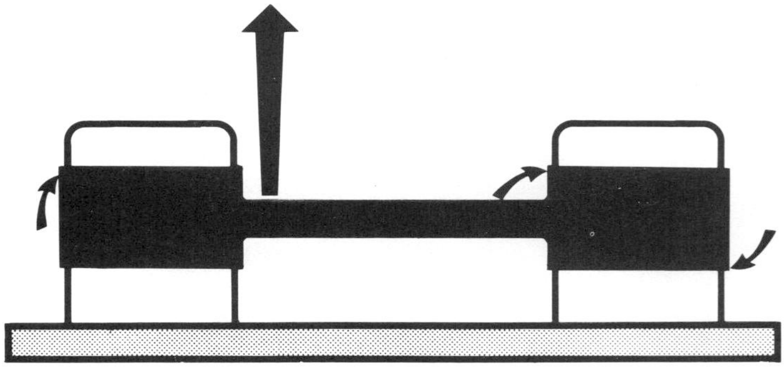

Fig. 5.15. Diagram of parallel abutments, showing how a displacing force (*large arrow*) puts unfavourable torsional and wedging stresses on abutments at the opposite end of the saddle or at the opposite side of the arch. (*See* text.)

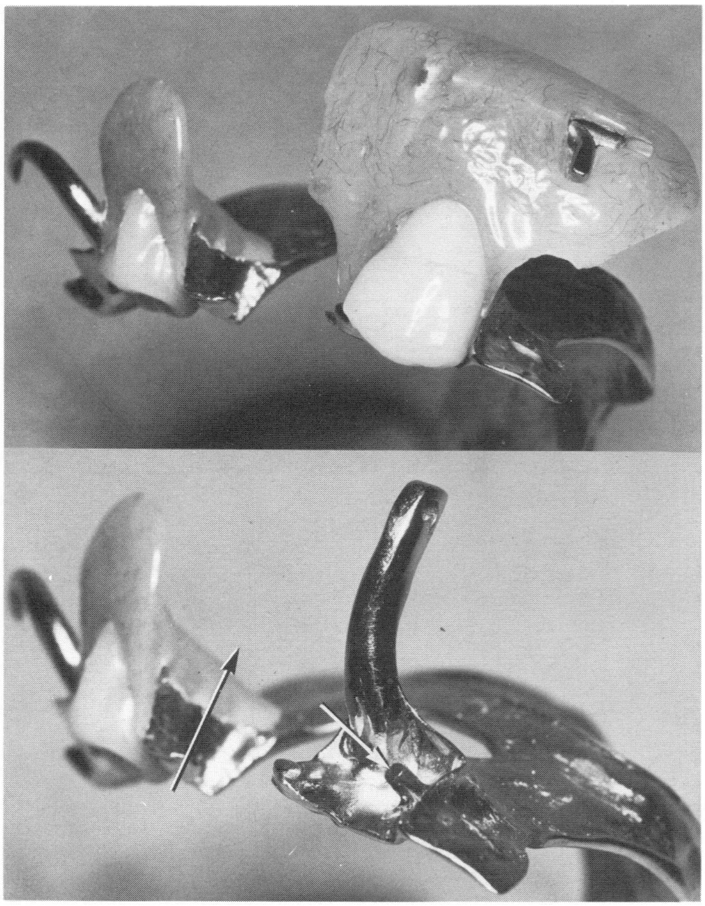

Fig. 5.16. A two-part cobalt-chromium partial denture which has a bolt-on flange with a horizontal path of insertion to use the labial undercuts. The guide pin (*white arrow*) defines the path of insertion of the flange. The guiding surfaces of the posterior teeth define the path of insertion (*black arrow*) of the main part of the denture base.

because wedging effects occur. For this reason, when surveying a cast before constructing a partial denture, use the analysing rod to identify as many parallel tooth surfaces as possible and choose a path of insertion and removal which is also parallel to these tooth surfaces. Some believe that the advantages to be gained by these parallel 'guiding surfaces' are such that the shape of teeth should be modified to increase their number and ensure as far as possible a single path of insertion and removal for all the saddles of the denture.

In a theoretical 'limiting case' in which the abutment teeth are cylindrical with their sides parallel to each other (*Fig.* 5.15) a displacing force at one end of a saddle results in torsional and wedging forces on the abutment at the other end and any attempt to remove one saddle results in wedging of the denture in the other saddles. Thus a certain amount of 'retention' might be thought to exist, although no actual retainers are used. There is no retention for the denture along the single path of removal, although wedging can occur when one part of the denture is displaced. Such wedging may be harmful to the teeth, since a displacing force on one saddle has a great mechanical advantage that produces large torsional forces on the abutment teeth on the opposite side. For this reason it is unwise to depend solely on the parallelism of guiding surfaces to provide the resistance of the denture to removal in an occlusal direction. In every case retainers should be placed as close to the saddles as possible to prevent these harmful forces.

In cases where many undercuts have been 'blocked out' the zone of displacement is invariably increased and this puts much heavier demands on the retentive devices that are used. It is often difficult to persuade patients to have teeth prepared to provide guiding surfaces for a removable partial denture. It is unwise to insist, as patients may feel that tooth preparation is unnecessary in the absence of caries and they may resent the treatment. Our usual advice is that if guiding surfaces are present they should be used. If they are not present, it is usually unwise to prepare them unless the teeth have already been restored or require restorations on which guiding surfaces can be built. In some cases extraction might be considered if a tooth has a poor prognosis and is misplaced or over-erupted.

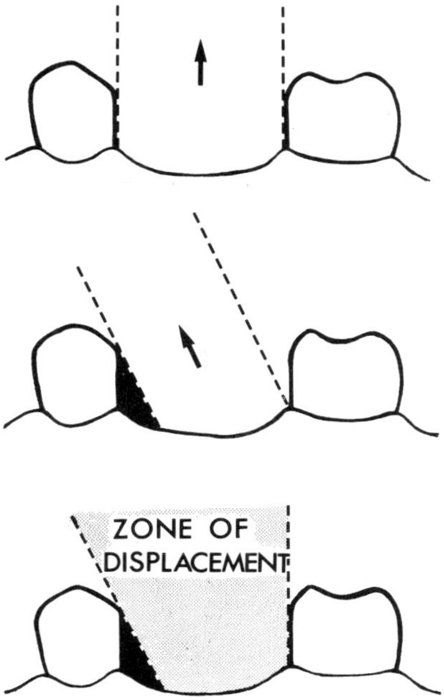

Fig. 5.17. Blocking out undercuts increases the zone of displacement.

Is a Labial Flange Required?

You may find suitable guiding surfaces for the posterior saddles of the denture, but if a labial flange is required an oblique path of insertion may be necessary to enable the labial flange to restore the lost gingival tissues (*see Fig.* 2.7). Sometimes a two-part denture can be made with a flange that has an almost horizontal path of insertion for the anterior saddle, while the path of insertion for the posterior saddle aligns with the guiding surfaces (*Fig.* 5.16). When the two parts of the denture are locked together in the mouth, firm retention is provided by the labial flange, making anterior clasp arms unnecessary. A less elaborate solution is to survey the whole cast in the oblique path of insertion for the anterior saddle and block out the unwanted posterior undercuts. This simplifies the design, but complicates the problem of retention by increasing the zone of displacement. Any blocking out of undercuts increases the zone of displacement (*Fig.* 5.17) as it makes a wedge-

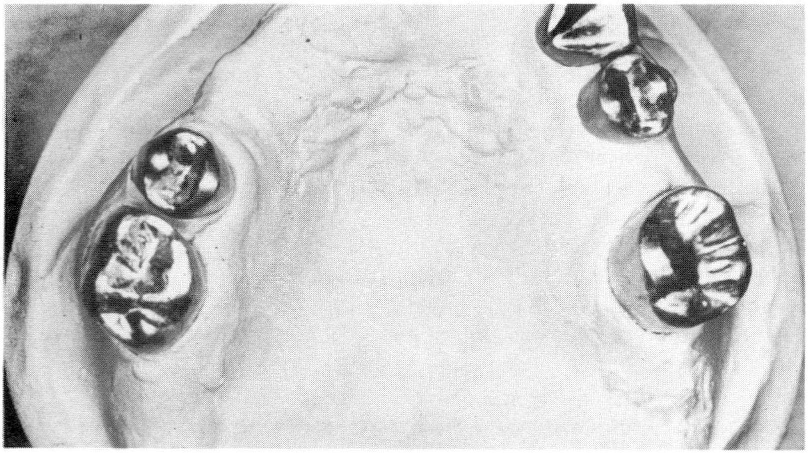

Fig. 5.18. When the remaining teeth are few in number the teeth may be crowned and guiding surfaces prepared. The path of insertion and removal is then made parallel to these surfaces.

shaped saddle that can be displaced from the saddle area along a greater number of paths than if its ends were parallel. In addition, blocking out undercuts produces unhygienic food traps between the denture and the abutment teeth. The method of blocking out unwanted undercuts is described in Appendix III.

The decision as to which path of insertion and removal is used depends upon whether or not the dentist decides to prepare guiding surfaces on the teeth (Smith and Turner, 1979). If he does, the path of insertion and removal will be parallel to the guiding surfaces (*Fig.* 5.18). If he does not consider preparation of the teeth, the path of insertion and removal may be tilted, possibly to accommodate an anterior flange. Thus a rigid portion of the denture can slide into the anterior undercut and also into the undercut at the distal end of the posterior saddle, while any undercut at the mesial end is blocked out (Appendix III, *Fig.* III. 33). In any decision as to which path of insertion and removal will be chosen for the denture, the following must be considered together as they all interact: the guiding surfaces, the presence or absence of a labial flange, the undercuts to be blocked out, and the type and position of retainers.

These matters are further discussed in chapter 6 and more details on the technique and basic principles of surveying can be found in Appendix III.

Chapter 6

Retention of partial dentures

Retention is defined in the BSI Glossary (1983) as 'the resistance of a denture to movement away from the tissue in a vertical direction'. With the exception of some simple mucosa-borne dentures retained by physical surface forces and forces within the saliva film, partial dentures depend on mechanical devices for their retention. These devices are called 'retainers' and may be in the form of clasps, prefabricated attachments, or extensions of the denture base into undercuts. The abutment pieces for fixed partial dentures (bridges) are sometimes called retainers, but the use of this term can be misleading because, although the crowns and inlays on the abutment teeth provide retention, they also provide support for the appliance. For this reason we prefer to use the term 'abutment piece' for the 'retainers' of fixed partial dentures. Before discussing these matters, let us first consider how much retention a patient really needs for a removable partial denture.

We have all met versatile lingual gymnasts who can converse perfectly intelligibly while simultaneously patting their upper dentures back into place with their tongues. We are also familiar with the traditional stiff upper lip, the reason for its stiffness being that its owner is keeping his upper denture in position by contracting his orbicularis oris against the labial flange. We can possibly count amongst our acquaintances charming individuals who have an undeserved reputation for grimness because they speak through clenched teeth in order to keep their dentures in place. All these people would probably tell you that their dentures are satisfactory, because they have accommodated to dentures that have no retention but when such patients are supplied with really retentive dentures their delight is apparent.

Apart from mechanical retention, the physical forces involved in the retention of dentures can be roughly divided into three groups: the surface forces associated with the adhesion of saliva to the denture and to the mucosa; atmospheric pressure; and fluid forces, such as the surface tension of saliva, the cohesive forces within saliva film, and the viscosity of the saliva. These groups of forces interact to a greater or lesser extent and contribute in varying degree to the retention of dentures (Roydhouse, 1960; Avant, 1973a, b; Driessens, 1977; Wright, 1981).

In order to use atmospheric pressure to resist a displacing force on a denture, it is necessary to maintain an intact peripheral seal round the denture. Skinner et al. (1953) showed the enormous importance of this. They found the retention of base plates was greatly reduced when the peripheral seal was absent. The difficulty or impossibility of maintaining a peripheral seal in partial dentures reduces the importance of atmospheric pressure as a factor in their retention.

We believe with Roydhouse (1960) that factors in denture design that impede fluid flow across the denture margins contribute most to the retention of complete dentures and also to the retention of mucosa-borne partial dentures that do not have clasps. *Fig.* 6.1 (after Brill, 1967) shows in diagrammatic form the factors on which denture retention depends. Imagine two tanks filled with fluid. The block on the left can be removed from the tank more easily than that on the right, not necessarily because it is lighter, but because it does not fit the sides of the tank and as it is pulled out of the tank the liquid can flow down its sides to fill the space beneath it. The closely-fitting block on the right cannot be withdrawn so quickly as the fluid takes longer to pass through the narrow gap between the block and the sides of

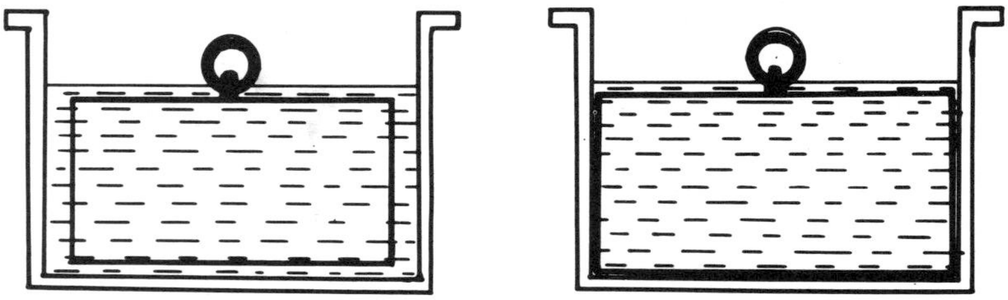

Fig. 6.1. Diagram (after Brill, 1967) illustrating the factors affecting retention. The block in the tank on the left can be easily withdrawn as the fluid can flow easily between its sides and the walls of the tank. The block on the right cannot be withdrawn easily as the flow of fluid is restricted by the narrow gap (analagous to a peripheral seal) between it and the tank. Increasing the viscosity of the fluid would also increase the 'retention' of the block, provided the gap was unchanged. This diagram has most relevance to complete denture retention. Partial denture retention without mechanical retainers could be compared to the condition where only the bottom of the tank was covered by a thin fluid film.

the tank. If the tanks are emptied, the blocks can be removed relatively quickly because air can pass beneath them much more easily than water. If the tanks are filled with sticky bitumen instead of water, it might be virtually impossible to remove the block on the right, whereas the block on the left could perhaps be withdrawn slowly. If both blocks fitted the bottom of the tank equally well, and if there was a thin layer of fluid between each of them and the bottom of the tank, the larger block would have the greater resistance to removal because of its greater area and the factors in Stefan's formula (1874) would operate (*Fig.* 6.2), but it is apparent that air would soon get under both blocks and the retention would be very much less than when the tanks were full.

We believe that the factors illustrated in *Fig.* 6.1 are the most important factors related to retention of dentures that do not have clasps or other mechanical retainers. Atmospheric pressure does not contribute to retention unless there is an adequate peripheral seal analogous to the contact of the block against the sides of the tank. It is virtually impossible to make a peripheral seal along the complex outline of partial dentures, the only exception being overdentures, which have a peripheral form similar to complete dentures. Thus, apart from mechanical retention, the forces that retain partial dentures are related to the factors in Stefan's formula and are analogous to the situation when a thin layer of fluid covers the bottom of the tank.

$$f = \frac{2\pi r^4 c}{4h^2 t} + \frac{2y}{h}$$

f force
r radius of plate
c viscosity
h distance after time t
y surface tension

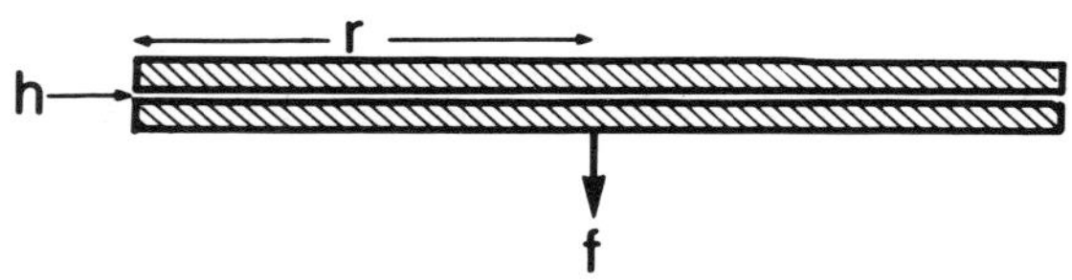

Fig. 6.2. The force required to separate two circular flat glass plates with a fluid film between them is related to the factors expressed in Stefan's equation (1874). The retentive force varies directly as the area of the plates, the viscosity and surface tension of the fluid film and varies inversely as the square of the distance between the plates.

Retainers for Partial Dentures

Mechanical retainers for partial dentures may be classed as follows:

Clasps. These usually lie on the surfaces of the tooth outside the normal contour of the anatomical crowns, but may lie in prepared recesses within artificial crowns or restorations of abutment teeth (*Fig.* 6.3).

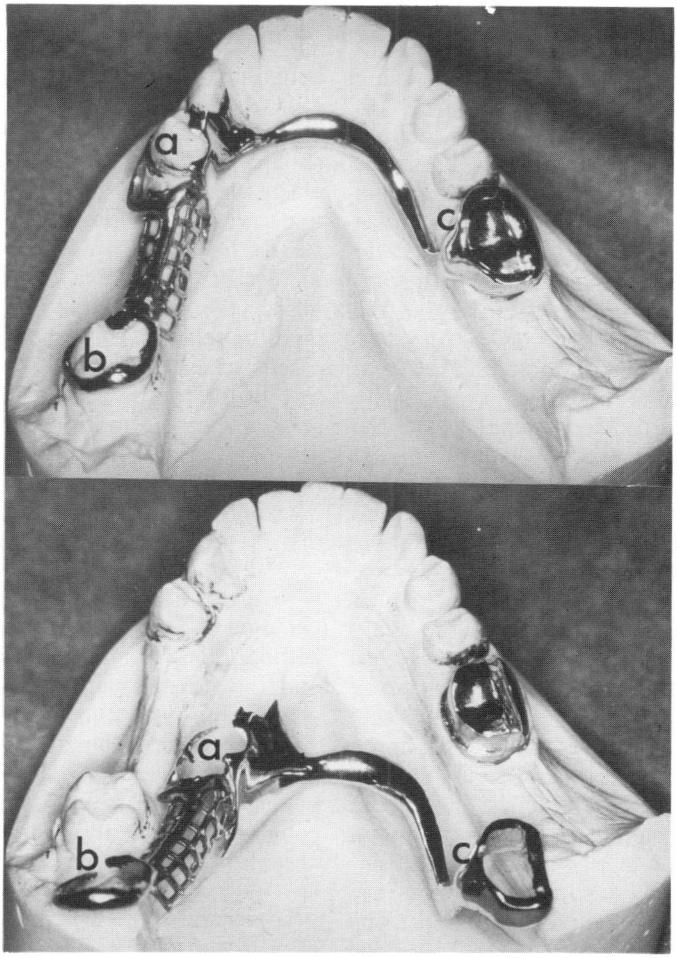

Fig. 6.3. Cast partial lower denture base illustrating three types of retainers: 'a', Gingivally-approaching clasp; 'b', Occlusally-approaching circumferential clasp; 'c', Channel shoulder pin retainer.

Extensions of the denture base into undercuts (*see Figs.* 2.6, 2.7, 5.16).

Prefabricated attachments. These may be classified as follows:

Intra-coronal (within the anatomical contour of the crown of the natural tooth, e.g. Chayes, McCollum, Schatzmann) (*see Figs.* 2.17, 7.2, 7.4).

Extra-coronal (beyond the anatomical contour of the crown of the natural tooth, e.g. Dalbo) (*see Figs.* 8.9, 8.10).

Studs (e.g. Gerber) (*see Fig.* 7.16).

Bars (e.g. Dolder) (*see Figs.* 7.10, 7.13, 7.14).

Miscellaneous. Channel shoulder crowns (*see Figs.* 7.22, 7.23), telescope crowns (*see Figs.* 11.7, 11.8), spring and friction devices (*see Figs.* 7.18, 7.19, 7.20), screws and bolts (*see Fig.* 7.21).

Many of these retainers provide support as well as retention for partial dentures (Nally, 1961; Preiskel, 1979).

Clasps

Clasps are the commonest type of retainer for partial dentures. There are several mechanical principles on which clasp design depends. The alloys used for making wrought clasps should be easily bent in the annealed condition, but should be stiff in the heat-treated or cold-worked condition. Type IV cast gold alloy clasps should be heat-treated in order to provide adequate stiffness. Cast cobalt-chromium alloys cannot usually be hardened by heat treatment unless they contain molybdenum. They have a very high modulus of elasticity and can be used only in comparatively shallow undercuts. A disadvantage of cast cobalt-chromium alloys is that the grains tend to be large. There may be only two or three grains across the whole thickness of an alloy clasp and therefore it is easily distorted or broken. Measurements of the mechanical properties of cobalt-chromium alloys, using conventional test pieces, can be quite misleading since they do not take into account the size and shape of the clasp or the types of stress encountered in clinical use (Lewis, 1978; Bates, 1980). The presence of 0·25–0·5 per cent molybdenum in the alloy refines the grain size and increases the strength of thin sections; it also produces a solid solution hardening effect. Nickel increases the ductility of cobalt-chromium alloys, but decreases their strength. The method of cooling after casting also influences the strength and structure of cobalt-chromium alloys.

The action of a clasp depends on the resistance of the alloy to deformation. The factors affecting this are length of arm, diameter, cross-section area, form, and the properties of the material, particularly its modulus of elasticity. An alloy with a low modulus of elasticity flexes easily while one with a high modulus is 'stiff'. The elastic limit (the point at which permanent deformation occurs in a loaded beam) should be high to prevent permanent distortion of the clasp. In a beam of constant cross-section, fixed at one end, the maximum stress occurs at the fixed end. If the beam is tapered, stress is distributed along its length. The conventional clasp should be tapered with a circular or semicircular cross-section. The retentive force of a clasp should be about 1 kg (Bates, 1980). The horizontal undercut for a cobalt-chromium clasp arm tip is 0·25 mm. This means that the clasp will be deflected by this amount on insertion and removal of the denture. This deflection is within its proportional limit. Gold alloy or stainless-steel clasps are used in undercuts greater than 0·25 mm (Bates, 1980).

Some general principles of clasp design should be observed. The rigid portion of the clasp arm should be on or above the survey line, while the flexible tips of clasp arms should lie below it and provide retention. It is a mistake to make a clasp arm pass straight across the survey line (*Fig.* 6.4). As far as possible clasp arms should be bent in two planes when viewed from the buccal or lingual side of the tooth. The nearer a clasp arm is to an L-shape, the more effective it is, since the torsional elasticity of the metal in the more rigid upright part provides flexibility to the horizontal arm and a more effective distribution of stress throughout the structure (*see Fig.* 8.6).

Straight clasp arms tend to flex at their 'shoulders' and stress is concentrated in a comparatively small area between the rigid and the flexible portions of the arm. Straight clasp arms that enter the undercuts either vertically or horizontally are usually unsatisfactory. Cast clasp arms should be made as long as possible, particularly if cobalt-chromium alloy is used. A long cobalt-chromium arm with a large cross-section area is unlikely to be stressed beyond its proportional limit, whereas it is comparatively easy to stress a shorter, thinner arm, causing a loss of retention and possible fracture.

Clasps are extra-coronal retainers and fall into two main groups:

Occlusally-approaching clasps: the arms approach the undercut of the tooth from its occlusal surface (*Fig.* 6.5**A**).

Gingivally-approaching clasps: the arms approach the undercut of the tooth from the gingival surface (*Fig.* 6.5**B**).

Clasp arms should be on opposite sides of the teeth to provide reciprocal action. Clasps should be on opposite sides of the denture and if only two are used they should be placed so that a line joining them bisects the denture. In a three-clasp retention system the centre of the triangle formed by drawing straight lines between the clasps should lie near the centre of the denture. Two clasps are sufficient in many tooth-borne dentures, but wherever

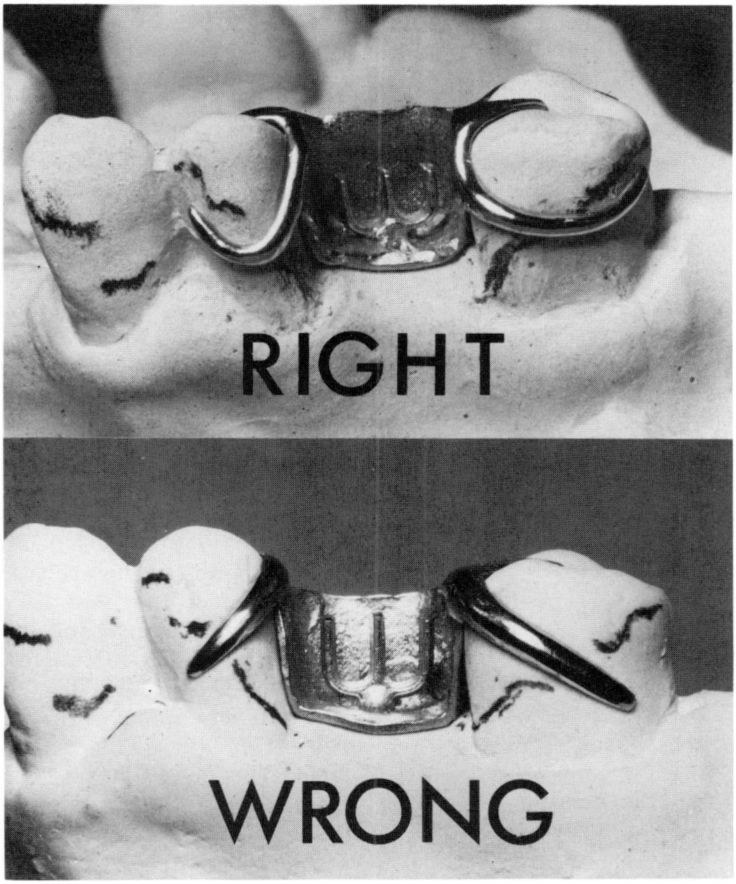

Fig. 6.4. It is a mistake to make a clasp arm pass straight across the survey line. As far as possible clasp arms should be bent in two planes to give more length and to take advantage of the torsional elasticity of the alloy. Straight clasp arms are more likely to break since the stress is concentrated at the junction with the connector.

possible three points of retention should be used on mucosa-borne and tooth-and-mucosa-borne dentures to prevent rocking when the mucosa-borne saddles move under load. Clasps should provide bracing for lateral thrusts transmitted to the teeth. As a general rule, clasps should be attached only to tooth-borne parts of a denture, and occlusally-approaching clasps should be used for tooth-borne designs as they provide the best bracing for lateral thrusts. Gingivally-approaching clasps are perhaps most suitable for mucosa-borne parts of dentures, as their greater flexibility enables some of the lateral forces to be borne by the mucosa. It is sometimes said that the clasp arms abrade enamel, but this is unlikely to happen unless the clasps are attached to mucosa-borne saddles. Damage to the enamel is usually initiated by other causes, such as acid degradation of food debris or plaque causing decalcification.

Occlusally-approaching Clasps

The parts of the clasp are as follows (*Fig.* 6.6):

the central part (body), which is the supporting element if it includes an occlusal rest;

the bracing part (shoulder), which transmits lateral thrusts to the teeth;

the distal third of the arm, which is the retentive element and lies in the undercut.

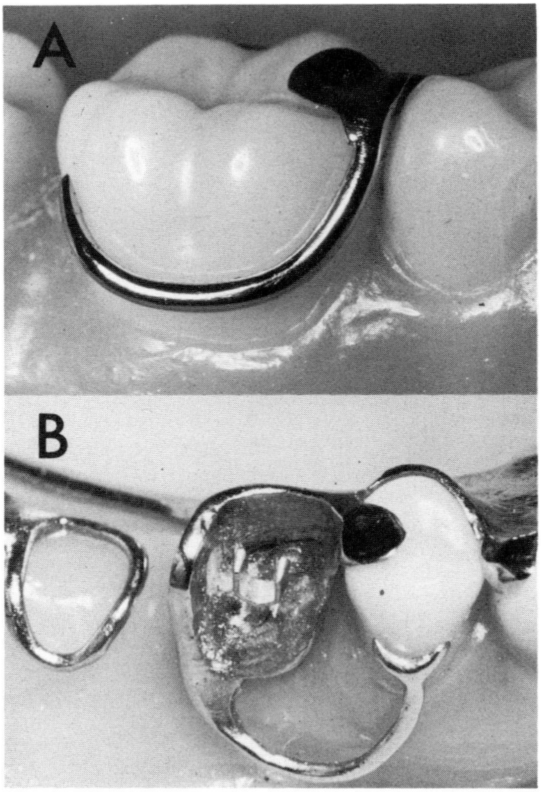

Fig. 6.5. **A**, Occlusally-approaching clasp on a lower right first molar. **B**, Gingivally-approaching clasp on a premolar.

Both the body and the shoulder of the clasp lie on or above the survey line, but never below it. The distance that the distal third of the clasp arm lies below the survey line depends on:

the bulbousness of the tooth—the more bulbous the tooth, the nearer the survey line;

the rigidity of the clasp alloy; with more rigid alloys the clasp tip should be nearer the survey line. The actual position of the clasp tip is determined by using the correct dimension of undercut gauge on the surveyor (*Figs.* 6.7, III.17).

It is very important that clasp arms should taper evenly in breadth and thickness towards their tips. A sudden decrease in section causes a concentration of stress at the narrow point, which results in permanent flexion and breakage (*Fig.* 6.8). Thin parts of clasps are most likely to be found opposite distobuccal or mesiobuccal angles of the teeth where the wax pattern may be thinned when being adapted to the investment cast.

Clasps on acrylic dentures that seem to be correctly positioned on the cast prior to flasking sometimes move during packing and processing, so that the bodies of the clasps lie in undercuts below the survey lines when the dentures are finished (*Fig.* 6.9). This is usually because the clasps have not been properly luted to the casts before flasking. The displacement also causes the arms to rise above the survey lines, rendering the clasps useless, since the bodies of the clasps have to be cut away to insert the dentures and the arms are not retentive.

Gingivally-approaching Clasps

Gingivally-approaching clasp arms should be constructed so that they do not press against the gingival margins (Roach, 1930). They can be cast in cobalt-chromium alloy or can be made of 0·8 to 1·2 mm diameter stainless steel, cobalt-chromium or gold alloy wire, the end of which is flattened by hammering on an anvil. The flattened end is then ground to fit the curvature of the tooth at the point selected for retention (*Fig.* 6.10**A**). Wrought prefabricated clasps can also be used, but the ends of some prefabricated designs are too large. The contact area between clasp and tooth should be as small as possible and in this respect wrought clasps are usually better than cast clasps (Fig. 6.10**B**). Wrought clasp arms have little bracing effect and put very little torsional stress on the clasped teeth and are therefore particularly suitable for mucosa-borne saddles.

A comparison between a gingivally-approaching clasp and an occlusally-approaching clasp is shown in *Fig.* 6.11. The gingivally-approaching clasp is made to lie at the margin of the flange and approach the distobuccal undercut in an inconspicuous way. Such a clasp aids streamlining of the denture and does not cause a food trap. It is easily tolerated by the patient. A conventional occlusally-approaching clasp arm on the same tooth does not provide as good retention. It is bulky and mars the appearance of the patient and occupies more extra-anatomical space

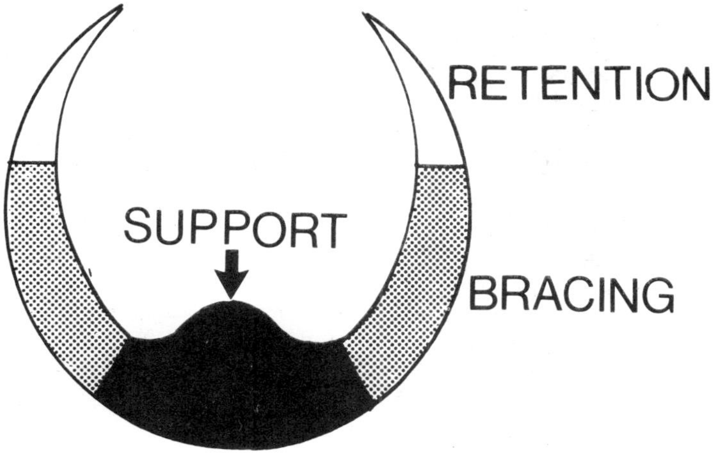

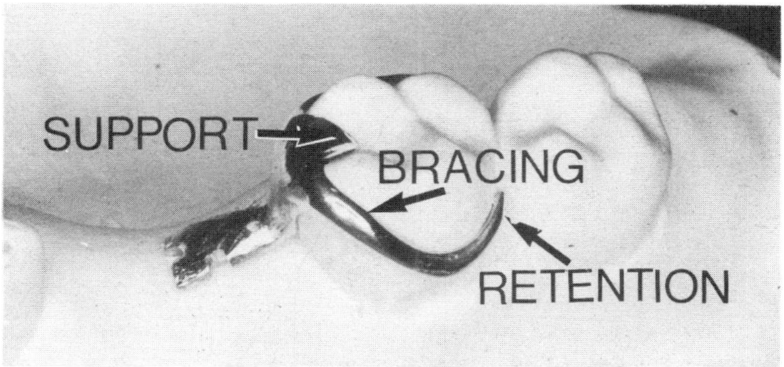

Fig. 6.6. The parts and functions of an occlusally-approaching clasp.

than the gingivally-approaching arm. A gingivally-approaching clasp provides better retention because its tip wedges against the tooth when the clasp is withdrawn. An occlusally-approaching clasp does not have this 'trip action'. With an occlusally-approaching clasp arm the patient may be more conscious of the food sticking round the arm and tending to displace the denture than with a gingivally-approaching clasp arm, but much depends on the method of construction (cf. *Fig.* 6.10**A** and 6.10**B**).

Gingivally-approaching clasps are unsuitable in positions in which there is a marked soft-tissue undercut, as the arms cannot enter the undercut without traumatising the tissues, with the result that they lie some distance away from the mucosal surface and trap food (*Fig.* 6.12). This is a fault of many gingivally-approaching clasps, but it can be avoided to some extent by making the clasp arm approach the tooth along the margin of the saddle (*Fig.* 6.12). Clasps designed in this way are inconspicuous and provide good retention. Greater flexibility of these arms can be obtained by extending the exposed part of the clasp further along the margin of the saddle.

Reciprocal Action of Clasp Arms

It is necessary to place clasp arms on opposite sides of a tooth so that the masticatory thrusts on the partial denture are transmitted to the tooth both buccally and lingually. A buccal clasp arm by itself tends to act like an orthodontic appliance and moves the tooth lingually, out of contact with the clasp, and retention is lost.

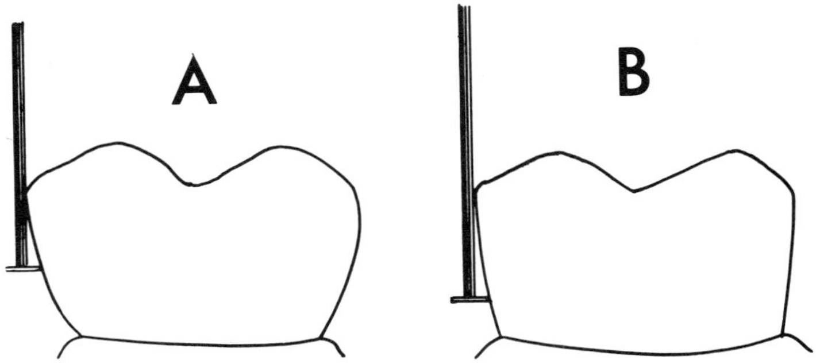

Fig. 6.7. The position of the retentive tip of the clasp arm is indicated by the undercut gauge (in this case 0·5 mm). On a bulbous tooth with a curvature of short radius (**A**) the tip of the clasp arm lies nearer the survey line than when the curvature of the tooth is of long radius (**B**).

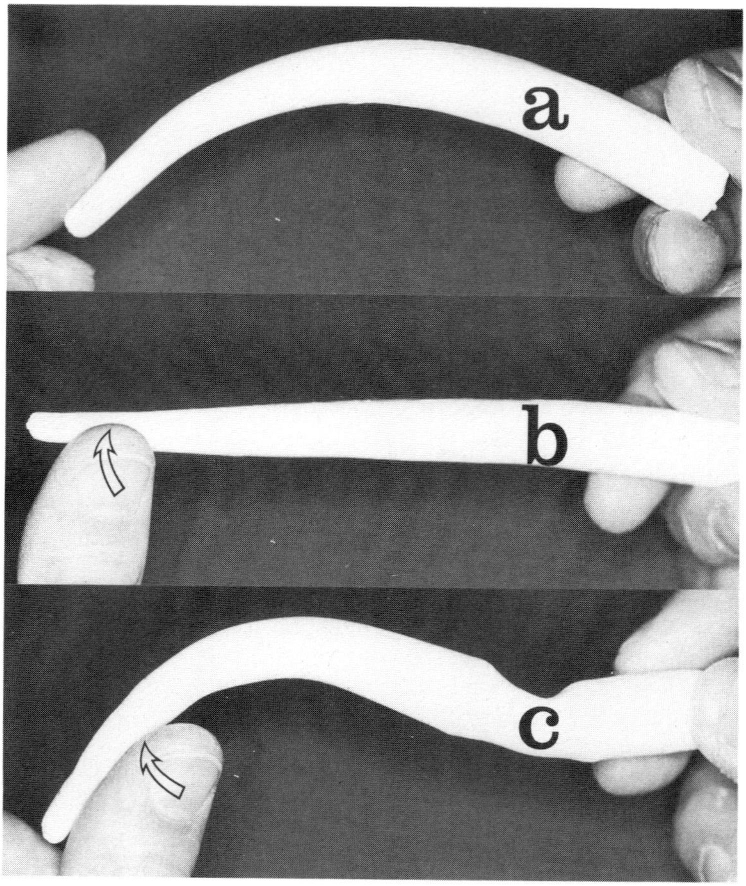

Fig. 6.8. These clay models illustrate the importance of an even taper on clasp arms and show how thinning in one area is likely to lead to a concentration of stress and fracture. '**a**', an evenly tapered curved rod; '**b**', pressure applied with the thumb to the end of the rod straightens it, indicating that the stresses and strains are distributed evenly along the rod; '**c**', stresses are concentrated where there is a narrower part of the tapered rod and the rod remains curved when displaced by the thumb.

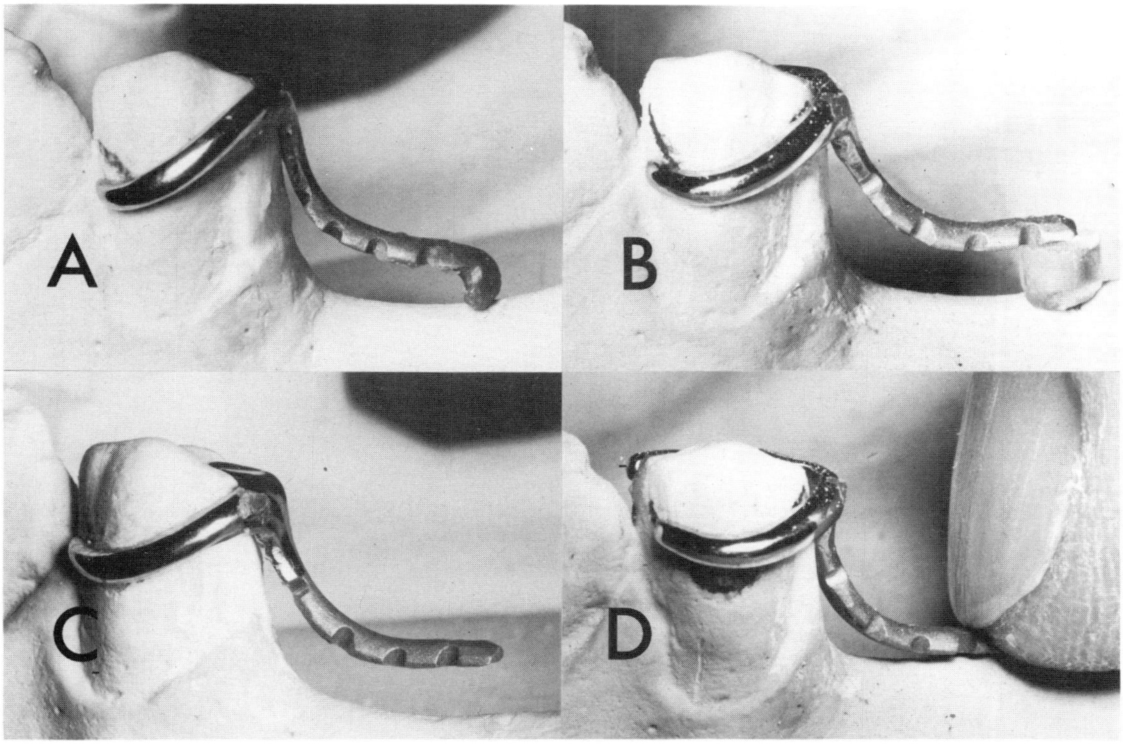

Fig. 6.9. Displacement of clasp during packing and processing can be prevented by (**A**) extending the cast tag to contact the ridge, or (**B**) propping the tag with a small piece of acrylic. Where no prop is made, the clasp can be displaced (**C** and **D**).

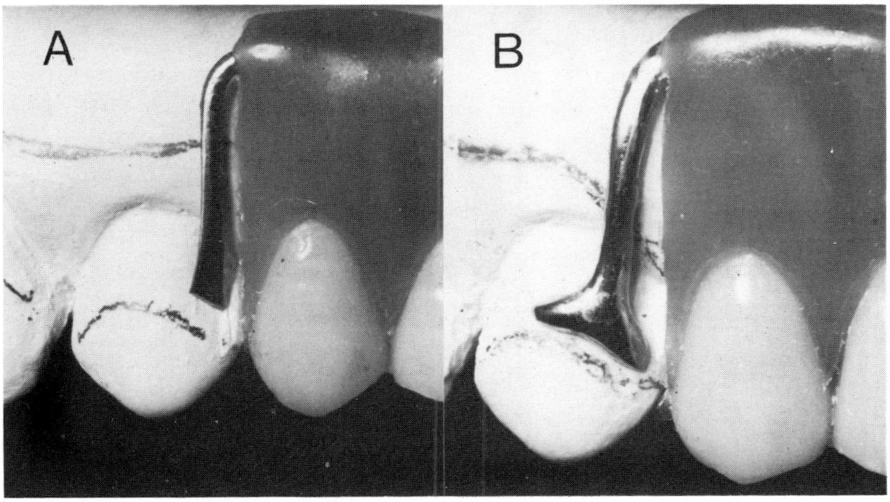

Fig. 6.10. **A,** Wrought stainless-steel wire clasp (1 mm diameter). The end of the wire has been flattened and ground to fit the contour of the tooth. **B,** Cast gingivally-approaching clasp occupies more space, is more rigid, and covers more tooth surface than the wrought clasp.

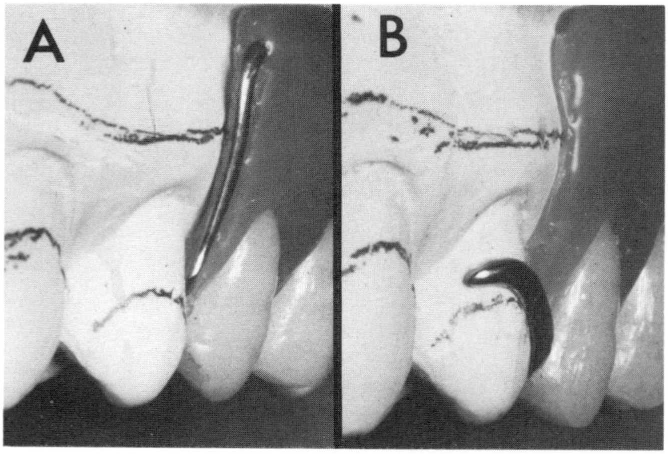

Fig. 6.11. **A**, Gingivally-approaching clasp. **B**, Occlusally-approaching clasp for same tooth. By making the gingivally-approaching clasp follow the margin of the saddle, the 'streamlining' of the denture is maintained. More 'extra-anatomical' space is occupied by the occlusally-approaching clasp.

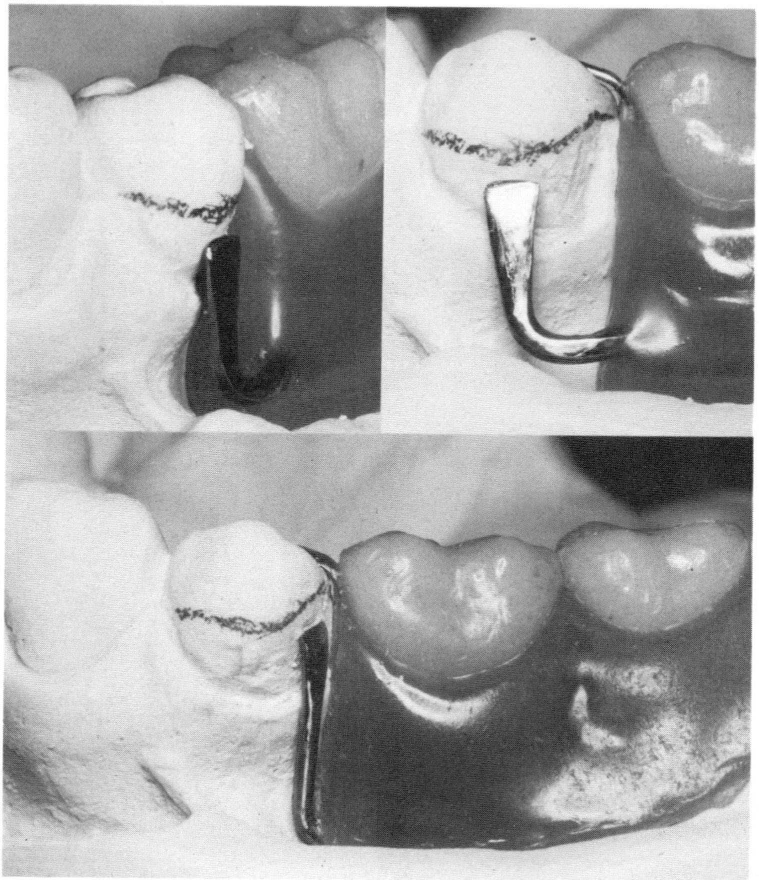

Fig. 6.12. *Upper,* Gingivally-approaching clasps should not be used in this case where there are large soft-tissue undercuts. A large gap between the clasp arm and the mucosa results. *Lower,* The problem can sometimes be resolved by making the clasp arm follow the margin of the saddle, thus aiding the 'streamlining' of the denture.

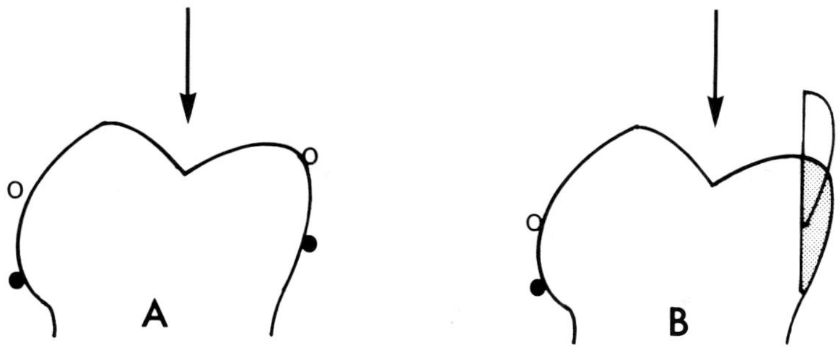

Fig. 6.13. Circles represent sections through clasp arms. Open sections: positions of clasp arm and lingual plate at first contact on insertion. Solid sections and stippled area: positions of clasp arms and lingual plate when denture is completely seated. **A**, It is seldom possible to make the buccal and lingual arms of a clasp contact the tooth at the same time during insertion and removal of the denture. **B**, Modification of the tooth does make it possible, but has some inherent disadvantages. (*See* text.)

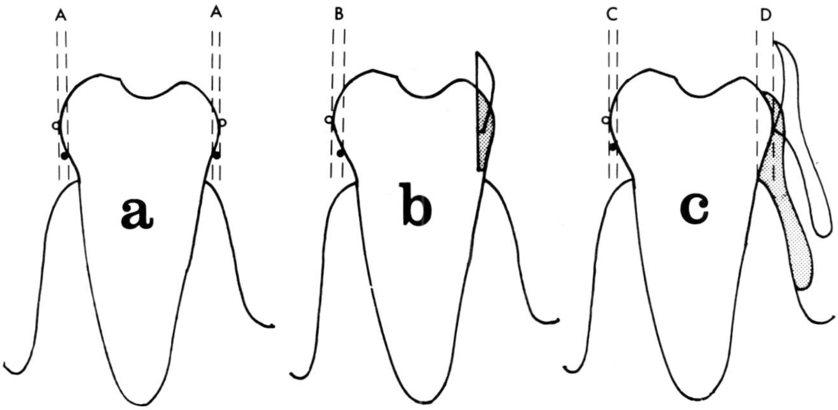

Fig. 6.14. The solid dots represent cross-sections of clasp arms in undercuts with the dentures seated. The open dots represent the same clasp arms fully deflected as they pass across the survey lines. The shaded areas are cross-sections of the denture bases seated, and the open outlines are the denture bases as they pass across the survey lines. **a,** Flexible clasp arms in opposite undercuts. The retentive force equals the force required for deflecting A + A. **b,** Flexible clasp arm opposite rigid denture base lying in a prepared guide plane parallel to the path of insertion and removal. The retentive force equals the force required for deflecting B. **c,** Flexible clasp arm opposite a rigid denture base lying in an undercut. The deflection of the clasp arm during insertion and removal is C + D since no deflection of the rigid base is possible.

It is sometimes supposed that the object of placing reciprocal arms on a clasp is to ensure that equal thrusts occur on both sides of the tooth when the denture is inserted, but this is seldom possible (Bates, 1980) (*Fig.* 6.13). Indeed, it is a minor matter if the tooth is slightly displaced by a clasp arm when the denture is inserted or removed. Such transient forces on a tooth frequently occur during mastication and are unlikely to have any lasting effect on the tooth or periodontium. A much more important aspect of reciprocation appears when we consider the relative rigidity of clasp arms on the opposite sides of a tooth. *Fig.* 6.14**a** shows a tooth with equal clasp arms on opposite sides lying in equal undercuts. When the denture is inserted each clasp arm is displaced 0·5 mm as it crosses the survey line and springs back into a 0·5 mm undercut, where it remains passive against the tooth. Thus the total retention provided by such a clasp is equivalent to the force required to displace two clasp arms 0·5 mm each. Let us suppose that the lingual arm is replaced by

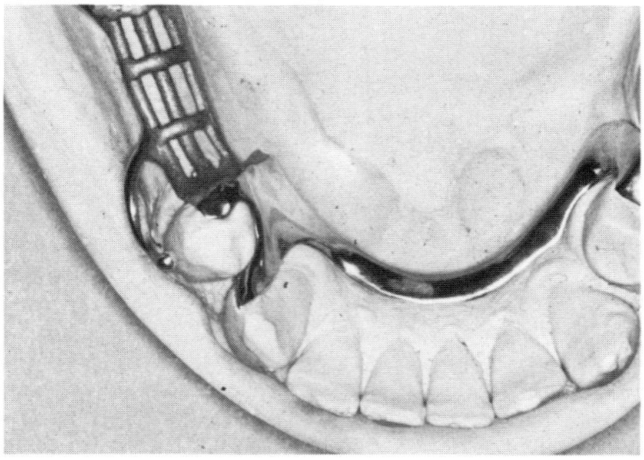

Fig. 6.15. A rigid part of the denture base provides reciprocation for a flexible clasp arm on the premolar. The theoretical implications of this arrangement are discussed in Chapter 3 (*see Fig.* 3.5).

a rigid part of the denture base, which enters a prepared seat. Then only the buccal arm is displaced 0·5 mm as the appliance crosses the survey line, because the rigid portion of the denture base does not flex at all (*Fig.* 6.14**b**). The buccal clasp arm then provides the only retentive force as it displaces 0·5 mm to enter the undercut. The total retentive force is thus halved compared to the situation in *Fig.* 6.14**a**. However, if a badly constructed denture is snapped into an undercut (*Fig.* 6.14**c**), the single clasp arm is deflected twice as much. It thus provides a greater retentive force, but is much more liable to break.

Consider the forces upon the tooth in *Fig.* 6.15. When a lateral masticatory force on the denture moves the denture buccally, the total force is transmitted to the tooth through the rigid portion of the denture base and the tooth moves buccally as far as the periodontium allows it. When a masticatory force tends to move the denture lingually, the flexible buccal clasp arm is displaced and absorbs some of the energy before the tooth is moved in a lingual direction. The periodontium on the lingual surface of the root is less compressed, while the buccal surface is under a greater compressive load. Normal adaptive processes (already discussed in Chapter 3) tend to equalize the movement of the tooth. Thus, the periodontium on the buccal side thickens to compensate for the lack of flexibility of the lingual denture base, while the periodontium on the lingual side of the tooth requires less adaptation, since part of the movement of the denture is taken up by the flexibility of the buccal clasp arm (*see Fig.* 3.5). However, it may be argued that lateral thrusts towards one side are transmitted to the tooth by the rigid part of the denture on the opposite side and the flexibility of the clasp arm is not used. Nevertheless, the situation remains that where rigid parts of the denture provide reciprocation on the lingual side of the teeth, thickening of the buccal periodontium is likely to occur, and where there are flexible buccal arms of clasps the lingual periodontium is unlikely to thicken as much.

The foregoing statements are obviously an over-simplification of the true situation within a three-dimensional periodontal membrane, since the complex viscoelastic forces cannot be easily resolved by a simple geometrical model, but there is ample evidence that the kind of changes described do take place when teeth are subjected to extrinsic loads (Waerhaug, 1955; Wentz et al., 1958; Ramfjord and Kohler, 1959; Glickman, 1963; Svanberg and Lindhe, 1973; Lindhe and Svanberg, 1974; Lindhe and Nyman, 1977; Nyman et al., 1978; Galler et al., 1979; Moss 1980a,b; Polson, 1980).

An additional complexity is that the occlusal forces on the remaining teeth are altered by the loss of teeth in partially edentulous patients, so that the teeth may not be in a state of stable equilibrium. It cannot be emphasized too strongly that occlusal stability should always be established before any partial denture is constructed (*see* Chapter 3).

Cast and Wrought Clasps

The following guidelines may help when deciding whether to make a clasp of cast or wrought metal:

1. Make clasps of wrought metal if the undercuts are deep and the clasp arms are likely to be subject to much displacement on insertion and removal.

2. If undercuts are shallow, a stiff clasp with a high modulus of elasticity is required; thus a cast clasp is generally indicated.

3. The 'trip action' of gingivally-approaching clasps provides firmer retention than

occlusally-approaching clasps of equivalent length and section.

4. When the denture base is made of acrylic, wrought clasps are cheaper and easier to use than cast clasps.

5. When it is not possible to make a clasp arm more than 10 mm long, wrought metal usually produces the best results, but cast alloy clasp arms can be used when it is possible to make them long enough to give the desired displacement without permanent distortion.

6. When it is necessary to clasp a tooth in the middle of a row of teeth, wrought embrasure hooks generally provide the best and simplest form of retention (*Fig.* 6.16) (Witt, 1981). However, when the occlusion is intact it is seldom wise to bring clasp connectors across occlusal embrasures because the supporting cusps of the opposing teeth occlude on the marginal ridges. If these are ground to make room for the clasp, it is not long before the opposing tooth moves and its cusp comes into firm contact with the ground marginal ridges. This explains the frequent finding that although a partial denture with embrasure hooks may seem to be all right at the trial stage, occlusal interferences with the clasp arms may become evident by the time the denture is fitted.

7. When it is essential to make a clasp cross the occlusal embrasure, it is wise to prepare crowns or inlays in the teeth to be clasped and to provide a well-defined channel for the clasp (*Fig.* 6.17). This channel must be constructed so that the supporting cusp either straddles the channel or firmly occludes on one or other side of it. The clasps in this case are made of cast alloy.

8. Where long mucosa-borne saddles are present on a denture, wrought clasps may be used to reduce the lateral thrusts on the abutment teeth. These clasps have sufficient 'give' to allow the mucosa of the ridge to accept part of the lateral thrust. Rigid cast clasps on such dentures transfer all the lateral load to the abutment teeth, with the result that they become traumatised, but well-designed cast clasps can reduce the risk of periodontal trauma (*see Fig.* 6.20).

9. Cast clasps should be used on cast tooth-borne dentures when the clasps and denture base can be cast together. This simplifies denture production, but casting shrinkage must be carefully compensated to avoid badly-fitting clasps.

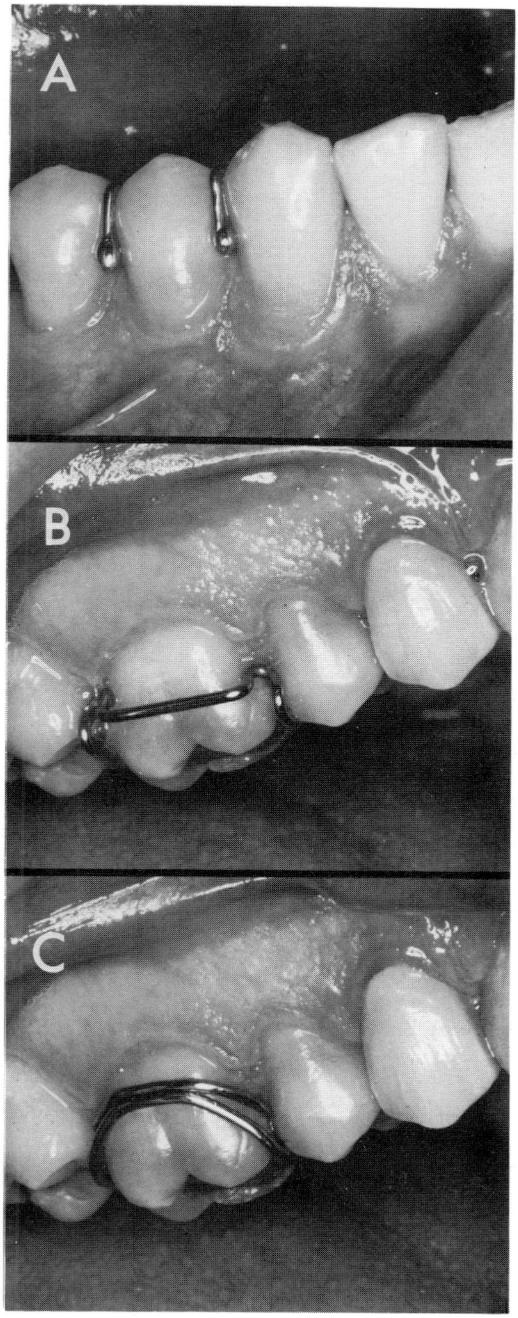

Fig. 6.16. **A,** Wrought wire embrasure hooks provide the simplest form of retention on teeth within intact portions of the dental arch, but crib clasps may also be used. **B,** Adams. **C,** Crozat.

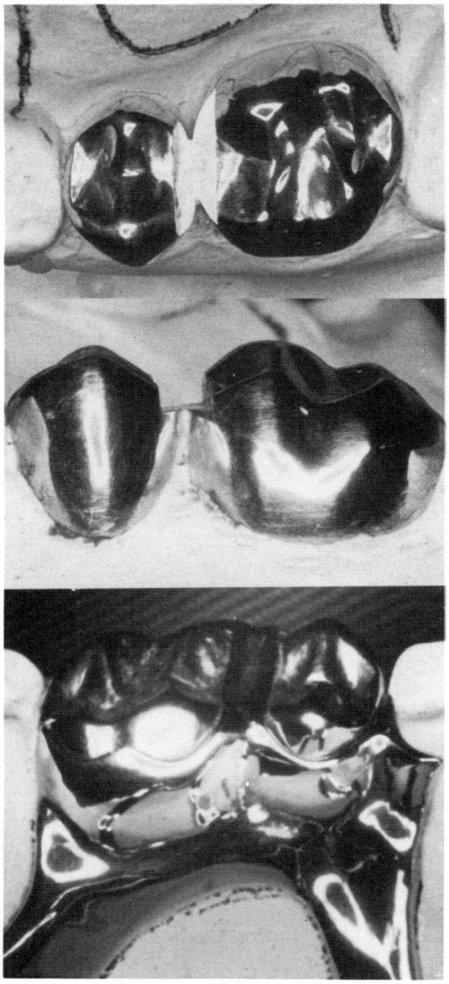

Fig. 6.17. Where a cast clasp must cross the occlusal embrasure, a well-defined channel should be prepared in the restorations to accommodate it. *Upper,* Occlusal view of channel. *Middle,* Buccal view. *Lower,* Lingual view with removable partial denture in place.

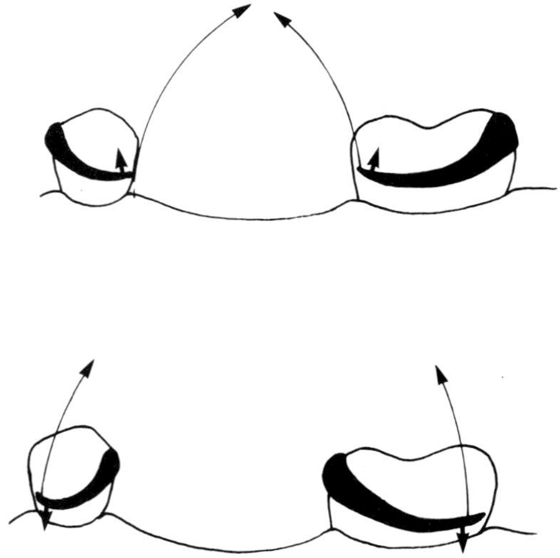

Fig. 6.18. The long arrows represent rotational displacement of the ends of bounded saddles; the short arrows represent the movements of the clasp arms at the ends of the saddles opposite those being displaced. Note that in the upper diagram rotational displacement at the molar end of the saddle is resisted to some extent by the premolar clasp pressing more firmly against the tooth in the undercut, whereas in the lower diagram rotational displacement of the molar clasp causes the premolar clasp arm to go deeper into the undercut; thus it does not resist displacement. Similarly, when the premolar end of the saddle is displaced, the molar clasp arm does not resist this displacement in the lower diagram, but does resist the displacement in the upper diagram.

10. The use of gold alloys for clasps near the front of the mouth is recommended for patients who are prepared to tolerate the glint of gold on smiling, but who would reject the flash of cobalt-chromium.

11. The attachment of wrought clasps to cast partial dentures can present problems. Some wrought alloys can be incorporated in the casting or can be soldered directly to the cast bases. If this is done and the joint is not covered with acrylic, the clasp arm may fail because of recrystallization of the wire at the site of the attachment to the cast base. Therefore wrought clasps should only be attached to cast bases if the junction can be covered by the acrylic of the saddles. To a lesser extent the same applies to gold, but the problem can sometimes be overcome by incorporating a tunnel in the casting to house the wrought wire at its point of exit from the casting. The wire is then soldered to the casting at a point distant from the tunnel. In this way the recrystallized portion of the wire is not subject to stress when the clasp is in use in the mouth.

12. Clasp arms at the ends of bounded saddles are sometimes placed so that their tips do not resist rotational displacement of the denture, although they may resist removal in the common path of displacement (*Fig.* 6.18). Clasp arms resist rotational displacement if their tips are placed in undercuts on the parts of the teeth furthest from the saddle but, as

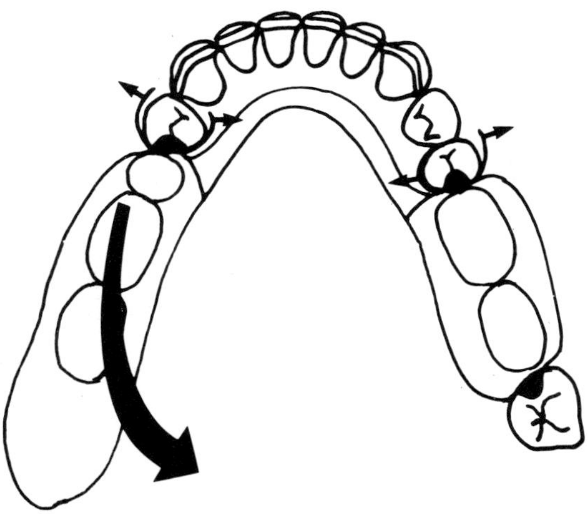

Fig. 6.19. A partial lower denture with insufficient bracing can be displaced posteriorly and rotated horizontally (*large arrow*). This may distort the wrought clasp arms (*small arrows*).

pointed out by Walter (1980), clasp arm tips facing towards the saddle provide more resistance to displacement if in adequate undercuts. Jacobson and Krol (1982) have systematized the use of rotational paths in removable partial denture designs. With extended occlusal rests and careful surveying techniques they reduce the number of conventional clasps on the denture and gain retention by placing rigid parts of the base in undercuts.

13. In addition to considering rotational displacement of dentures in a vertical plane, we must also consider the effect of rotational displacement in a horizontal plane. Such displacement is most likely to occur in dentures with unilateral or bilateral free-end saddles when medial and lateral chewing thrusts on the denture may distort and displace clasp arms if bracing is insufficient (*Fig.* 6.19). In some cases it may be wise to design the denture so that the bracing arms are rigid, although this has the disadvantages previously mentioned, and like all other design decisions it is probably the lesser of two evils.

As an aid in the choice of clasps for mandibular dentures with bilateral free-end saddles, the clasps are graded as shown in *Fig.* 6.20.

The clasps numbered I to VI have been graded for Appearance, Comfort, Efficiency and Hygiene on a scale 1–3, 1 being best and 3 worst. Under the general heading 'Efficiency' the clasp is rated for retention and for the way in which it transmits the masticatory forces to the teeth. For example, clasps IV and VI are graded 3 for Efficiency because, although they are retentive, they may traumatise the abutments when used on free-end saddles, but they would be quite satisfactory on bounded saddles. Clasps IV and V have a low Comfort grade as the lingual clasp arms tend to irritate the tongue, but clasps I, II and VI with lingual plates are graded 1 for Comfort but grade 3 for Hygiene. The Rest-Plate I-bar System III rates highly for Comfort, as the rest connector is tucked into the embrasure and out of the way of the tongue. The Hygiene rating is good as the gingival margin of the premolar is uncovered and this also is true of clasps IV and V. However, the absence of a lingual clasp arm in III makes the lingual gingiva more accessible to the tongue than in IV and V where food trapping might occur. They are therefore graded 2 for Hygiene.

The Rest Plate I-bar (RPI) System III seems to the best of this group of clasps, but the teeth must be suitably shaped to prevent trauma and to resist backward movement of the appliance. If that is not possible, then the efficiency of the retainer is lost. This is also true of V. The difficulty can be overcome, however, by extending the buccal retentive arm into the embrasure (dotted line V) and placing it near the fulcrum axis through the mesial occlusal rests. This puts much less stress on the teeth than the clasp system IV or VI. In VI the presence of the distal occlusal rest would cause the mesial rest to rise from the tooth when the free-end saddle was loaded. Removal of the distal occlusal rest would improve the design as the mesial rest would then transmit the load more favourably to the tooth. The buccal clasp arm would then lie behind the fulcrum axis and would not put tilting forces on the teeth. It is possible that the lingual plates in clasps I and II might also transmit unfavourable forces to these teeth and for this reason their Efficiency grade is 2.

Clasp I is graded 3 for Appearance as the buccal arm, where it crosses the embrasure, would show at the corner of the mouth. Clasps

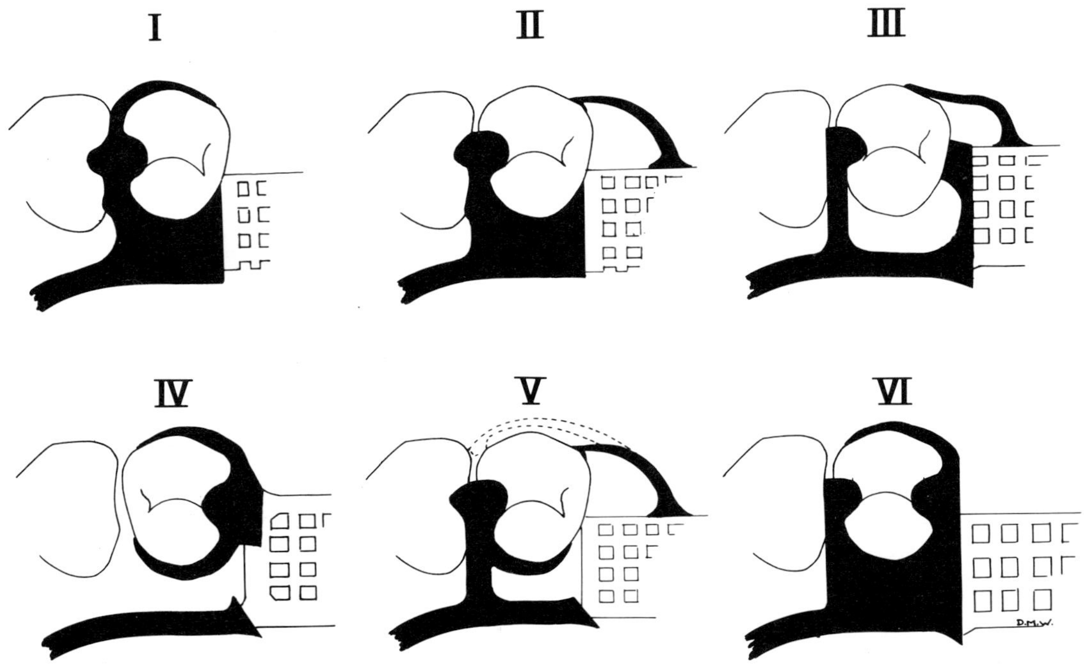

Fig. 6.20. Clasps for bilateral free-end saddle lower dentures are numbered I to VI and are graded for Appearance, Comfort, Efficiency and Hygiene. the grading is 1 to 3 (1 = best and 3 = worst).

	Appearance	*Comfort*	*Efficiency*	*Hygiene*
I	3	1	2	3
II	1	1	2	3
III	1	1	1*	1
IV	2	3	3	2
V	1	3	1*	2
VI	2	1	3	3

*provided the teeth are suitably shaped to prevent trauma and to resist backward displacement of the denture, but the dotted extension shown in V would overcome this difficulty.
(*See* text for discussion.)

IV and VI are graded 2 for Appearance as their buccal arms are less conspicuous than that of clasp I. Clasps II, III and V are all inconspicuous and are graded 1 as they have the best Appearance. A glance at *Fig.* 6.20 shows that the RPI system is clearly ahead of the others provided there is adequate resistance to backward movement of the denture.

It is obvious that this grading system is somewhat subjective and many other factors operate in the final choice of clasps for individual patients. The type and position of the survey lines have perhaps the greatest influence and have tended to give rise to hard and fast rules that ignore the other factors. We hope this discussion will help in your choice of appropriate clasps to meet your patients' needs.

Summary

Thus, when designing retention for dentures, careful consideration must be given to the shape and position of the individual teeth, to the requirements for reciprocally-acting clasp arms, and to the comfort and appearance of the patient. Avoid placing clasp arms on the anterior teeth. Patients don't like them and will seldom wear a denture that has such arms. Even patients who have lips that are

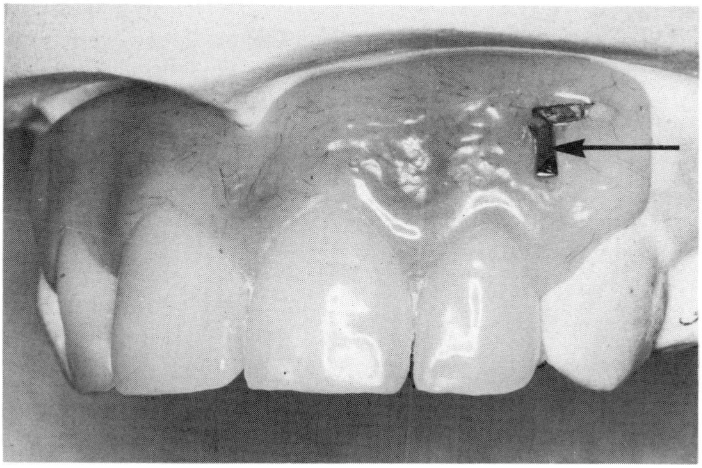

Fig. 6.21. An acrylic hinged flange locked in position with a bolt (*arrowed*) provides retention for a partial denture.

apparently long enough to cover these clasp arms can usually retract their lips sufficiently to see the clasp arms; although the arms are not visible in normal function, their very presence embarrasses such patients. In these cases other means of retention should be used. The appearance of partial dentures is further discussed in Chapter 15.

Extensions of the Denture Base into Undercuts

Use of Oblique Paths of Insertion and Removal

Some acrylic dentures that fit around gingival margins are made without any prior survey of the cast. Such dentures are retained by forcing rigid portions of the denture into undercuts and causing displacement of the teeth as the undercut portions pass over their widest contours. After much chairside trimming, the dentures go in with a snap and are very often difficult to remove. This type of denture should not be made. The average width of the periodontal membrane is 0·2 mm, and the amount of displacement of the teeth can approach this figure when such dentures are forced in. The result is that the periodontal membrane is crushed between the teeth and their bony sockets. The gingival margins are also damaged because such dentures are usually mucosa-borne. Hence, both deep and superficial periodontal lesions are produced.

Retention of partial dentures in relation to the common path of displacement can be obtained from extensions of the denture base into undercuts by using an oblique path of insertion and removal. In bounded saddles usually one undercut can be engaged while the other undercut is blocked out (*see* Chapter 5). Undercuts are to be found on both the soft and hard tissues and the most obvious ones are those on the labial side of the incisor region. These can be engaged by labial flanges that are rigid or hinged (*Fig.* 6.21) or entirely separate and bolted in position. Anterior flanges engage buccal and proximal undercuts and provide the necessary retention without clasps showing at the front of the mouth, giving the denture a pleasing appearance.

Occasionally, soft-tissue undercuts alone can be used to provide anterior retention. *Fig.* 6.22 illustrates a simple acrylic design for this method of anterior retention, which is particularly suitable for patients who are very intolerant of anything covering the front of the palate and who refuse to wear partial dentures that show clasps at the front of the mouth. Extension arms are placed on the labial alveolar mucosa to provide retention in relation to the common path of displacement (Tuerkheim, 1933). The base does not cover the anterior part of the palate and thus does not interfere with the tongue. The denture may

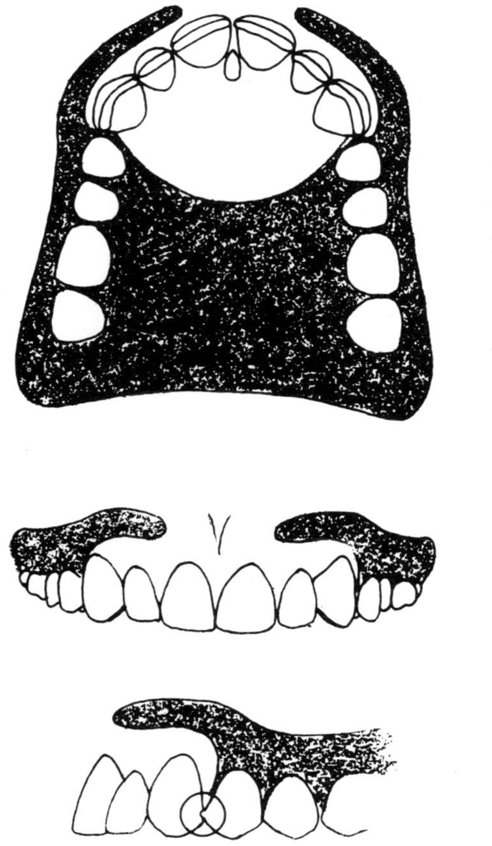

Fig. 6.22. Mucosa-borne acrylic partial denture with extension arms into labial undercuts. These provide direct as well as indirect retention.

be rather fragile, but patients are usually willing to accept this because of the increased comfort and improved appearance. These acrylic partial dentures often give many years of service provided oral hygiene is maintained.

When we examine more closely the way in which these dentures function, it is evident that some 'gum-stripping' is likely to occur at the distal gingival margin of the canine teeth, but this does not always occur, probably because the denture rotates around a soft-tissue fulcrum when loaded and thus does not necessarily damage the gingival margin (*see* 'Realities of gum-stripping' in Chapter 4).

One problem that can arise in designing this type of denture is that when the labial undercut is very deep it may be necessary to block out a large undercut distal to the canines and this tends to produce a food trap. This can also destroy the contact points and thus the axis of rotation. Fitting a second canine tooth against the mucosa distal to the natural canine reduces the danger of food lodgement, but increases the problem of developing an adequate axis of rotation and it is sometimes necessary to cut a small groove at the contact point on the natural tooth to provide a fulcrum and ensure adequate retention of the appliance (*Fig.* 6.23).

Sectional Dentures

Sectional dentures are usually used for short bounded saddles. The dentures are tooth-borne and are made in sections that are put in the mouth and are then locked together by a mechanical device. The sections are usually buccal and lingual or mesial and distal and the locking devices may be bolts, spring-loaded clips, magnets, split pins or posts that enter tubes in the opposite section. In some cases the sections are completely separate, but in others they are hinged together in such a way that the appliance can be inserted when open and locked in position when closed. The general principles underlying the design of these dentures and the details of their construction are clearly described by Pullen-Warner and L'Estrange (1978). More details of sectional dentures are given in Chapter 12.

Swinglock System

The swinglock system provides a flange or bar that swings horizontally round a vertical hinge and locks on the other side of the arch (*Fig.* 6.24) (Simmons, 1963; Antos et al., 1978; Schulte and Smith, 1980; Becker and Bolender, 1981; Bolender and Becker, 1981; Gomes et al., 1981). The flange may cover the labial gingivae of the anterior teeth, or spurs from a swinging bar may engage the teeth and provide firm retention for the appliance (*Fig.* 6.25). These flange retention systems require a high level of oral cleanliness to prevent gingival damage. It is essential that in all hinge-flange or swinglock systems the denture is adequately tooth-supported to avoid damage to the soft tissues. When the

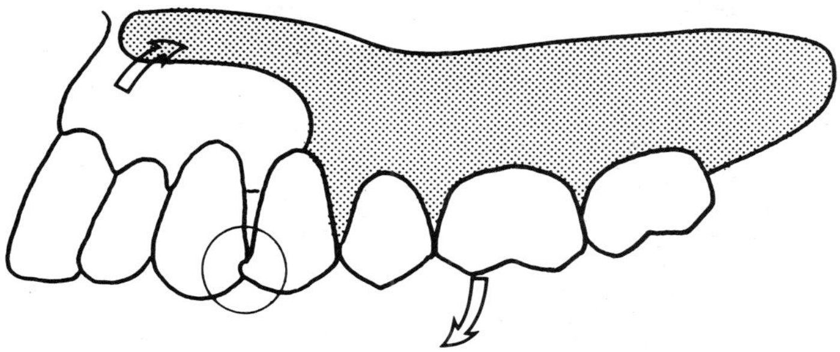

Fig. 6.23. A second canine in place of the first premolar improves the hygiene of the denture but a notch must be cut at the contact point to provide an axis of rotation. The labial extensions give indirect retention to the appliance. (*See also Fig.* 6.22).

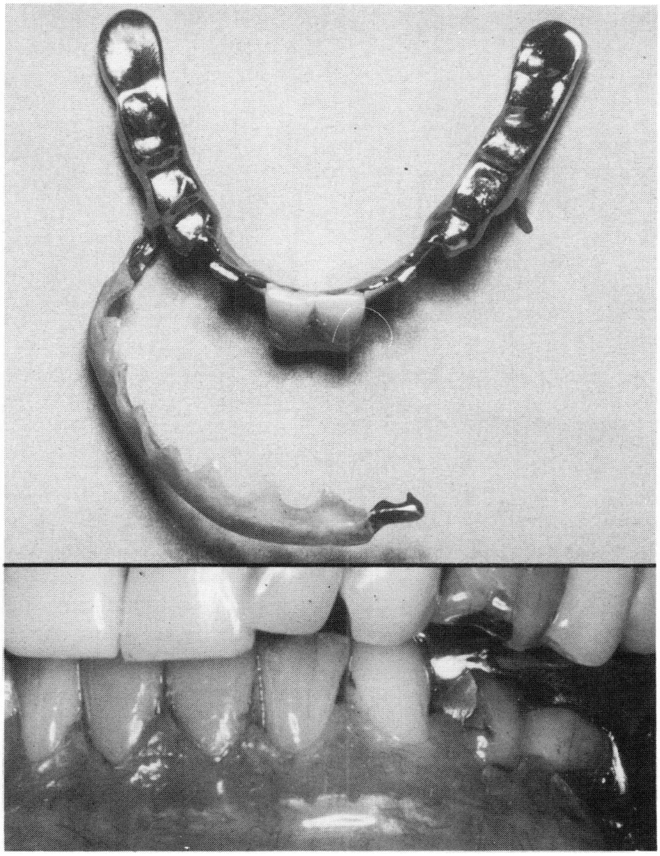

Fig. 6.24. The swinglock system provides retention for an occlusal corrective appliance. In this case the unconventional acrylic flange effectively hides the replacement of the lower central incisors.

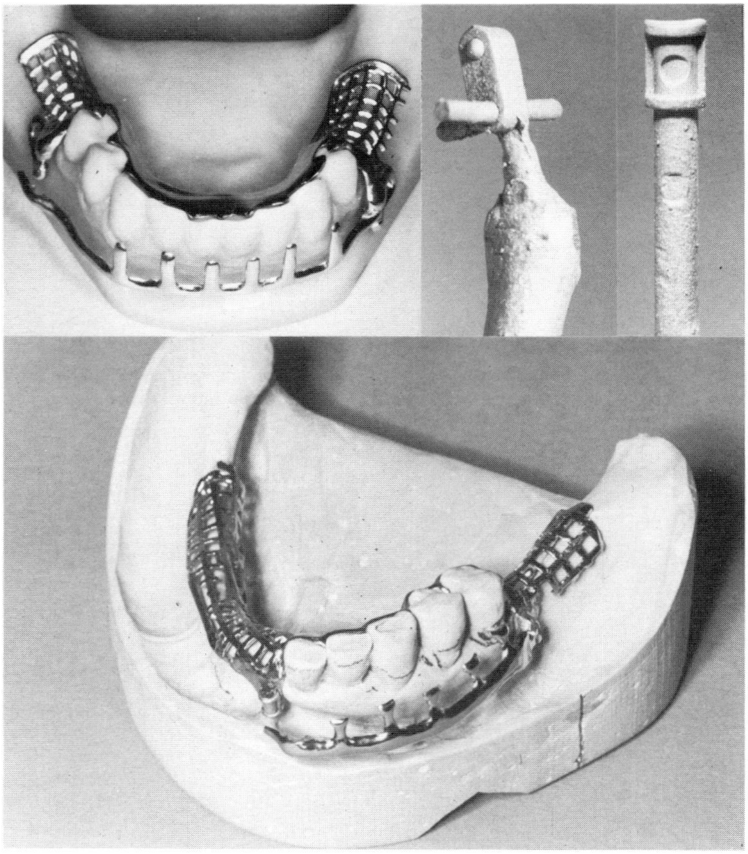

Fig. 6.25. Two examples of swinglock bars with retentive spurs. The upper right photographs show the hinge and latch as cast from plastic patterns.

swinglock system is used as retention for bilateral free-end saddle lower dentures, the effectiveness in providing indirect support depends largely on the distance between the anterior spurs and the occlusal rests. The greater the distance, the more effective are the spur-like retainers in providing indirect support for the saddles (*Fig.* 6.26). However, it must be accepted that this type of support may produce damaging extracting forces on the teeth carrying the retaining spurs, and regular relining of the saddles is essential in these cases.

Indirect Retention and Indirect Support

Indirect Retention

When a supporting element of a denture lies on one side of a line drawn between the direct retainers of the denture, it provides indirect retention for the part of the denture on the opposite side of the line. Any attempt to displace that part of the denture tends to make the denture rotate around the line drawn between the clasp arm tips. This rotation is opposed by the pressure of the supporting element (indirect retainer) against the oral structure on which it rests (*Fig.* 6.27). The indirect retainer can be an occlusal rest or continuous clasp resting against the tooth or it might be an extension of the denture base that rests against the mucosa. As the distant part of the denture is displaced, the fulcrum round which the denture tends to rotate moves from the line between the clasp arm tips to the position of the indirect retainer, converting the denture into a third class lever, whereby the direct retainers resist the displacing force

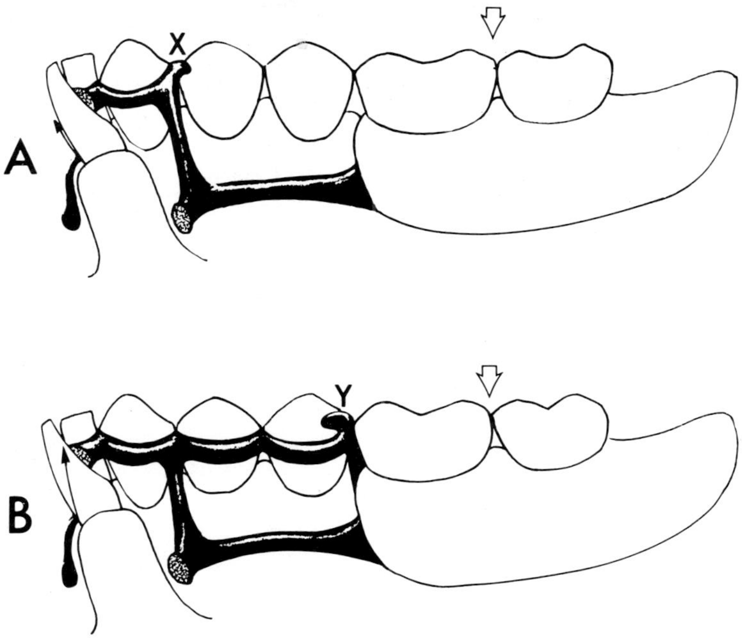

Fig. 6.26. **A**, An occlusal rest placed on the mesial marginal ridge of the first premolar (X) makes the retentive spurs of a swinglock denture less effective for indirect support than in '**B**' when the rest is placed on the distal part of the occlusal surface of the second premolar (Y). The *open arrows* indicate the point of application of the masticatory loads. The *small black arrows* indicate the arc of rotation of the spurs round the occlusal rests. Note that in '**A**' the spur loses contact with the tooth when the saddle sinks.

around the fulcrum provided by the indirect retainer. The indirect retainer by itself does not provide retention.

Indirect Support

When a load is applied to a mucosa-borne saddle the denture tends to rotate towards the mucosa round a fulcrum passing through the occlusal rests nearest the mucosa-borne saddle. This rotation can be resisted by a retainer placed on the side of the fulcrum axis opposite the point of applied load. That retainer provides indirect support. This indirect support is sometimes known as 'cantilever support' and is a converse of indirect retention as the retaining element produces indirect support while a supporting element produces indirect retention. The cartoon of children on a seesaw helps to illustrate the point (*Fig.* 6.28). In the upper illustration the boy cannot raise his end of the seesaw from the ground as long as the girl has her legs extended and firmly supported on the ground. In this respect she is providing indirect retention for the boy's end of the seesaw. We must assume that the real retention comes from the hoop of metal that crosses the plank of the seesaw at its fulcrum and is equivalent to the direct retainer. In the lower illustration the girl provides indirect support for the boy, as he cannot make his end of the seesaw touch the ground as long as she has her toes hooked under the stone. Her toes then act as a retainer, providing indirect support for the boy, but the direct support comes from the log, which supports the seesaw at its fulcrum.

In practice, indirect support is seldom effective for removable partial dentures, since it is seldom possible to make a retainer sufficiently rigid to provide it. Nevertheless, in fixed partial denture work cantilever bridges are frequently used as the abutment pieces firmly cemented on the teeth can provide the necessary indirect support. Unfortunately, however, where indirect support is used the teeth carrying the retainers have extracting

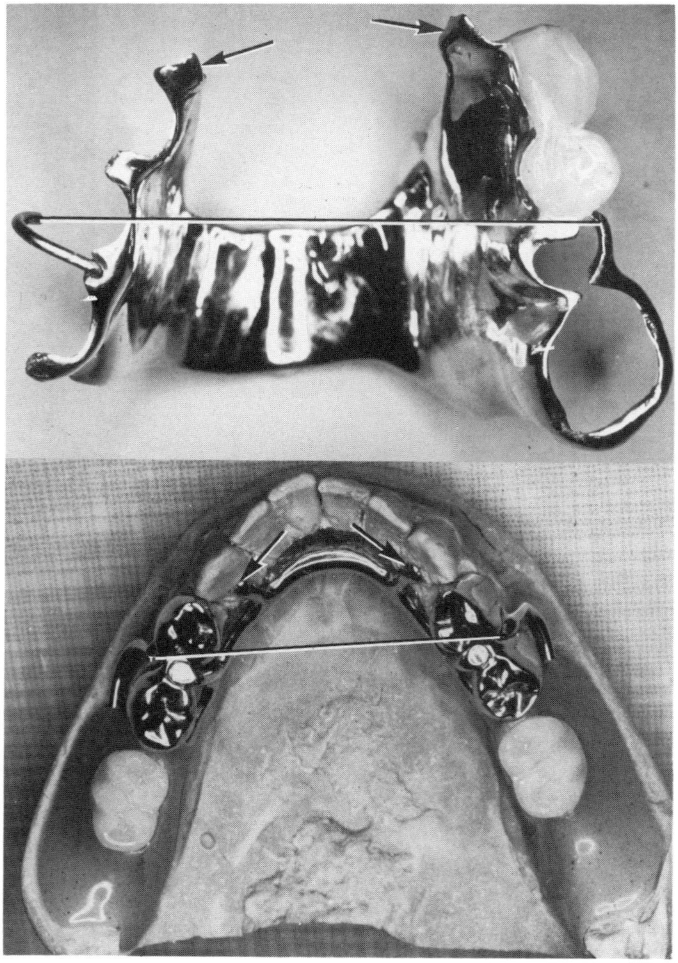

Fig. 6.27. Examples of indirect retainers (*arrows*) on upper and lower dentures. The lines join the direct retainers and represent the axis round which the denture would rotate if displaced. The indirect retainers prevent this rotation.

forces placed on them every time the patient bites upon the cantilevered pontics. This may damage the periodontium of these abutment teeth. Amongst others Izikowitz (1976) has suggested that fixed free-end saddle dentures can be made entirely tooth-borne using the cantilever principle of support. A minimum of two or three abutment teeth are required to support the anterior part of these 'extended bridges', but when the extended pontics are loaded there is a great risk that the anterior abutment piece will be pulled loose from its abutment tooth. For this reason pin retention is sometimes used for these crowns. While this may prevent them being loosened, it does not prevent extracting forces being placed on the anterior abutment teeth when the cantilever pontics are loaded. Most dentists who advocate this type of prosthesis recommend that a maximum of two pontics should be cantilevered out beyond the last abutment tooth. The mechanical disadvantages of such appliances are such that one would not expect them to succeed, but nevertheless it has been claimed that they have been worn successfully for many years. Presumably the muscle force on the appliance is limited by the nociceptors in the periodontium of the abutment teeth

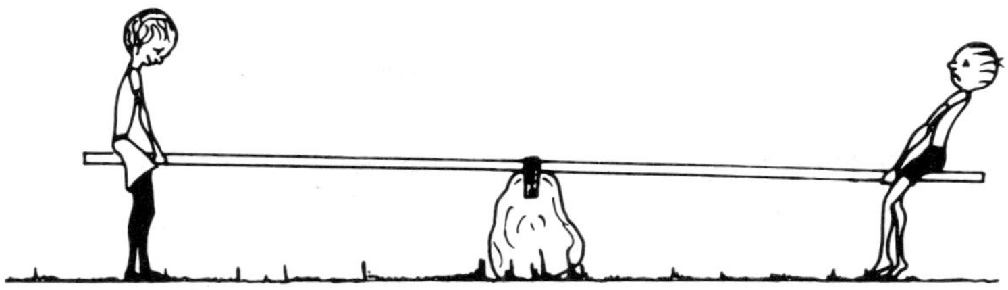

INDIRECT RETENTION

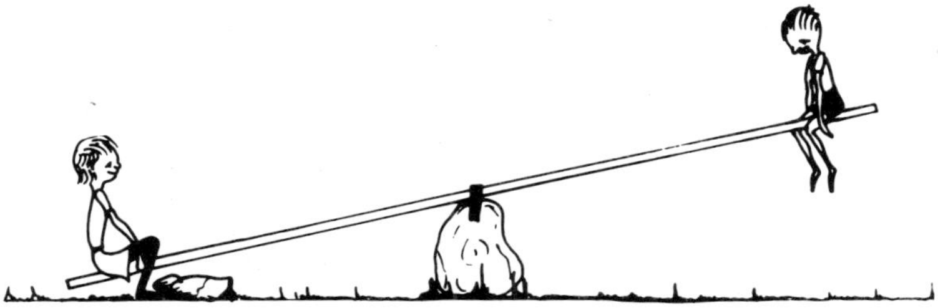

INDIRECT SUPPORT

Fig. 6.28. Indirect retention and indirect support. *Upper diagram,* By keeping her feet firmly on the ground, the girl on the left prevents the boy on the right from raising his end of the see-saw. Her feet represent the supporting element, providing indirect retention for the boy, although the direct retention is provided by the band of metal over the see-saw. *Lower diagram,* Indirect support; the girls's feet hooked under the stone constitute a retaining element which provides indirect support for the boy, although the direct support is provided by the log on which the see-saw rests.

when subjected to extracting forces. The survival of such appliances may depend upon this and also on the fact that the cantilevered pontics are avoided when chewing.

Relationship between Retention and Occlusion

Many of the lateral forces of occlusion are transmitted to the teeth through the clasp arms, particularly the bracing parts, and if saddles are mucosa-borne it is wise to make these retainers sufficiently flexible so that lateral occlusal thrusts on the teeth are diminished. Therefore when choosing retainers the cusp height and the number and position of the natural teeth must be considered and the retainers must be arranged so that the lateral forces of occlusion are directed to the tissues that can support them. In these cases the use of a functionally-generated occlusal surface reduces the lateral loads and increases the comfort of the patient.

Chapter 7

Prefabricated attachments

There are many different kinds of prefabricated attachments, but all have this in common: they enable us to design streamlined partial dentures. Regardless of whether the attachments are intra-coronal or extra-coronal, they are enclosed within the form of the dental arch of natural or artificial teeth and do not go beyond the denture space, so that they are not 'extra-anatomical' (*Fig.* 7.1). In discussing these attachments we have limited our consideration to those of which we have personal experience in clinical cases and which we have found to be useful. The omission of a number of attachments does not necessarily mean that they are unsuitable.

Intra-coronal Attachments

Attachments that lie within the anatomical contour of the crown of the abutment tooth are called intra-coronal attachments (Preiskel, 1979). Two that we have found useful are McCollum and Schatzmann (*Fig.* 7.2). These can also be attached to the surface of the abutment piece, i.e. used as extra-coronal attachments (*Fig.* 7.3). When designing a denture that incorporates these retaining elements, it is important to ensure that adequate bracing is provided. Parts of the rigid portion of the removable denture base provide this bracing by extending buccally and

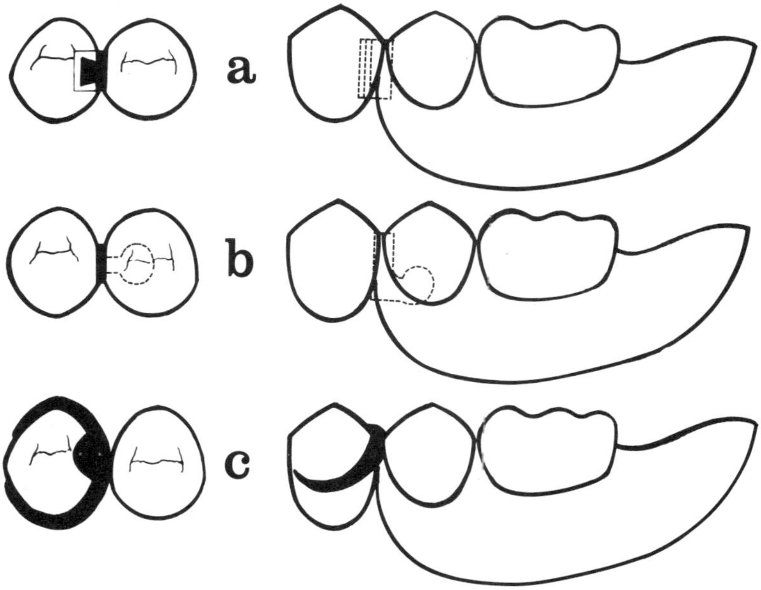

Fig. 7.1. Internal and external prefabricated attachments (**a, b**) lie within the confines of the denture, but clasps (**c**) are 'extra-anatomical'.

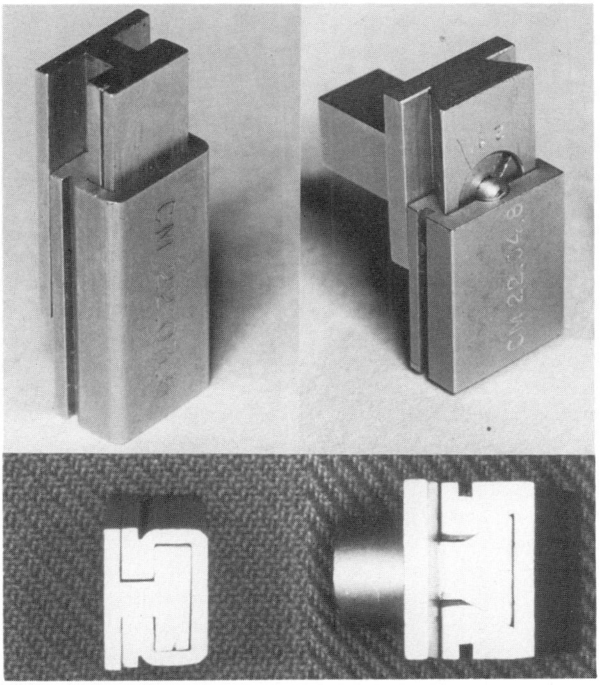

Fig. 7.2. Intra-coronal prefabricated retainers. *Left,* McCollum. *Right,* Schatzmann.

lingually on the abutment teeth to prevent lateral thrusts being transmitted directly to the attachments (*Figs.* 7.4, 7.9). Some dentists believe that the reduction of the lower part of the attachment ('bottoming out') further protects it against breakage, but if this is done the attachment no longer provides support for the saddle (*Fig.* 7.5). The chief difficulty in using prefabricated attachments is to find enough room for them when preparing the abutment teeth, and it is essential that a sufficiently long clinical crown is available so that the retention is adequate (*Fig.* 7.6).

Extra-coronal Attachments

Fig. 7.3 shows how an intra-coronal attachment can be used extra-coronally, but some attachments are specifically designed to be soldered on to the surface of a crown on an abutment tooth and these are classified by Preiskel (1979) as extra-coronal attachments. One of the most useful of these is the Dalbo attachment (*Figs.* 7.7, 8.9, 8.10, 10.9, 11.6) which is particularly suitable as a retainer and supporting element for mandibular free-end saddle dentures. Although the attachment itself is extra-coronal, it falls entirely within the dental arch and does not encroach on the surrounding soft tissues (*see Fig.* 7.1). This attachment incorporates a spring in the matrix so that a degree of stress-breaking occurs (*see Fig.* 8.9). The ball on the patrix forms a fulcrum around which the denture can rotate as the mucosa is compressed. Since the ball is close to the gingival margin, this fulcrum is low, and the tendency for the saddle to rise when the patient is chewing sticky food is resisted by the mesial surface of the matrix of the attachment contacting the distal surface of the abutment tooth and thus providing indirect retention. No spurs or other indirect retainers need be placed on the anterior teeth and so the denture design is streamlined. A disadvantage of the appliance is that the force of occlusion is not directed down the long axis of the abutment tooth, but tends to tilt it distally. For this reason it is best to use two abutment teeth

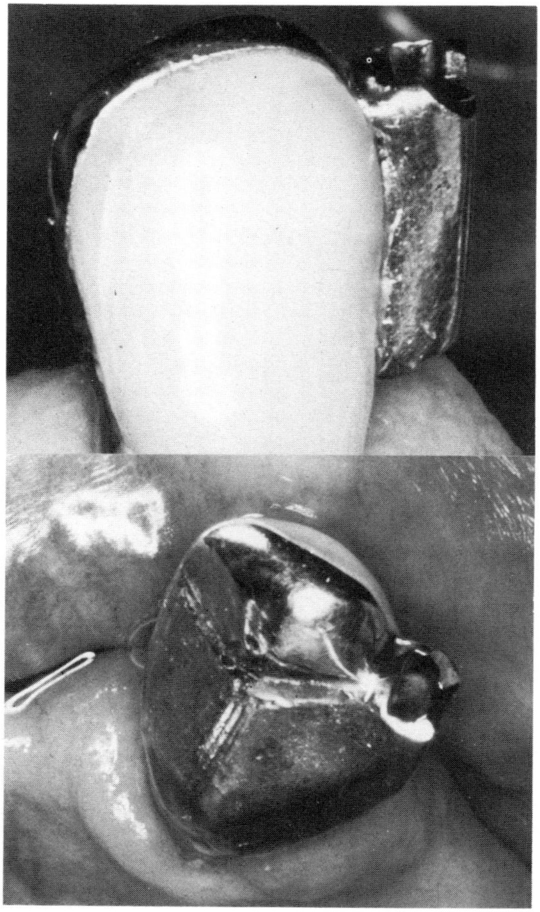

Fig. 7.3. Where there is insufficient space, a McCollum 'intra-coronal' attachment can be attached extra-coronally. Note the lingual rest seat on the full veneer crown.

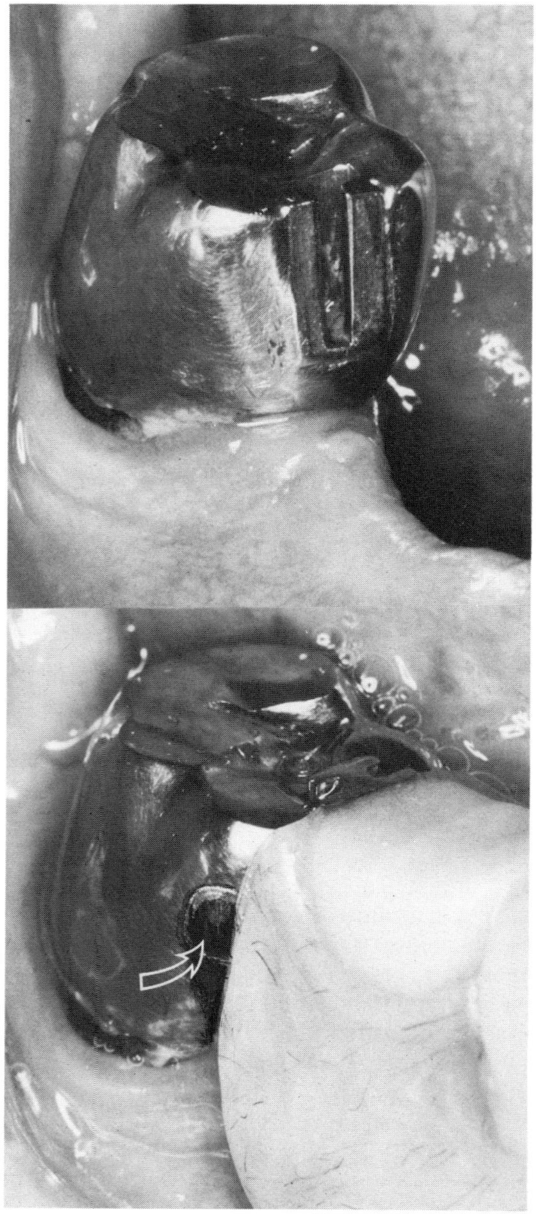

Fig. 7.4. When prefabricated attachments are used, bracing elements (*arrow*) on the denture help to prevent damage to the attachment. The denture has not been completely seated in order to show the patrix of the attachment. Although the bracing element is 'extra-anatomical' in this case provision should be made to keep it within the normal contours of the abutment tooth. (*See Fig.* 7.9**A**, **B**.)

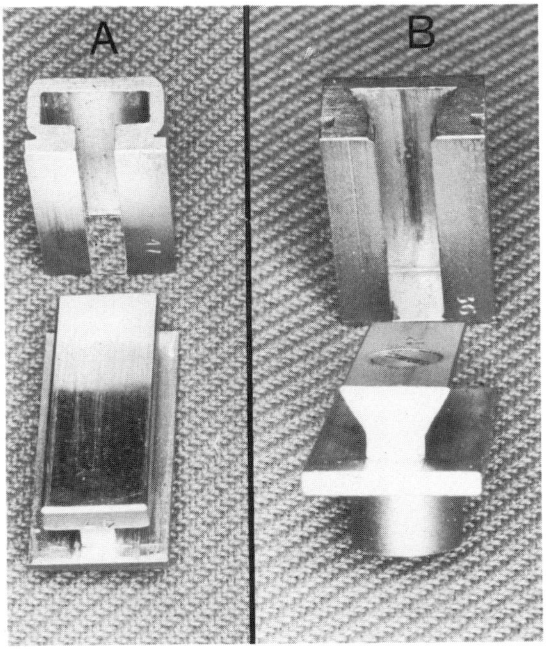

Fig. 7.5. Rigid and 'bottomed out' intra-coronal retainers. **A**, The lower part of the attachment has been removed to protect it against breakage. This 'bottoming out' reduces the tooth support of the appliance. **B**, Intra-coronal retainer that has not been 'bottomed out' provides tooth support for the appliance.

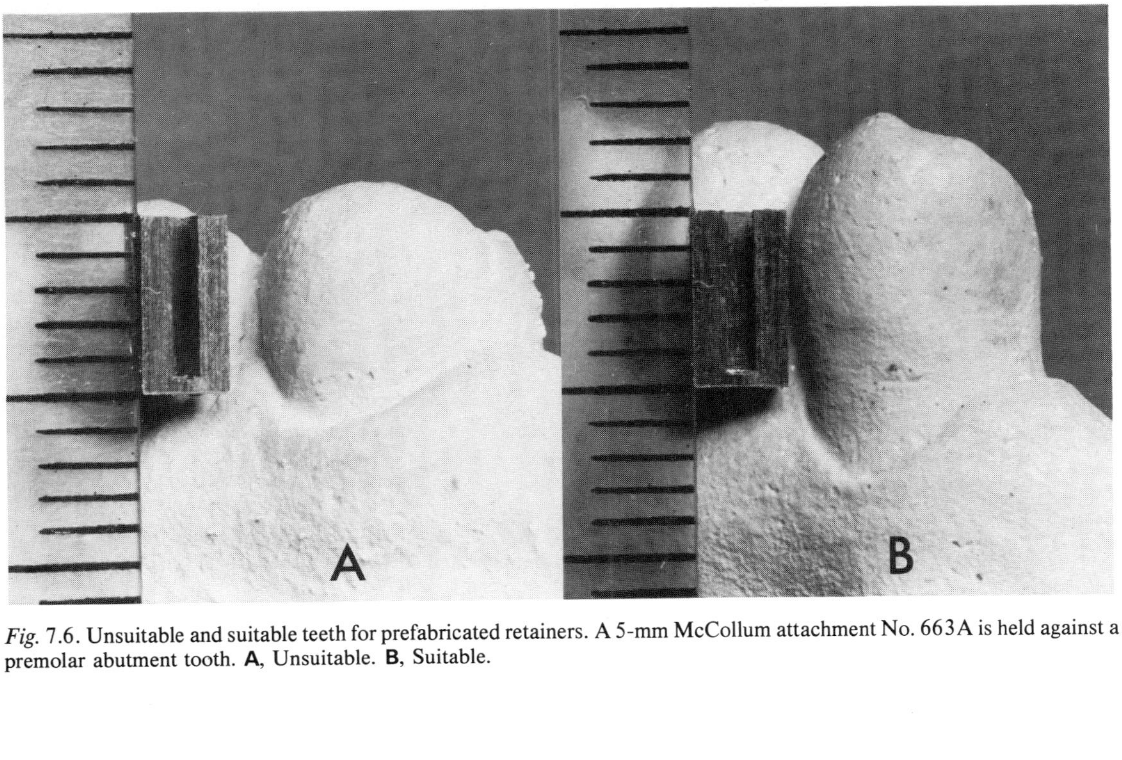

Fig. 7.6. Unsuitable and suitable teeth for prefabricated retainers. A 5-mm McCollum attachment No. 663A is held against a premolar abutment tooth. **A**, Unsuitable. **B**, Suitable.

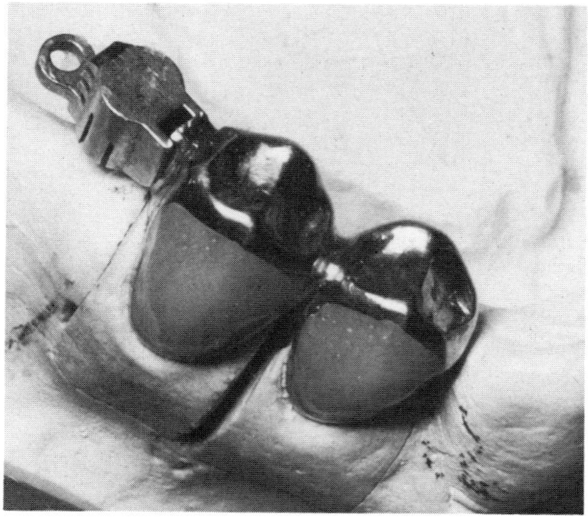

Fig. 7.7. Dalbo extra-coronal attachment incorporates a hinge and stress-breaking spring. It is best to use double abutment pieces with this attachment.

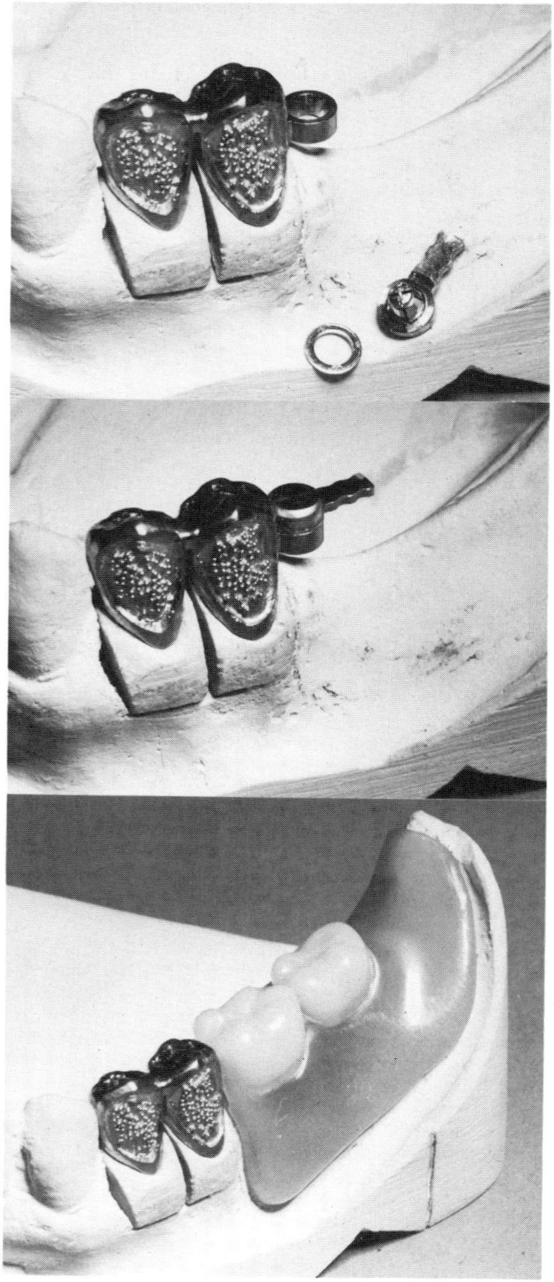

Fig. 7.8. The CEKA attachment (No. 696 KS) used as a retainer and supporting element for a mandibular bilateral free-end saddle denture.

for Dalbo attachments (*Fig.* 7.7). Another disadvantage of this extra-coronal attachment is that food is trapped beneath the ball where it projects over the gingival margin. The patient's attention should be directed towards careful cleaning of this area with dental floss.

The Universal CEKA Attachment System is very versatile. It can be used on teeth with shorter crowns than those required for the Dalbo attachment. The extra-coronal attachment for bilateral free-end saddle dentures has a ring that projects from the distal surface of the abutment tooth. The patrix of the attachment is fixed to the denture base and enters the ring from above (*Figs.* 7.8, 7.9). It is a split cone with an expanded end that engages the ring, the splits making it elastic enough to clip into the ring. It allows some rocking movement, but has not the stress-breaking springs that characterize the Dalbo attachment, but by using a washer to create space between the two parts of the attachment (CEKA No. 696 KS) it allows mucosal compression of the free-end saddles (*Figs.* 7.8, 7.9). CEKA attachments can be incorporated in bars to provide positive retention and can also be used as stud retainers.

Bar-supported Prostheses

Various bars are available to support prostheses for bounded saddles (e.g. Dolder, Andrews, Ackermann) and since they lie under the denture, they provide hidden retention and support for the appliance (*Figs.* 7.10, 7.11). The CEKA retainer used with a bar has already been mentioned. Most of the other bar prostheses are retained by means of clips engaging the buccal and lingual surfaces of the bars, but other types of precision retainers can be used in conjunction with bars to provide retention (*Figs.* 7.12, 7.13). Full veneer crowns were made for the central incisors for the patient illustrated in *Fig.* 7.13 and in order to avoid sacrifice of tooth substance in the preparation of the parallel premolar abutments, extra-coronal slots were prepared parallel to the incisor preparations.

In the patient illustrated in *Fig.* 7.14 the whole procedure was simplified as the teeth were non-vital; all that was necessary was to place posts and caps in position and attach the bars by means of Schubiger screws. The prosthesis was then placed over the bars and a satisfactory appearance was achieved. Retention in this case was by means of clips on the bars. In some cases bars with parallel milled sides are used without clips, since the precision fit of the milled surfaces provides sufficient retention for the appliance (*Fig.* 7.15) but, as already discussed in Chapter 5, this has the disadvantage of putting torsional stress on the teeth.

Stud and Clip Retainers

When an abutment tooth for a removable partial denture is devitalized and root filled, its crown should be removed and a post and diaphragm placed to carry the patrix of a stud retainer (e.g. Dalla Bona, Gerber) (*Fig.* 7.16). The matrix of the attachment should be embedded in an artificial tooth on the denture, so that the means of retention cannot be seen when the denture is inserted in the mouth (*see Fig.* 10.12).

The Rothermann clip retainer has a flat stud that needs little vertical space (*Fig.* 7.17). The encircling clip engages a groove around the stud and so does not add to the height required. Although sufficient buccolingual width is needed to accommodate the clip, this does not usually present much of a problem. The studs should be positioned so that the marks on them, representing the deepest part of the groove, lie opposite the gap in the clip when the retaining tag of the clip is in a suitable position for embedding in the denture. There are two types of Rothermann attachment. One type is rigid and the clip fits the groove accurately and is firmly retained in it. In the other type the groove is wider than the clip and allows vertical movement of the appliance. This provides some stress-breaking and reduces the risk of the clip breaking when the adjacent saddles are mucosa-borne. When using Rothermann clips or stud attachments on partial dentures, it is wise to cement the studs to the abutment teeth first and finish the denture with holes opposite the studs. Then position the finished denture in the mouth and firmly press it against the tissues and attach

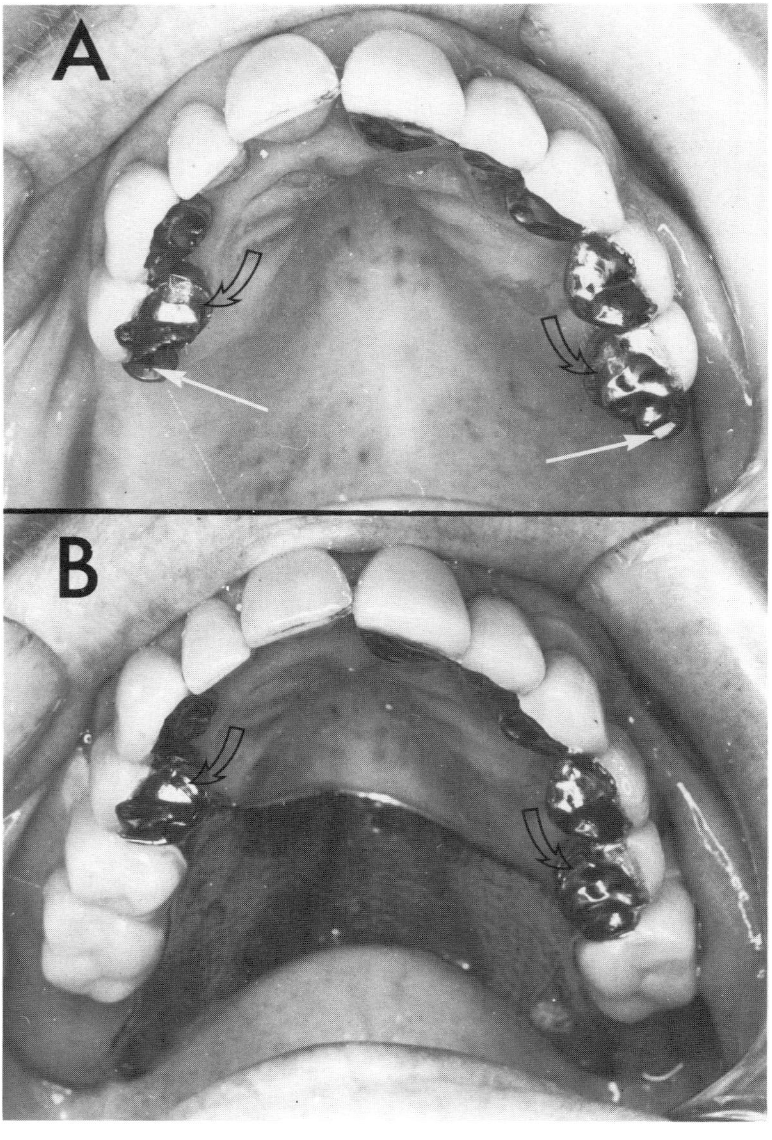
A
B

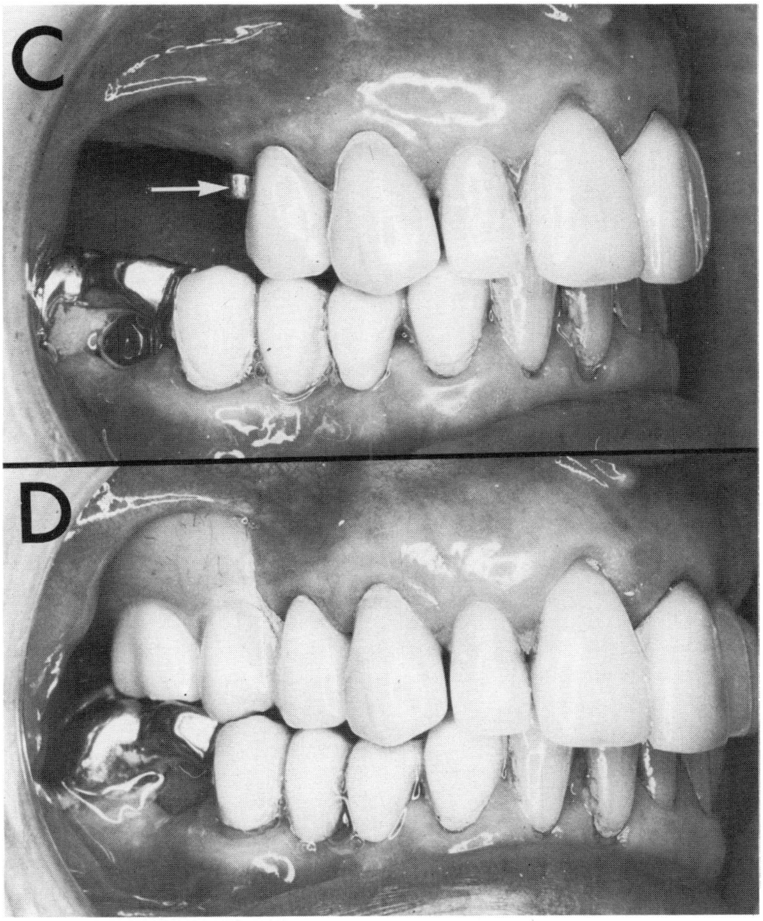

Fig. 7.9. CEKA OL 696 KS resilient attachments (*white arrows,* **A** and **C**) provide retention and stress distribution for a removable partial denture for maxillary free-end saddles. Note the milled recesses in the abutment teeth (*open arrows* **A**) and the extensions of the denture (*open arrows* **B**) to provide bracing and to protect the CEKA attachments. The denture is 'streamlined' and the appearance is not marred by clasps (**D**).

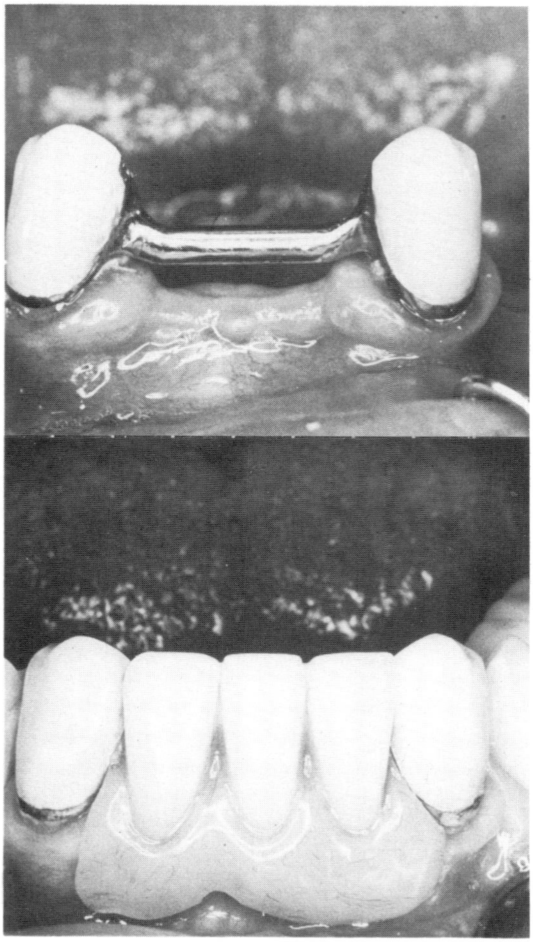

Fig. 7.10. Dolder bar provides support and retention for a partial lower denture which clips over it (*see Fig.* 7.11).

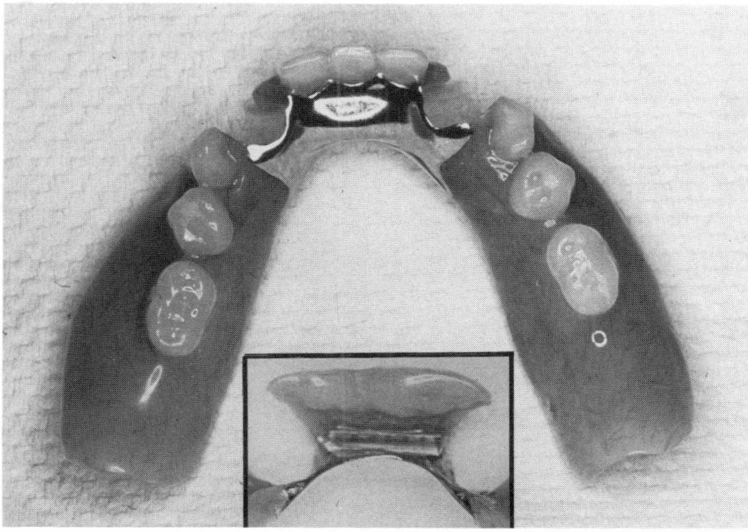

Fig. 7.11. Bar-supported partial denture is retained by a clip (*insert*). Note the narrowness and reduced number of the posterior teeth. This reduces the masticatory load on the saddle areas.

the clips or studs by placing self-curing resin in the holes. Remove the denture and add more acrylic to complete the attachment of the clips. There are other methods whereby the clips can be attached to the denture, but we prefer the method described as it ensures most accuracy. Positioning the clips in relation to the studs on the cast, for example, can sometimes have disappointing results as slight changes in the position of the studs takes place when they are being cemented to the teeth and the denture position may alter with compression of the mucosa. Further details of technique may be found in Rudd et al. (1981) and Stewart et al. (1983).

Spring-loaded Attachments

Spring-loaded attachments are particularly useful when there are short bounded saddles near the front of the mouth, as they can be embedded in the mesial and distal aspects of the saddles and engage dimples in small restorations on the distal surface of the anterior abutment and the mesial surface of the posterior abutment. The saddle clicks into place and can be relatively easily removed by the patient, provided the dimples have been properly constructed. It is essential that the depth of the dimple should be less than the radius of the rounded end of the plunger of the attachment (*Fig.* 7.18). When placed at the end of a bounded saddle, the attachment used should have the screw (that closes the housing for the plunger) at the plunger end of the housing so that it can be removed and the spring renewed when required. Attachments such as the Ipsoclip 102.02.2 (*Fig.* 7.19) and the Pressomatic 115B (*Fig.* 7.20), with the screw cap at the opposite end of the housing, cannot be used at the ends of bounded saddles. These attachments should be used only where access to the screw can be obtained, usually on metal dentures. *Fig.* 7.20 illustrates the use of Pressomatic 115B. When these are fitted the plungers and springs are removed and the housings are soldered to the casting. The plungers and springs are then replaced. The dimples are not usually cut in

(*continued on p. 108*)

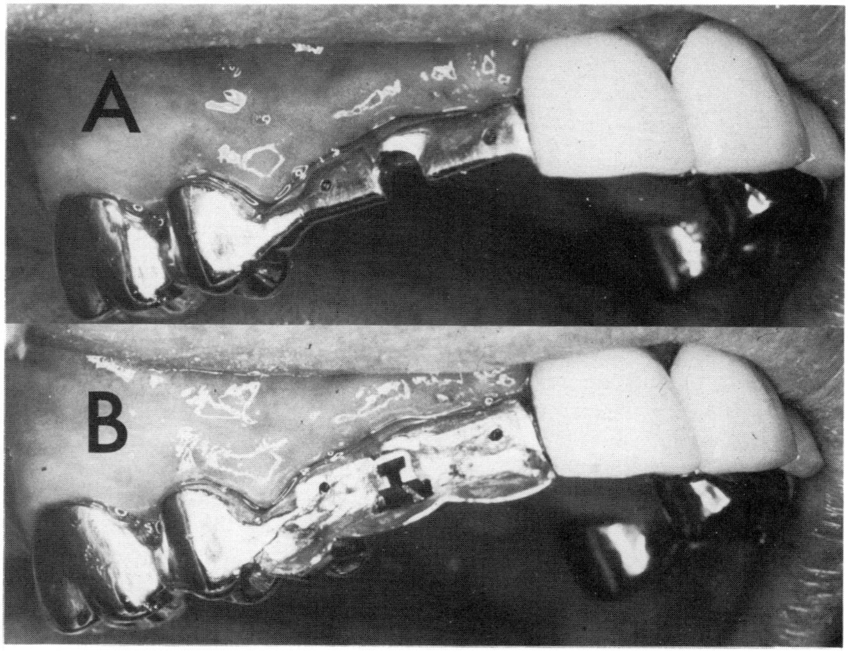
A
B

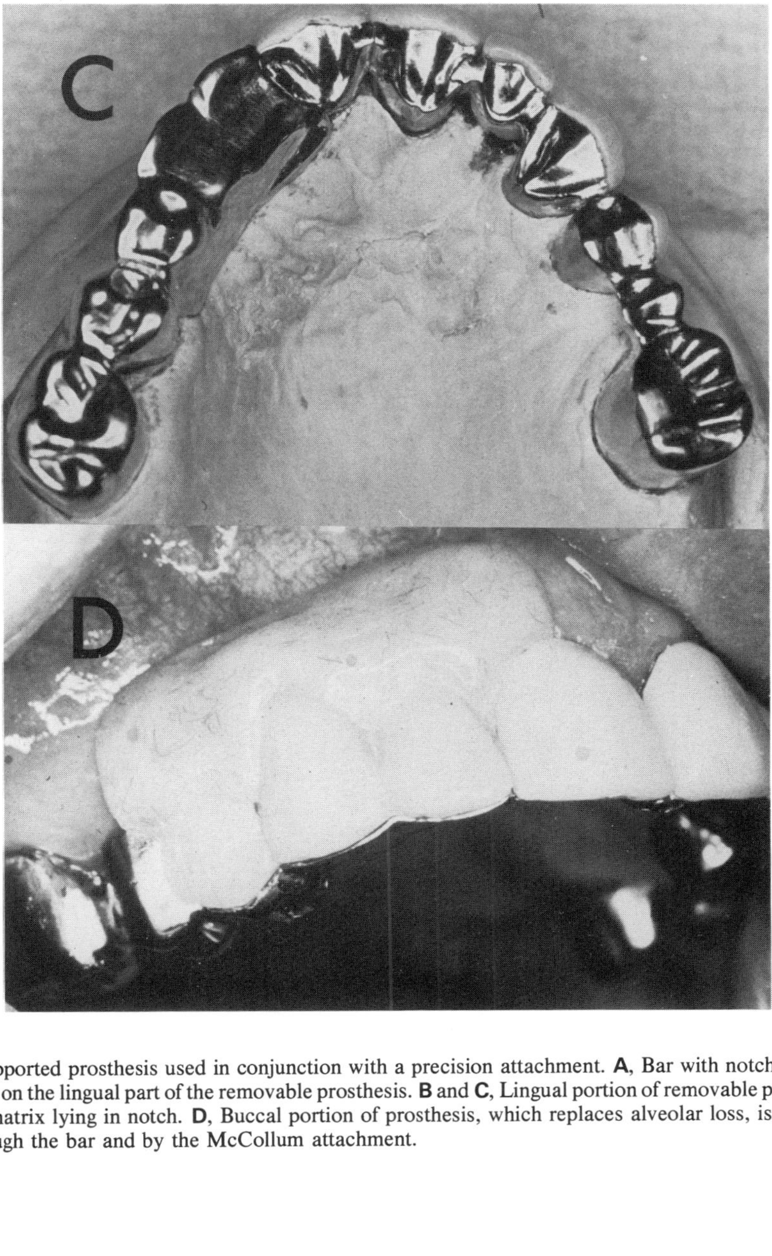

Fig. 7.12. Bar-supported prosthesis used in conjunction with a precision attachment. **A**, Bar with notch to accommodate a McCollum matrix on the lingual part of the removable prosthesis. **B** and **C**, Lingual portion of removable prosthesis in position with McCollum matrix lying in notch. **D**, Buccal portion of prosthesis, which replaces alveolar loss, is held in position by parallel pins through the bar and by the McCollum attachment.

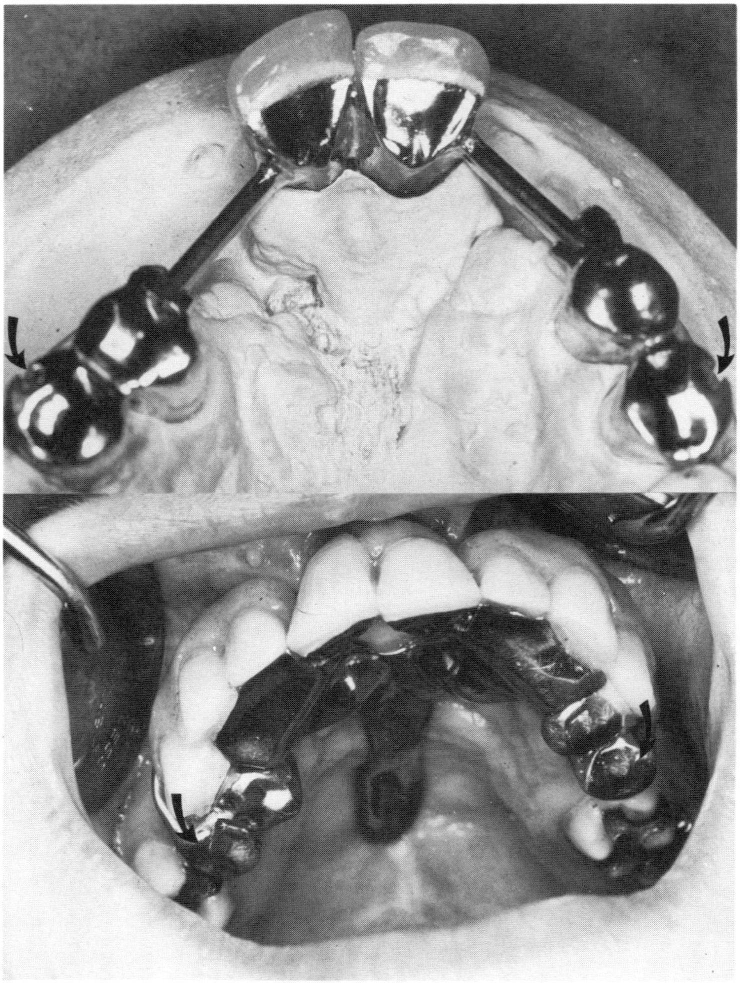

Fig. 7.13. Dolder bars provide stability for a mobile premaxilla in a patient with a Class IV cleft. The difficulty of making the preparations parallel has been reduced by fixing extra-coronal slots on the premolar abutment pieces; these slots are parallel to the path of insertion of the incisor portion of the appliance. Additional retention is provided by intra-coronal Chayes attachments (*arrowed*) on the second premolars.

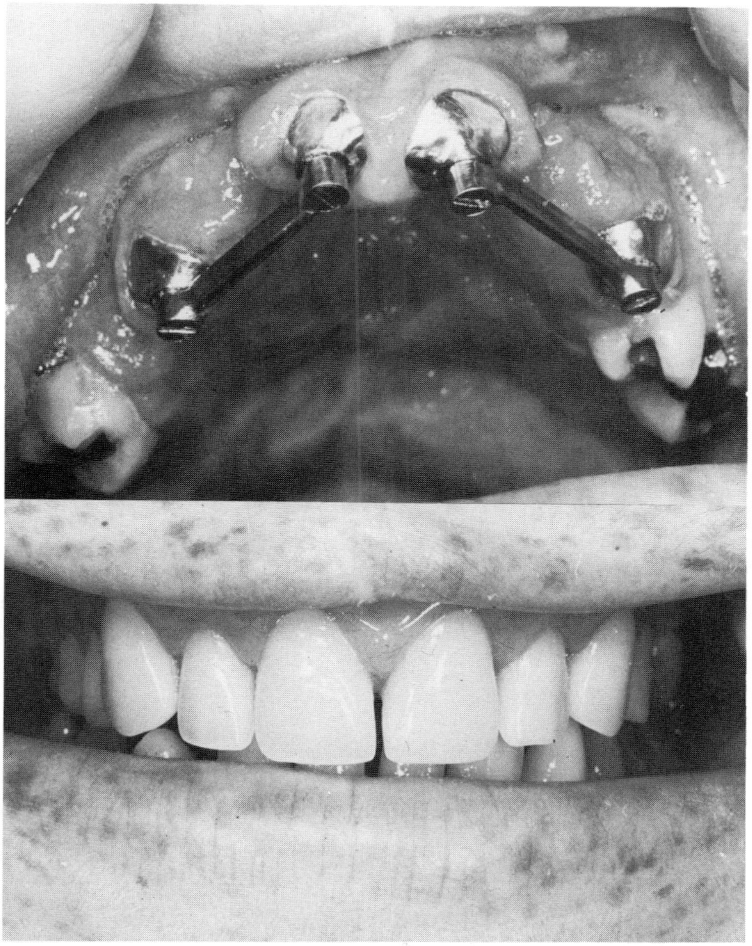

Fig. 7.14. *Upper,* Bars attached to devitalized abutment teeth by means of Schubiger screws simplify the problems of parallelism and also make it possible to replace the bar with a Gerber stud retainer should one of the abutments fail (*see Fig.* 7.16). *Lower,* The finished prosthesis in the mouth.

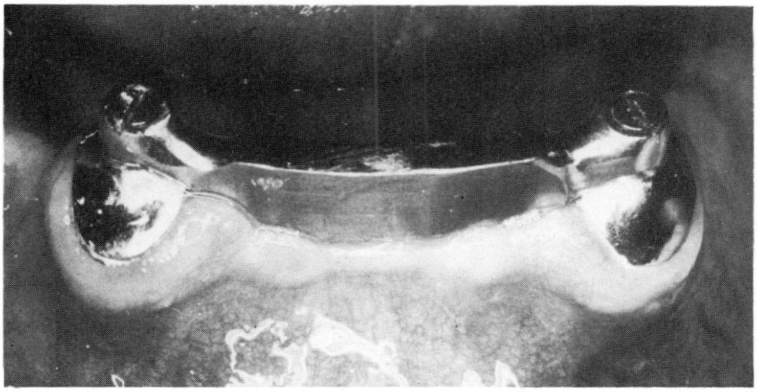

Fig. 7.15. A milled bar with parallel sides attached by Schubiger screws to the canine teeth is used without a clip retainer on the appliance.

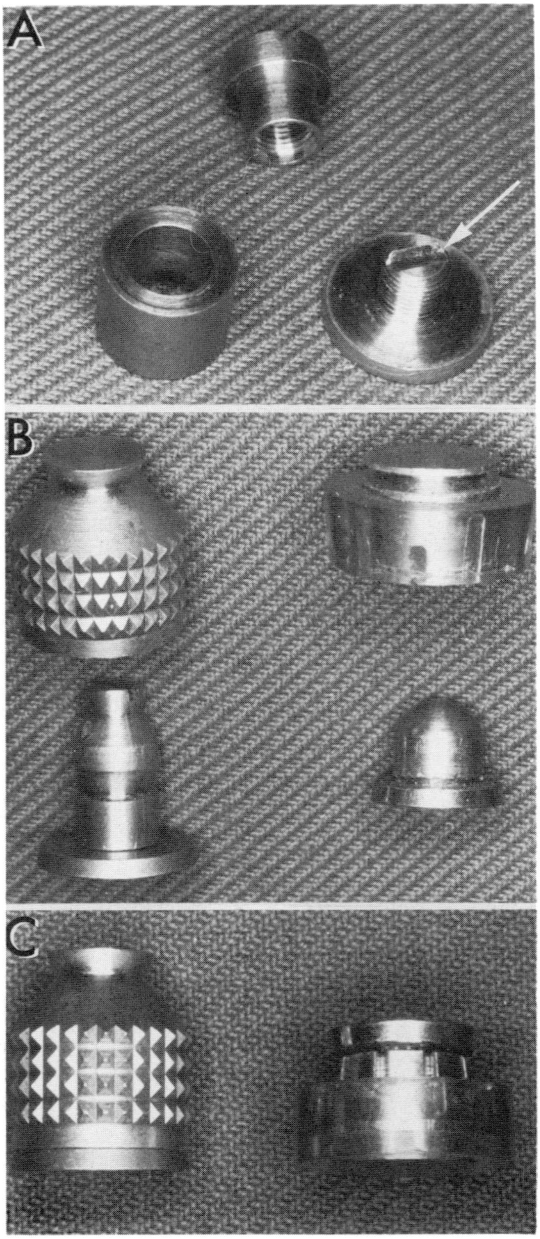

Fig. 7.16. **A**, Exploded view of a Schubiger screw attachment which incorporates the base of a Gerber stud retainer (*arrow*). **B**, Exploded view of stud retainers: Gerber (*left*), Dalla Bona (*right*). **C**, Assembled stud retainers.

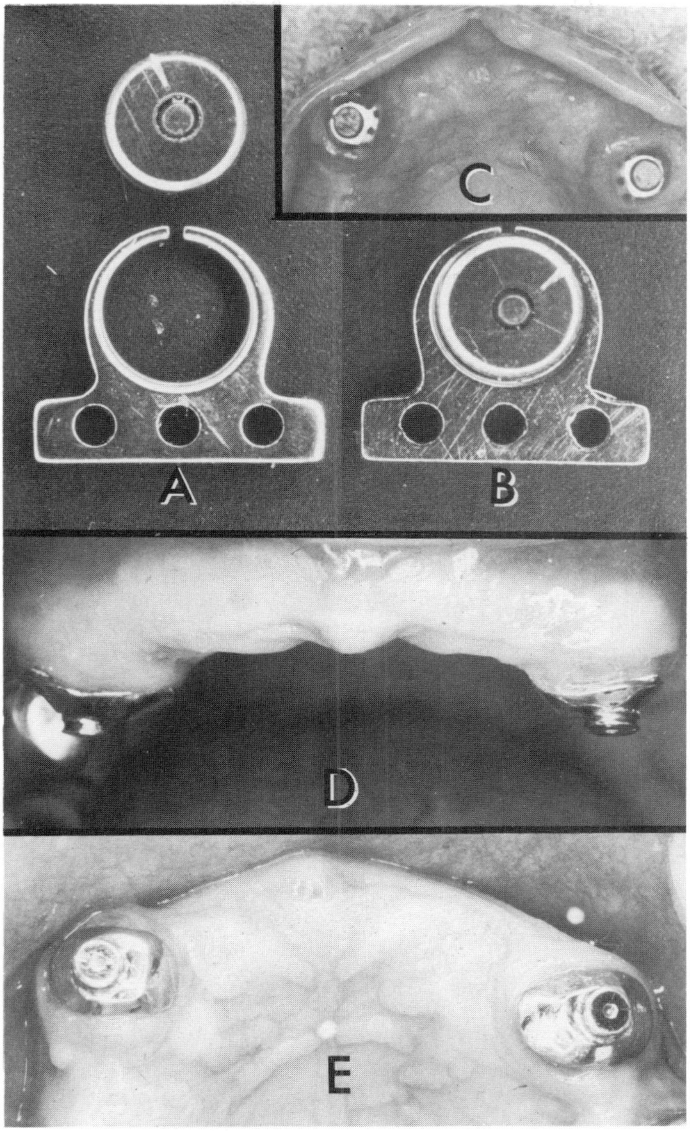

Fig. 7.17. Rothermann clip retainer (Cendres et Metaux: Rothermann retainer 32.01.5—rigid; 41.01.5—movable). **A**, Clip matrix) and stud (patrix) separate. **B**, Clip and stud assembled; the mark on the stud should be opposite the gap in the clip. **C**, Denture with Rothermann clips in position. **D**, Studs in the mouth, showing retentive grooves. **E**, Studs (occlusal view).

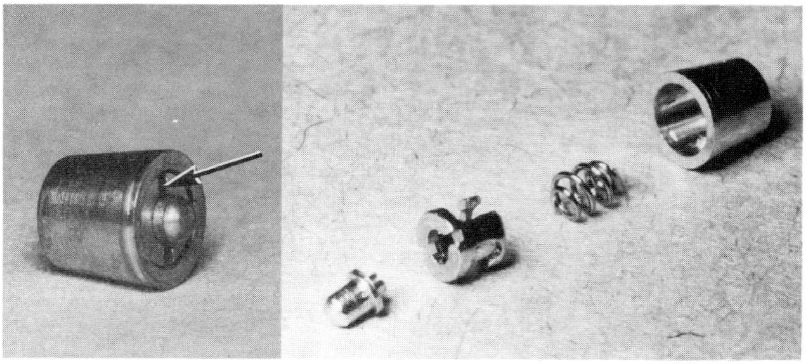

Fig. 7.18. Ipsoclip 102.03.2 (Cendres et Metaux): assembled and exploded views. The spring-loaded plunger engages a dimple in the surface of the abutment tooth and provides retention for a partial denture. The depth of the dimple should be less than the radius of the rounded end of the plunger. The screw cap (*arrow*) that closes the housing for the spring of this Ipsoclip retainer gives access for its replacement. This type is suitable for use at the end of bounded saddles.

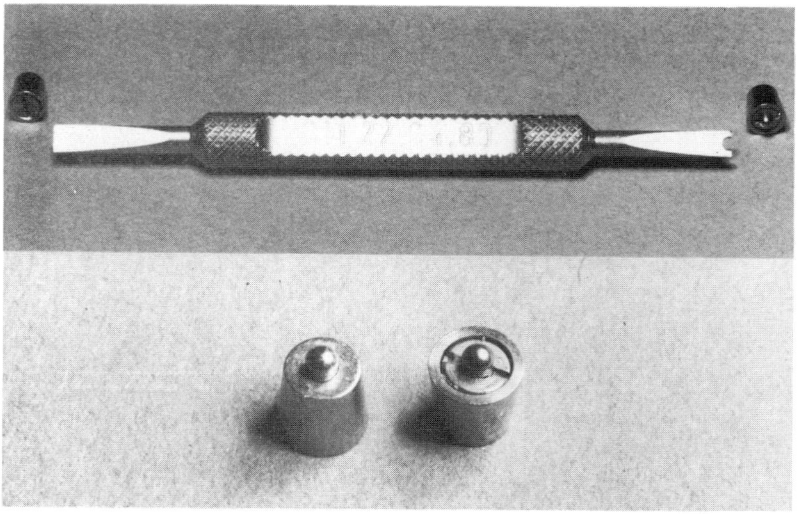

Fig. 7.19. Two types of Ipso clips and the screwdriver used to dismantle them. *Left,* Ipsoclip 102.02.2 cannot be used at the ends of bounded saddles, as the screw is at the end of the housing opposite the plunger. *Right,* Ipsoclip 102.03.2 can be used, as the screw is at the plunger end of the housing.

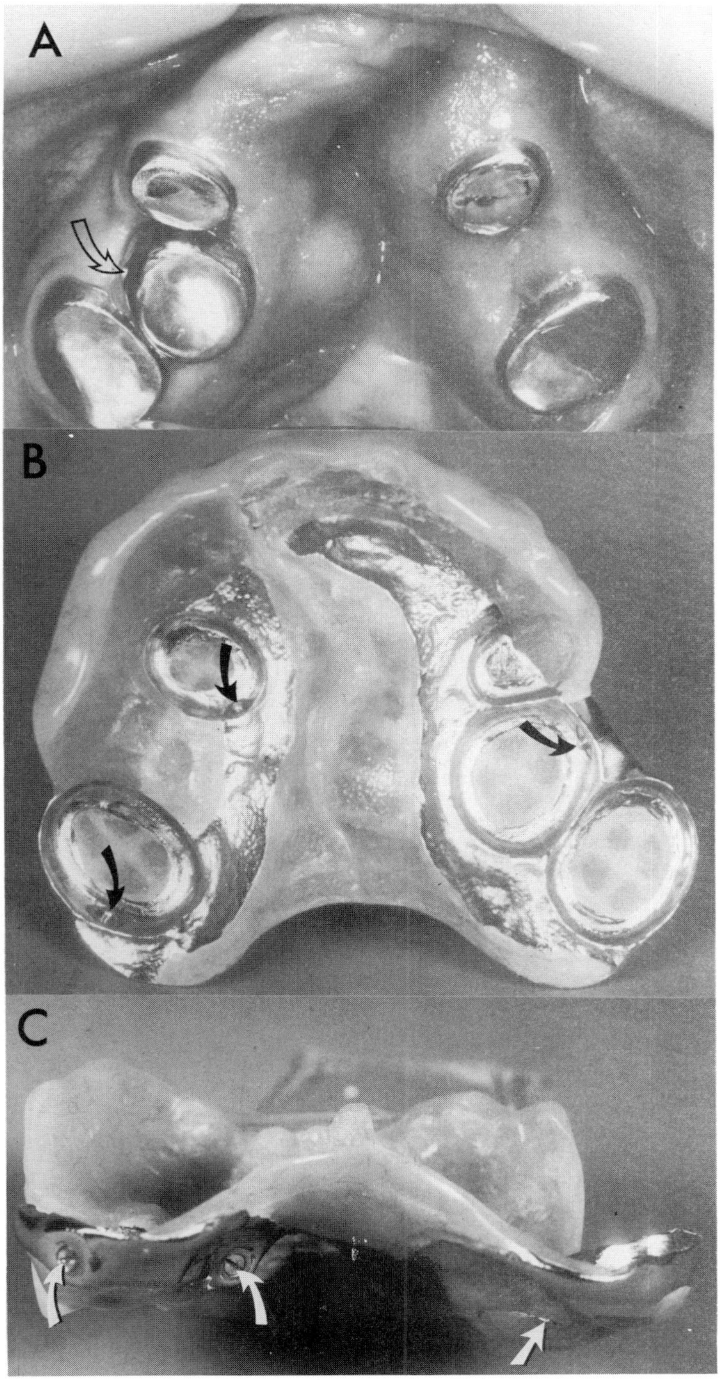

Fig. 7.20. **A**, The maxillary arch of a patient with congenital cleft palate. **B**, The overdenture is retained by the spring-loaded plungers (*black arrows*) of Pressomatic 115B attachments (Metaux Precieux, Neuchatel) which are soldered to the cast denture base. The plungers engage dimples on the crowns (*open arrow in* **A**). **C**, The screw caps (*white arrows*) can be removed when the springs of the attachments have to be replaced.

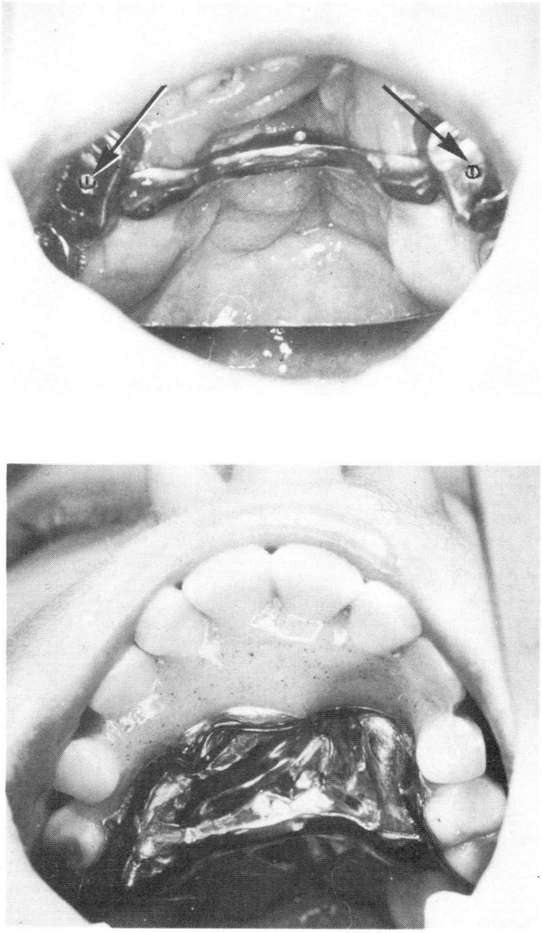

Fig. 7.21. In special circumstances when an appliance should not be removed by the patient, screws (*arrowed*) are used to retain it. In this case a transverse bar was used to hold the segments of a rapidly expanded cleft palate. A dimple in the middle of the bar provided retention for the removable part of the appliance, which carried an Ipsoclip. After 6 months of retention of the cleft segments the transverse bar was fixed to the removable part of the appliance and the screws were removed.

the abutment teeth until the appliance is ready for fitting in the mouth. The position of the dimples is marked by using indicator paste.

Screw Retainers

Various types of prefabricated screw retainers are available (Matsuo and Shimegi, 1981). They are used to retain parts of fixed

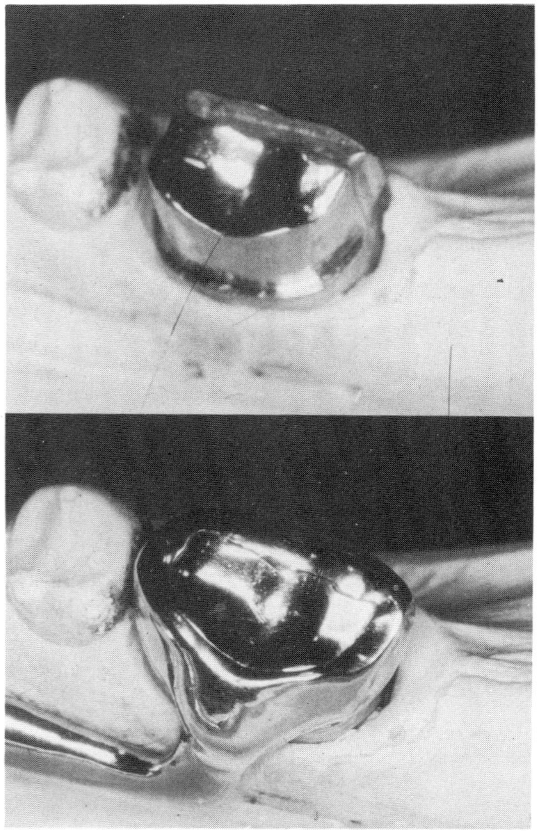

Fig. 7.22. Channel shoulder crown attachment provides retention for a partial denture.

prostheses that cannot be removed by the patient, but may be removed by the dentist. They are also used to isolate abutment teeth that might give trouble after a fixed prosthesis has been cemented. Should the abutment tooth have to be extracted at a later date, an additional pontic can be locked in its position without requiring the total replacement of the prosthesis. A less conventional use of screws to retain a portion of a prosthesis is illustrated in *Fig.* 7.21. In this cleft palate case the transpalatal bar was fixed by screws to prevent the segments of the arch collapsing after rapid expansion. An Ipsoclip was used to retain the removable part of the prosthesis on the transverse bar which was screwed firmly in position. After a suitable time had elapsed the screws were undone and the bar was incorporated in the removable prosthesis.

Milled Attachments

Milled attachments are not prefabricated attachments, but are included in this chapter for convenience. The channel shoulder crown (*Fig.* 7.22) is an example of a milled retainer that depends on friction for the retention of the appliance (Steiger and Boitel, 1959). Full veneer crowns are milled with almost parallel sides, and shoulders and channels are milled to accommodate the removable parts of the attachments fixed to the removable partial denture (*Fig.* 7.23). In addition two parallel holes are drilled in the crowns to accommodate parallel pins that are fixed to the removable part of the attachment. The friction of the pins in the holes provides additional retention. The fabrication of these retainers is time-consuming and the result is not as strong as simple telescope crowns (*see Figs.* 11.7, 11.8), which also provide retention through friction. The disadvantage of the telescope crown is that the abutment teeth may change position if the removable part of the appliance carrying the crowns is left out for any length of time. This is because there is no occlusion on the cemented part of the crown.

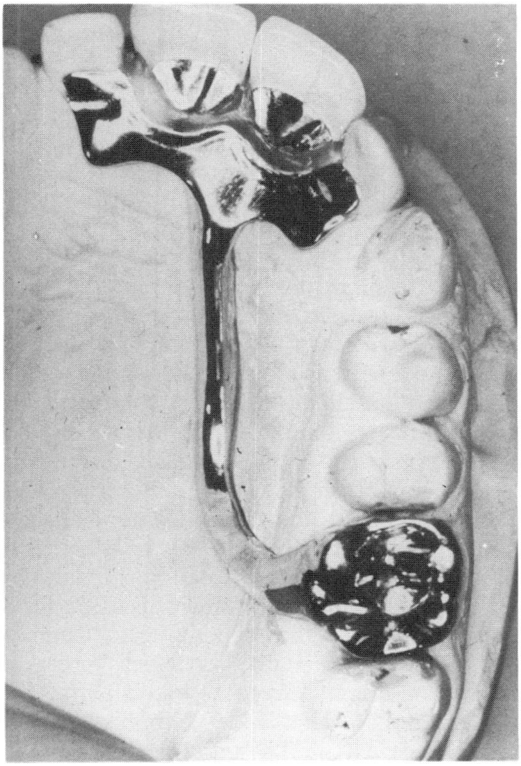

Fig. 7.23. A novel use of a channel-shoulder pin-crown retaining a 'posterior milled retained anterior prosthesis' (McCarron and Sharkey, 1977) replacing two central incisors. While at first glance this may look like a spring cantilever bridge, it is in fact an appliance that can be removed by the patient. It is entirely tooth-borne and is more hygienic than a spring cantilever bridge.

Magnetic Retainers

Cobalt samarium (Co_5Sm) has exceptional magnetic properties and has been used for the retention of partial dentures (Gillings, 1977, 1980; Cerny, 1978; Laird et al., 1981). Gillings has developed small magnetic units that can be inserted in prepared roots for the retention of overdentures. These magnetic appliances provide adequate retention in this situation, but are rather bulky for insertion into root ends and there is always a danger of fracture if the roots are not properly prepared. The magnets can also be used as locking devices in sectional dentures where considerations of bulk are less pressing (Ling, 1982).

Chapter 8

Connectors

Connectors that connect the saddles of a partial denture are called saddle connectors or major connectors. Connectors that connect the clasps or occlusal rests to the partial denture base are called clasp connectors, rest connectors or minor connectors (*Fig.* 8.1). Connectors may be rigid, hinged, or flexible. Saddle connectors between tooth-borne saddles should be rigid to transmit lateral occlusal forces to the teeth (*Fig.* 8.2). When some parts of the denture are tooth-borne and some mucosa-borne, provision must be made for the mucosa-borne saddles sinking up to 1 mm into the mucosa when the occlusal forces are applied to them. The tooth-borne parts of the denture do not sink under biting load to any appreciable extent. The difference in behaviour of the support for tooth-and-mucosa-borne partial dentures significantly affects the design of partial dentures. If a tooth-borne part of a denture is connected rigidly to a mucosa-borne part, the denture rocks round a fulcrum axis that passes through the occlusal rests nearest the mucosa-borne saddles, and harmful stresses may be placed on the clasped teeth unless special provision is made to avoid them. The provision of flexible connectors is one way of avoiding harmful stresses on the teeth and for this reason some flexible connectors are called 'stress-breakers' or 'stress-distributors' (*Fig.* 8.3). A general rule governing connectors is that 'like' saddles should be connected rigidly, but 'unlike' saddles may be connected flexibly, unless the partial denture has been designed so that it can rock round a fulcrum axis without damaging the remaining teeth. 'Like' saddles are saddles of the same type (e.g. all saddles tooth-borne) and 'unlike' saddles are of different types (e.g. some tooth-borne and some mucosa-borne).

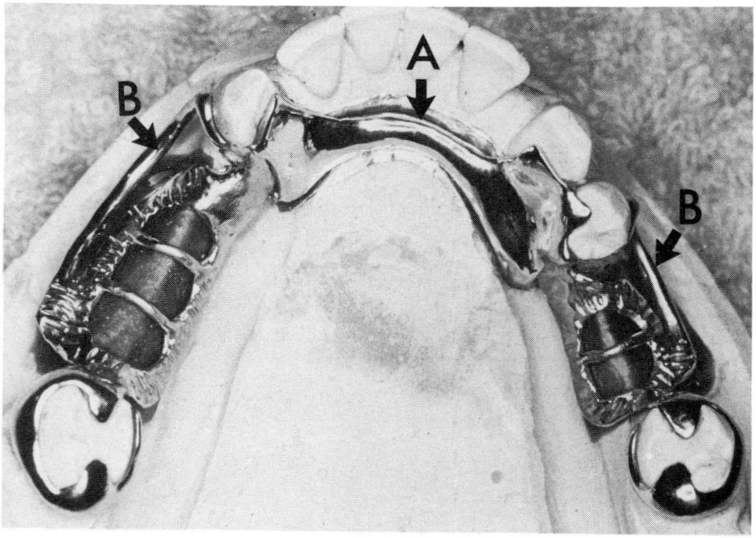

Fig. 8.1. Cast partial denture base showing saddle connector (A) and clasp connectors (B).

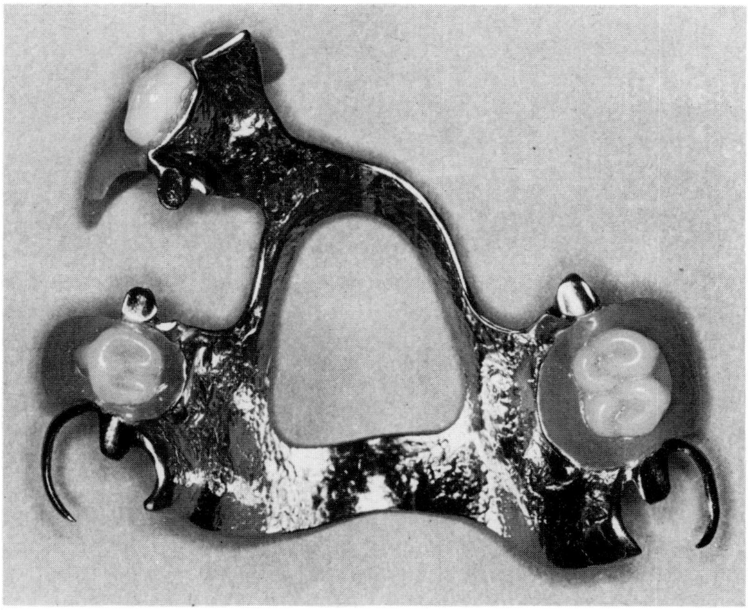

Fig. 8.2. Rigid connectors connecting the tooth-borne saddles of a partial upper denture. The labial flange enters the anterior undercuts on an oblique path of insertion and provides retention in the common path of displacement. Thus the clasps can be placed far back out of sight.

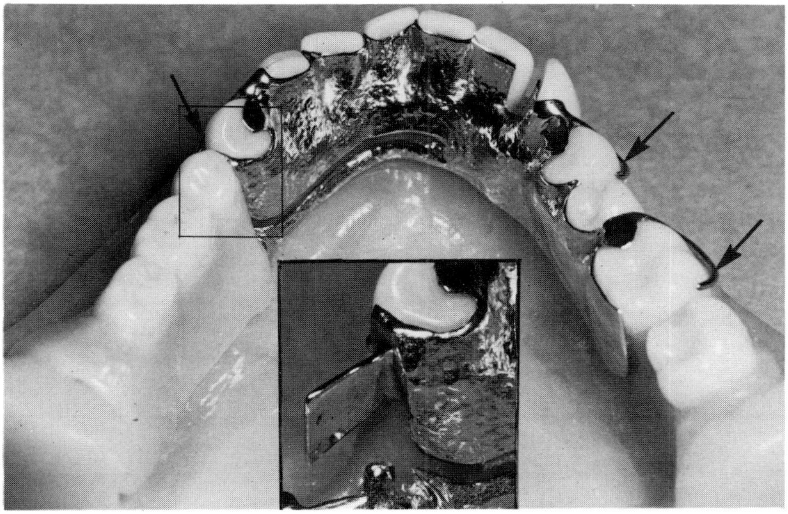

Fig. 8.3. Springy type of flexible connector connecting the left free-end mucosa-borne saddle to the tooth-borne part of the denture. The clasps (*arrowed*) must provide sufficient retention to prevent displacement of the tooth-borne part when the flexible connector bends. The fin (*insert*) slides in a groove in the mesial tooth of the free-end saddle and prevents lateral movement while permitting vertical movement.

Rigid Connectors

Rigid connectors are the most popular way of connecting saddles of partial dentures, whether they are tooth-borne, mucosa-borne, or tooth- and mucosa-borne. Rigid connectors transmit lateral loads to the teeth. Many practitioners believe that all connectors should be rigid. Rigidity is considered to be a desirable property in partial denture bases, as without a rigid base clasps and other retainers do not bear a constant relationship to each other and unpredictable forces can be placed on teeth if the denture base bends under transient load or even becomes permanently distorted.

There appears to be a considerable variation in viewpoint about the dimensions of rigid connectors. A review by Anderson (1958) showed that the dimensions used by prosthodontists were based more on use and want than on measurement of the mechanical requirements, although these have been investigated by Waters (1972) and by Waters and Nairn (1972). Wrought stainless-steel lingual bars are usually about 3 mm wide and 1·5 mm thick, but cast bars vary greatly in thickness, shape and length. The shapes of various connectors have been discussed by Basker and Tryde (1977), Henderson and Steffel (1981) and by Wagner and Traweek (1982). Farrell (1971) investigated the tolerance of patients to different partial denture bases and showed that the avoidance of the area of the rugae at the front of the palate was of the utmost importance to most patients wearing partial dentures.

While we agree that rigid connectors are desirable, we are also very much aware of the 'flexibility' of the supporting tissues on which the dentures rest. Our experience with nylon dentures taught us that flexibility of the denture base increased the comfort of the dentures (Watt, 1955). There is much evidence that the mandible distorts on movement (McDowell and Regli, 1961; Picton, 1962; Osborne and Tomlin, 1964). Gates and Nicholls (1981) reviewed the literature and added new evidence from 10 patients whom they studied. They showed that this distortion may be up to 0·5 mm on extreme movements, but is less (0·2 mm) in normal movements. The denture base should accommodate this distortion by being at least as flexible as the mandible. Patients who have worn acrylic partial dentures sometimes find cobalt-chromium alloy replacements are less comfortable. This might be related to the demands that such rigid structures place on the periodontium (*see* Chapter 3). Alloy dentures may transmit stresses to the teeth that were previously absorbed by the acrylic, but the discomfort caused by some alloy dentures is partly a result of the difficulties inherent in producing very accurate castings in high-fusing metals.

With regard to connectors between tooth-borne and mucosa-borne parts of dentures there are two schools of thought, rigid and flexible. The most 'rigid' school believes implicitly that anything other than a rigid connector is bound to be harmful to the tissues. Within the 'rigid' school there are some who believe that by using tissue-displacing impressions, altered cast techniques, and various other means, it is possible to modify the mucosa of the saddle area sufficiently to provide virtually the same resistance to displacement as the abutment teeth. This view represents a degree of self-deception that can easily be corrected by observing precisely the amount of rock that these dentures develop within a few weeks of their placement. It seems inevitable that rocking must occur shortly after the fitting of all rigid tooth-and-mucosa-borne dentures in view of the extensive research on mucosal displacement (Kydd and Mandley, 1967; Kydd et al., 1969; 1971; Wills and Manderson, 1977; Picton and Wills, 1978; Manderson et al., 1979; Kydd and Daly, 1982). Despite being well aware that rigid tooth-and-mucosa-borne dentures rock, many dentists believe that the advantages of rigid connectors outweight their disadvantages. The designs of such dentures are therefore modified to ensure that rocking can take place round a fulcrum axis of the rests nearest the mucosa-borne saddles without traumatising the teeth. This is further discussed in Chapter 10.

The rigidity of a connector is a relative state. Beams flex to some extent, the deflection varying directly with the cube of the length and inversely with the cube of the depth of the beam (Shillingburg et al., 1976).

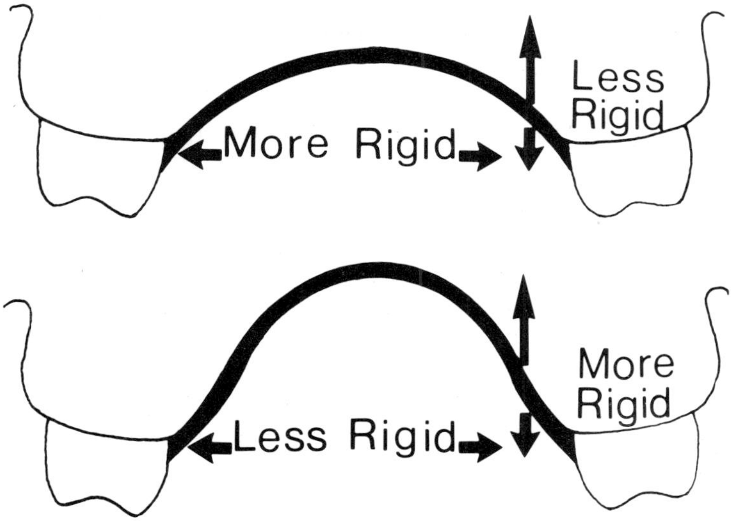

Fig. 8.4. Bars of equal cross-section area crossing shallow and deep palates. The shorter bar crossing the shallow palate is more rigid when loaded horizontally and less rigid when loaded vertically. The longer bar crossing the deep palate has less horizontal rigidity and more vertical rigidity.

According to McLean (1980), as the length of a beam changes, the transverse deflection increases as the cube of the length. Doubling the length of a span will allow eight times as much deflection for a given force. For example, if a one-tooth pontic bridge is compared with a two-tooth pontic bridge, and the design of the pontics and connectors remains unchanged, then the two-tooth bridge will bend eight times as much as the one-tooth bridge. The above statements are true for beams of homogeneous material and uniform cross-sections.

There is no such thing as an absolutely rigid beam; some slight movement is bound to occur under load. The movement of rigid connectors should be negligible and not more than the distortion of the mandible on movement. The amount of bending of connectors is a function of their cross-section area, their length, their shape, the material of which they are made, and of the magnitude and direction of the applied load. For instance, if loads were applied to the two bars in *Fig.* 8.4, the bar crossing the deeper palate would provide less rigidity to horizontal forces than the bar crossing the shallower palate, but the latter bar would offer less resistance to vertical loads than the bar crossing the deeper palate. Rigidity does not only depend on length, cross-section area and direction of load; it also depends on the shape of the bar. This is illustrated by the bars of equal cross-section area in *Fig.* 8.5. The bar on the right side of the diagram is more rigid in relation to vertical loads than to horizontal loads. It would be 'edge' bent in the long axis of the cross-section in relation to vertical loads, but horizontal loads would bend it 'on the flat' in the short axis of the cross-section. The bar on the left of the diagram offers the same resistance to both vertical and horizontal loads because its cross-section is circular.

Torsional Elasticity

When a metal bar is twisted at its ends, complex stresses are distributed along the whole length of the bar. This distribution of torsional stress within the bar is such that large stresses can be placed on a bar without it rupturing and quite large torsional deflections can take place. Thus, any L-shaped connector is unlikely to remain rigid as twisting can take place in one leg of the L when the other leg is deflected (*Fig.* 8.6). This can be used when designing flexible connectors for mandibular free-end saddle dentures. When a split lingual

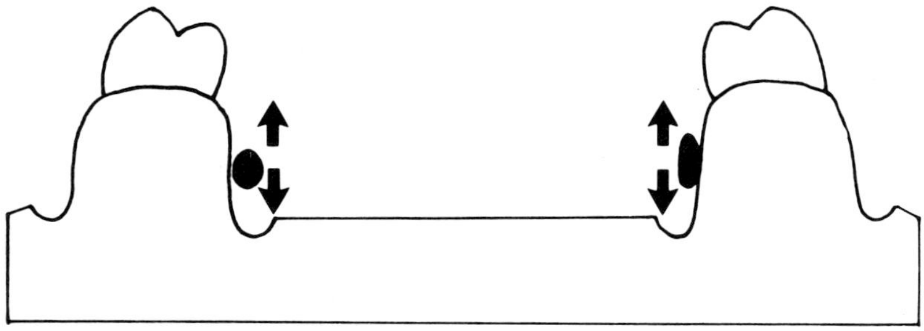

Fig. 8.5. Bars of equal cross-section area, but different shapes. The oval bar on the right of the diagram is more resistant to vertical bending.

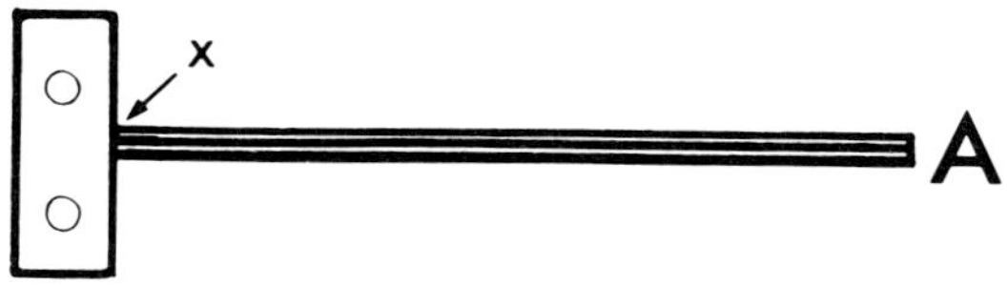

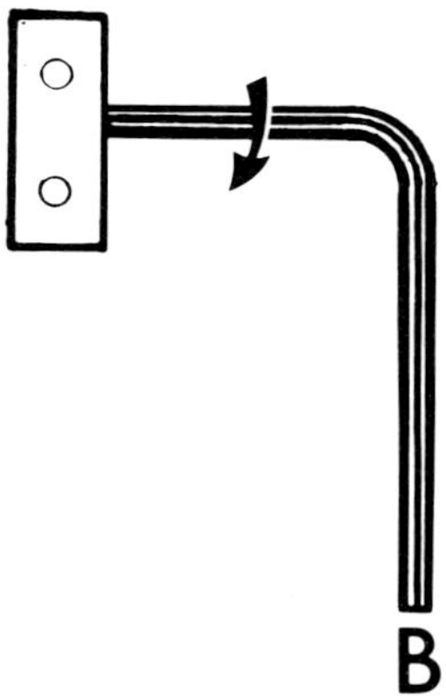

Fig. 8.6. A deflecting load applied at **A** to the metal bar whose end is firmly clamped will concentrate the stress (and hence the strain) at the point X. A deflecting load applied to the bent bar at **B** will cause torsion of the metal, indicated by the arrow, and thus distribute the stresses and strains over a greater region of metal.

plate is used, the split should be long enough to be L-shaped and thus provide a stress-breaking connector to the free-end saddle (*Fig.* 8.7). Quite a small force loading the saddle twists the part of the lingual bar indicated by arrows. This additional flexibility from the torsional elasticity of the metal can be put to advantage in flexible designs of dentures, but is a disadvantage when a rigid design is required. Rigid denture designs are usually simple and this is their main advantage as there are fewer edges for food to catch on or the tongue to play with.

Flexible Connectors

Flexible connectors or stress-breakers may be either saddle connectors or clasp connectors that join a mucosa-borne part to a tooth-borne part of a partial denture.

Types

Flexible connectors fall into two main groups, the springy type and the mechanical type. The springy type depends on the inherent flexibility of the material of which it is made (*see Fig.* 8.3). The mechanical type comprises movable joints, such as hinges (*Fig.* 8.8) or ball-and-socket joints, that allow a limited amount of movement to take place. Some prefabricated attachments incorporate springs in addition to mechanical joints to provide stress-breaking; for example the Dalbo 63.02.2 attachment (*Figs.* 8.9, 8.10).

Function

The function of stress-breaking connectors is to divide the load of mastication between the teeth and the mucosa in as favourable a way as possible and to help to direct occlusal forces down the long axes of the natural teeth and protect them from lateral and torsional stresses. Clearly most 'stress-breakers' do not fulfil all these functions.

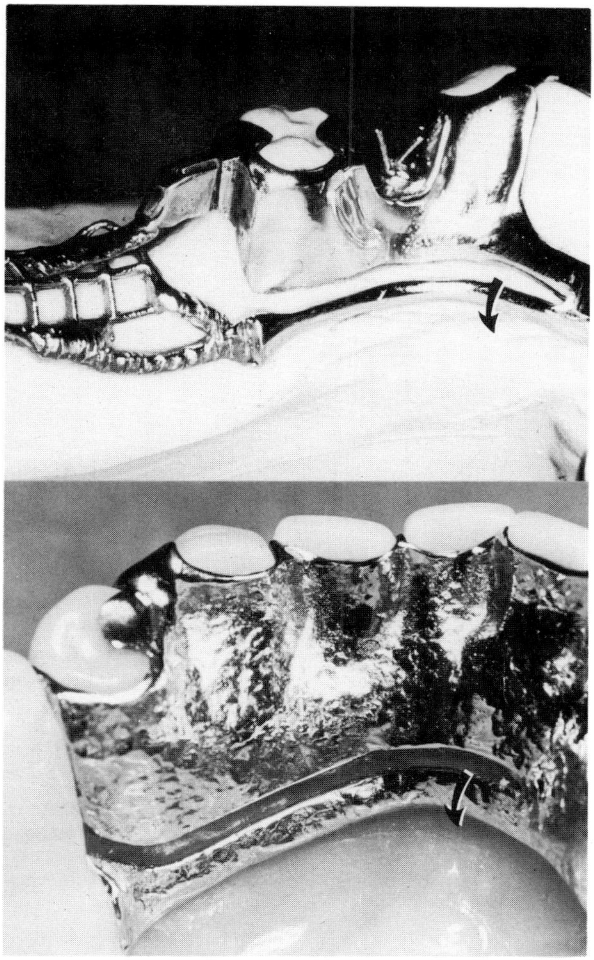

Fig. 8.7. Lower denture bases incorporating L-shaped stress-breaking connectors to free-end saddles. The *arrows* indicate the part of the connector where torsion occurs under load.

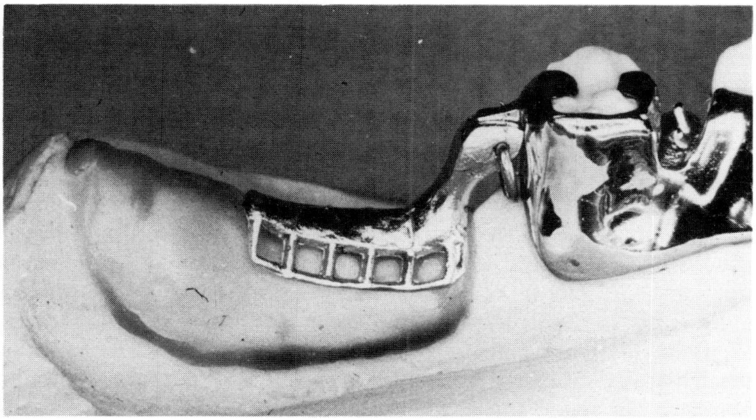

Fig. 8.8. Hinge connector joining free-end saddle to tooth-borne part of a partial lower denture. The pin can be withdrawn from the lingual surface of the acrylic saddle when relining is required.

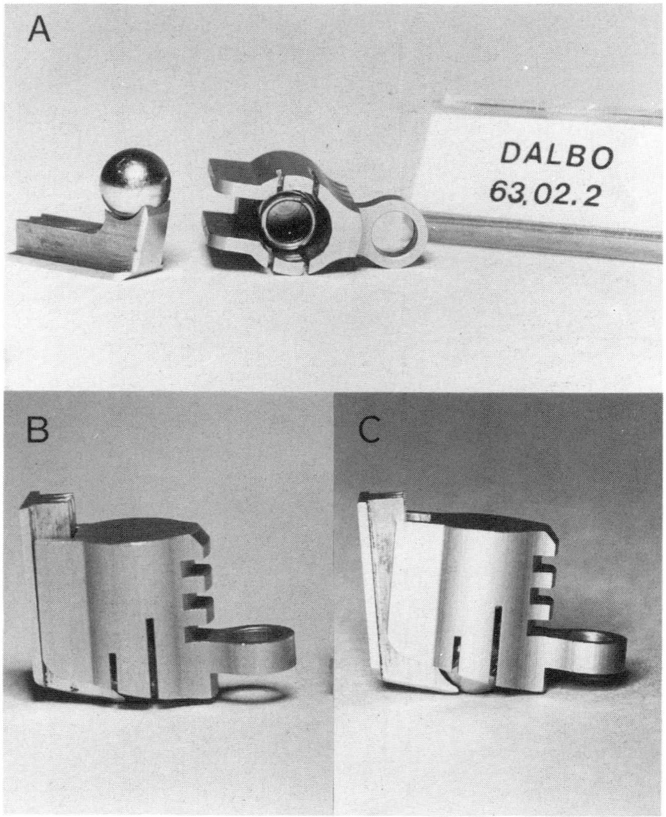

Fig. 8.9. Dalbo extracoronal attachment has a ball and spring mechanism that permits vertical as well as hinged movement. **A**, Dalbo attachment with patrix and matrix separated. **B**, Assembled attachment. **C**, Attachment showing hinge movement.

Design Implications

The springy type of stress-breaker depends on the flexibility of the alloy connector (*see Fig.* 8.3) and the retention of the tooth-borne part of the denture must be sufficient to ensure that it does not move while the springy stress-breaker bends. Thus, the force of retention must be greater than the force required to displace the stress-breaker to the extent of the compressibility of the mucosa. This implies that when the mucosa-borne saddle is bitten upon, an extracting force is put on the tooth carrying the retainer furthest from the point of the applied load. If the retainer is not strong enough or far enough away from the axis of rotation, the denture rotates round the fulcrum axis through the occlusal rests nearest the point of application of load and the stress-breaker does not function. The denture then acts as if rigidly connected.

Disadvantages of Stress-broken Dentures

Some consider the disadvantages of stress-broken appliances are as follows:

1. They put too much of the occlusal load on the mucosa and too little on the teeth. Hinged stress-breakers adjacent to the abutment teeth distribute most of the occlusal load on the mucosa at the distal end of the saddle and possibly less than half the load on the teeth, depending on the point of application of the load, but this is true only if a spring is incorporated in the hinge. Simple hinges placed distal to the abutment teeth distribute the load in the same way as rigid dentures (*see Fig.* 8.14), but distribute more

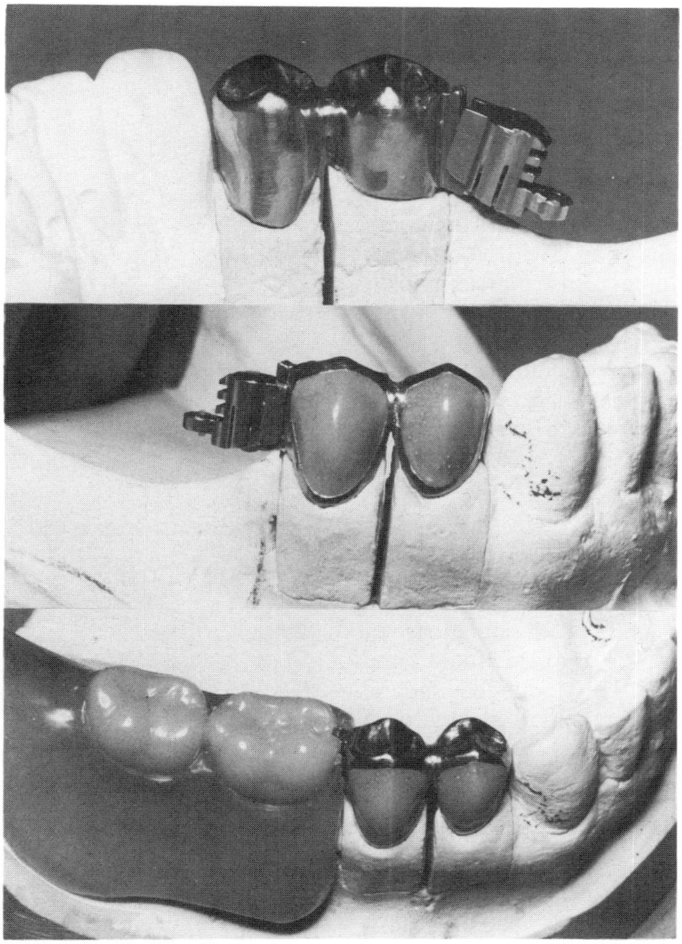

Fig. 8.10. *Upper,* Lingual view of double abutment pieces with Dalbo attachment, showing hinged movement. *Middle,* Buccal view. *Lower,* With free-end saddle attached.

load to the mucosa if placed anterior to the abutment teeth.

2. Stress-breakers that are stiff enough to distribute load between tooth and mucosa tend to put extracting forces on the clasped teeth of the tooth-borne part. These extracting forces may become unacceptably high if the retention is sufficiently good to allow a stiff stress-breaker to bend without displacing the tooth-borne part.

3. If the clasps on the tooth-borne part are arranged so that they do not provide 'indirect support', the denture rocks round an axis through the occlusal rests nearest the mucosa-borne saddle and the stress-breaker behaves as if it were part of a rigid denture base.

4. Stress-breakers may allow unacceptably high lateral loads to be transferred to the mucosa.

5. Stress-breakers increase the complexity of the denture and thus make the dentures less comfortable, more expensive and more difficult to keep clean.

6. Breakage is more likely with stress-broken designs than with rigid designs and maintenance costs are higher.

Advantages of Stress-broken Dentures

1. Stress-breakers distribute the load between the teeth and the mucosa so that the

mucosa takes a greater proportion of load when the periodontal condition is poor.

2. Stress-breakers may protect the teeth against lateral and torsional loads.

3. Stress-broken dentures are more comfortable as the patient does not feel that the abutment teeth are being tugged during mastication. For this reason many patients who are unable to wear rigid tooth-and-mucosa-borne dentures find stress-broken dentures acceptable.

4. Some hinged designs give the best distribution of load between teeth and mucosa when many posterior teeth are missing.

5. Stress-broken designs are best when the remaining teeth are of poor prognosis and cannot be used to provide support for conventional partial dentures.

Tooth-and-mucosa-borne Saddles

We shall now consider the implications of designing a denture to provide tooth and mucosa support for a long bounded saddle. *Fig.* 8.11 illustrates a maxillary dental arch with a long bounded saddle having the left canine and second molar as abutments. On the right there are full veneer crowns on the second premolar and first molar. The occlusal rests on the left canine and second molar distribute the load to these teeth, while split-bar stress-breakers (marked X and Y) allow some compression of the mucosa when the load falls on the saddle. Fine splits in the bars can best be produced by embedding strips of stainless-steel plate in the wax before investing. Thus, removal of the strip after casting leaves a fine split that is almost undetectable to the patient's tongue. If the bars X and Y (*Fig.* 8.11) were absolutely rigid the saddle would be entirely tooth-borne, while if they were completely flexible it would be mucosa-borne so, in theory at least, by altering the flexibility of the bars we can alter the proportion of load borne by the teeth and mucosa.

The point of application of the masticatory load on the long bounded saddle lies on a line between the occlusal rests on the abutment teeth on the left, so that there is little tendency for the base to tilt when under load. The stress-breakers are therefore effective and the

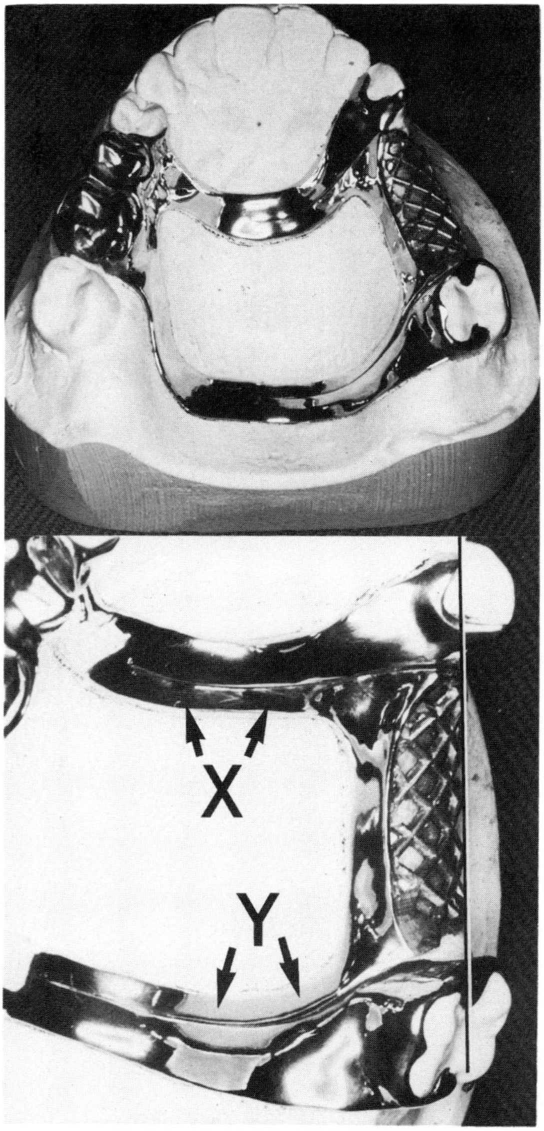

Fig. 8.11. *Upper,* Stress-distributing design for a long bounded saddle in the left maxillary arch. Split bar connectors allow compression of the mucosa. *Lower,* Enlarged view of split bar connectors (X and Y). The line drawn between the abutment teeth represents the fulcrum axis round which the denture might rotate when the saddle is loaded. However, as the point of application of masticatory load lies in this axis, no rotation takes place and the retainers on the patient's right prevent movement of the whole denture base.

retainers on the tooth-borne part of the denture easily hold it in place when the stress-breakers bend. Another important consideration is the degree of compressibility of the mucosa of the saddle areas. In order to use the mucosa for support, it should be compressed when under load. Thus the opposing teeth must meet the artificial teeth before the natural teeth come into occlusion. The amount of premature contact must be closely related to the degree of compression of the mucosa and must also be finely adjusted to the flexibility of the stress-breakers and the amount of load transmitted to the left canine and second molar.

The daunting task of adjusting these four factors (i.e. prematurity of occlusion; compressibility of mucosa; load-bearing capacity of mucosa; flexibility of stress-breakers) is often sufficient to discourage prosthodontists from using such stress-broken designs. Nevertheless it is possible to make approximate estimates of the forces involved. First, the compressibility of mucosa can be measured with the instrument shown in *Fig.* 4.13, and when the area of the saddle is known the amount of force for a specified degree of compression can be calculated. It is also possible to calculate the amount of load necessary to deflect the stress-breakers through the distance the mucosa is compressed and relate their length and cross-section area to the force required.

Associated with a design of this sort there is the insuperable difficulty that occurs when very hard food is bitten on the saddle. For instance, suppose that a denture has been designed so that, when a load of 30 kg is applied to the centre of the saddle, 10 kg is transmitted to the mucosa and 10 kg to each of the abutment teeth through the bars X and Y. Suppose that the load is increased to 50 kg. The dimensions of bars X and Y are unchanged and so only about 10 kg is transmitted to each of the two abutment teeth, as before, and the extra 20 kg is transmitted almost entirely to the mucosa, which now receives 30 kg. Not quite all the additional load falls on the mucosa, however, because the increased deflection of the bars X and Y transmits slightly more than 10 kg to each of the teeth, but the amount is likely to be only a small proportion of the total increased load. In these overload conditions there is another factor that has not yet been considered: the periodontal afferents of the opposing teeth limit the load to within the capacity of the periodontal support. The same problems that have already been discussed with regard to mucosa-borne dentures (Chapter 3) apply to some extent in this case when the mucosa is overloaded.

The many variations in patients, such as the type of mucosa, direction of load and shape of palate, require individual attention, and the innumerable technical variations, such as differences in composition of alloys, method of laboratory construction and similar factors, defy precise analysis.

Role of Retention in Stress-broken Dentures

The stress-breakers in the foregoing design (*Fig.* 8.11) could be made quite stiff without the denture being displaced, as the load on the saddle is in line with the occlusal rests and thus the retainers can easily hold the denture in place, while the stress-breakers bend. Many other so-called 'stress-breaking' designs are unsuccessful because the fundamental importance of retention of the tooth-borne part is not appreciated. For example, *Fig.* 8.12 shows a design that is supposedly stress-broken, but when a load is applied to the

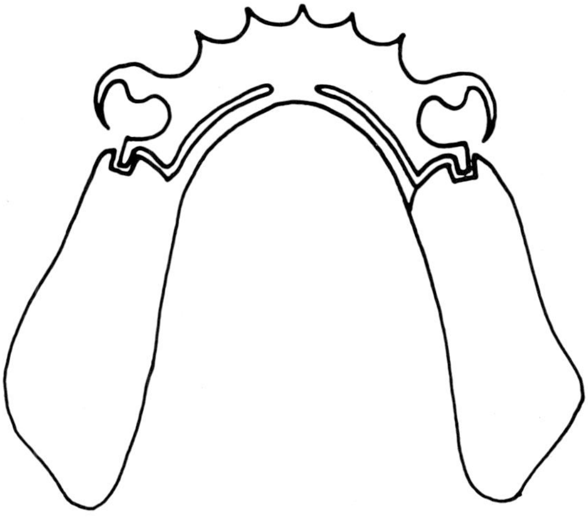

Fig. 8.12. A 'stress-broken' design which would not work since the clasps do not prevent the rotation of the denture round the fulcrum axis when the saddles are loaded. Thus, this denture acts in the same way as a rigid design.

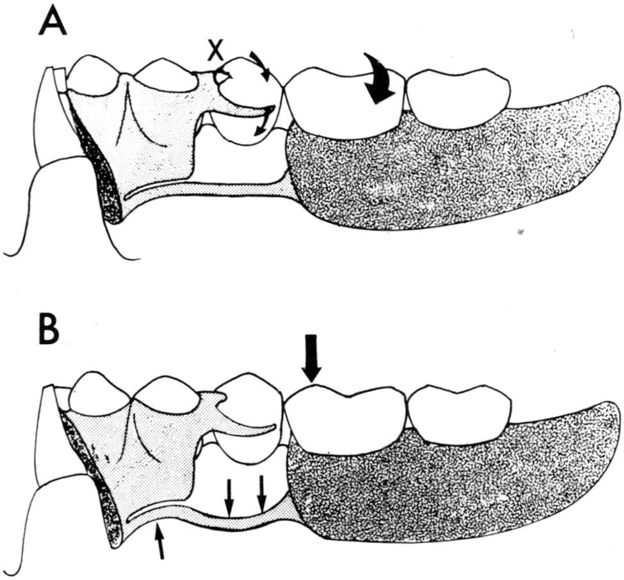

Fig. 8.13. **A**, Although a 'stress-broken' design, this denture rocks round the occlusal rest (X) when a load is applied to the saddle. This is because the retainers do not resist the rocking movement. **B**, It is possible that there might be an S-shaped deflection of the stress-breaker after the distal end of the saddle area reaches maximum compression from a load applied on the first molar (*arrow*). This deflection is exaggerated in the diagram.

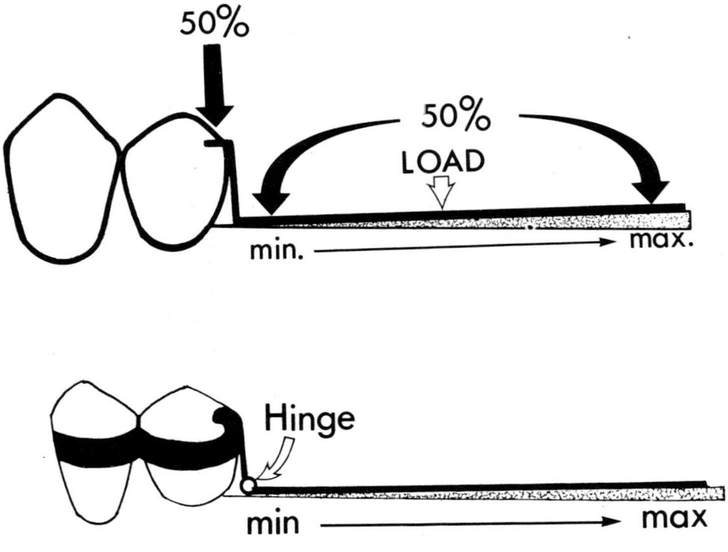

Fig. 8.14. The load on the tissues supporting a free-end saddle lower denture that is rigidly connected to the occlusal rests is distributed equally between the tooth and the mucosa if the total load is applied in the middle of the saddle. Immediately distal to the abutment tooth little or no load is accepted by the mucosa and the 50 per cent of the load that is distributed to the mucosa increases to a maximum in a wedge-shaped manner at the distal end of the saddle. The presence of a simple hinge has little effect on the distribution of the load between tooth and mucosa, but prevents the anterior part of the denture rising when the posterior part is depressed.

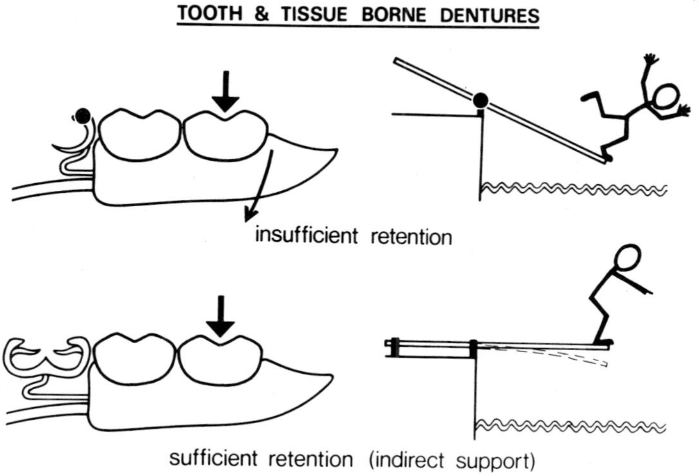

Fig. 8.15. Where there is insufficient retention the flexible stress-breaker, like the diving board, does not bend as tilting takes place, but if there is sufficient retention to resist tilting the stress-breaker bends.

saddle areas the denture rotates round the occlusal rests and the distally facing clasps go deeper into the undercuts, providing no resistance to this rotation. The thin 'stress-breaking' connectors are therefore unnecessary, as this denture behaves as if it was rigid and rocks round the fulcrum axis when the saddles are loaded. It could be argued that a load applied to the mesial end of the free-end saddle might produce an S-shaped deflection of the stress-breaker (*Fig.* 8.13) after the distal end of the saddle area has reached its maximum compression, but we consider that the probability of this making a significant contribution to the mucosal support is small and certainly does not justify the additional complexity of the design. It might be thought that the design shown in *Fig.* 8.3 would fall into the same category as that in *Fig.* 8.12, but in *Fig.* 8.3 sufficient retention is provided by the clasps (arrowed) to hold the tooth-borne part in place, while the stress-breaker bends, and therefore this design is acceptable while the one in *Fig.* 8.12 is not. The cartoon (*Fig.* 8.15) illustrates the point.

Purely mechanical stress-breakers that do not incorporate a spring allow a simple hinge movement. The position of the hinge determines the method of loading the saddles. If the hinge is immediately distal to the abutment tooth of a free-end saddle (*Fig.* 8.8) 50 per cent of the total load applied to the middle of the saddle falls on the abutment tooth and 50 per cent falls on the saddle, chiefly at its distal end and diminishing to zero towards its mesial end (*Fig.* 8.14). However, if a spring is incorporated in the hinge, the load falling on the abutment tooth is related to the amount of force required to compress the spring to the extent of the compressibility of the mucosa. The tooth is protected against any load beyond the compressibility of the spring unless (through failure to reline the saddle) the spring is compressed against itself and acts as a solid stop, in which case the stress-breaking connector acts as the simple hinge did. Dentures incorporating hinges are further discussed in Chapter 10.

Chapter 9

Discussion of design

Aspects of Design

So far this book has been devoted to the changes associated with partial loss of teeth and to a discussion of the components of dentures used to replace this loss. Separate chapters have been given to the discussion of support, retention and connectors. In this section of the book we put these theoretical considerations together, so that the practical business of designing partial dentures can be understood. We feel that the practice of designing partial dentures should be based on a sound knowledge, so that while opinions may differ as to how the denture should be designed, at least the theory on which the opinions are based is understood. Students who may be quite confused by different viewpoints on the design of a denture for a particular patient will be able to judge the viewpoints against the theory and decide their own priorities as to how much weight they should give to each part of the design. Show a patient requiring partial dentures to six dentists and it is likely that you will get six different designs, as each dentist will put a different amount of emphasis on the different aspects of the design (Frantz, 1975). These aspects of design are: appearance, comfort, hygiene, support, retention, occlusion, cost and technical resources.

Many dentists in general practice place most emphasis on appearance and comfort, as these are the patient's chief priorities. In other words, they want the dentures to look good and feel good, but these two aspects may conflict with the maintenance of good oral hygiene and dental health and with the other factors on the list. In the welter of conflicting opinions about denture design for any one case, there is usually a sensible balance that can be found by careful examination of the various factors. In this chapter we discuss these factors and decide their relative importance.

Appearance

The appearance of partial dentures is fully discussed in Chapter 15. We have shown that to make dentures virtually undetectable in the mouth it is necessary to provide a wide buccal flange for anterior saddles to restore the lost gingival papillae (*see Figs.* 2.3, 2.6, 2.7, 2.8). Such a flange endangers the health of the gingivae, and those who put appearance first are prepared to sacrifice hygiene, while those who put hygiene first might have to sacrifice the appearance. Dentists who put appearance first are often prepared to sacrifice retention as well, since they do not want clasps to show at the front of the mouth. However, retention does not necessarily have to be sacrificed, as a number of attachments can be used instead of clasps. These devices (*see Figs.* 7.2–7.9 and 7.16–7.20) provide good appearance and good retention, but are not particularly hygienic and are expensive and involve considerations of cost and technical resources.

In the conflict between considerations of appearance and of hygiene it is the dentist's duty to put the health of the remaining tissues first, but little is to be gained if the appearance is so unsatisfactory to the patient that he will not wear the denture. The decision must always be related to the individual patient and to his ability to keep the dentures clean.

Retention

Few dentists give retention over-riding importance in the design of partial dentures, since dentures with comparatively little retention can be accepted and tolerated by most patients. Dentures are often designed with retention entirely dependent on clasps, but in some cases the retentive qualities of the clasps fail a week or two after the denture is given to the patient. This failure may be the result of incorrect design, indifferent technology or mishandling of the materials used in the construction of the clasps. While the bracing aspect of the clasps is usually maintained, retention is diminished. In spite of this, however, most of these dentures continue to be worn with reasonable comfort. Some patients remove clasps from their dentures to improve the appearance and willingly sacrifice the retention by doing so. Thus, the retention of partial dentures is not usually given first priority, although it is undoubtedly important for the patient's comfort. The factors associated with the retention of dentures are fully discussed in Chapter 6 and 7.

Comfort

It is difficult to quantify the amount of retention that a patient requires for comfort. Certainly many patients believe that their dentures are comfortable with little retention. While some patients may remove clasps to improve appearance, others may remove clasps from dentures to improve comfort because they are conscious of the clasps tugging the teeth, particularly in tooth-and-mucosa-borne dentures of rigid design. Comfort is sometimes a measure of the adaptability of the patient rather than a quality of the design. However, if the design is kept simple, it is more likely to be comfortable and hygienic than if it is made too complicated. In designing partial dentures sufficient attention is rarely given to the adaptive response of the oral tissues. Different designs call forth different responses from the tissues and there is great variation in this from one patient to another. Poor designs may exceed the adaptive potential of the patient and result in rejection of the denture or damage to teeth and mucosa, whereas good designs help to preserve the remaining tissues and make the patient feel comfortable.

When receiving finished cobalt-chromium alloy cast partial dentures from laboratories, dentists assume that these castings will fit very accurately round the natural teeth. Undoubtedly many of them do fit well, but whenever a denture is cast in one piece there are inevitably unavoidable small dimensional errors. These inaccuracies are usually tolerated by patients, although quite frequently they complain that the denture 'feels tight' when it is first inserted. Dentists usually reassure patients that the feeling of tightness will soon disappear and it usually does after about one week of the dentures being worn. The feeling of tightness is most common in patients with bilateral bounded saddles, particularly when the teeth at each end of these saddles are clasped. These observations are made after reviewing partially edentulous patients in both our clinics. A review of this sort merely records the patients' reactions, but at least it gives an indication that this feeling is common in patients who have partial dentures fitted and is more commonly experienced with cast alloy dentures than with acrylic dentures. This might indicate that casting shrinkage and the rigidity of the metal contribute to the discomfort. In fixed bridges and gold alloy removable partial dentures casting inaccuracies can be considerably reduced by soldering the various cast components together with or without wedges that negate the effect of the shrinkage of the solder.

It is generally accepted that partial denture bases should be as rigid as possible, but clinical experience shows that patients sometimes prefer a flexible acrylic denture to a rigid metal one. An interesting clinical finding of some of those who have experimented with nylon partial dentures is that many of the patients said how comfortable these dentures were and preferred them to acrylic dentures (Matthews and Smith, 1955; Watt, 1955; Hallett and Farrell, 1956; Hargreaves, 1971; MacGregor and Stafford, 1983). This feeling of comfort was attributed to the flexibility of the denture bases. It would therefore be worth while examining the requirement of rigidity in partial denture bases which appears in the *Guides to Standards in Prosthetic Dentistry* published by the British Society for the Study of Prosthetic Dentistry (1981).

Patient comfort may not be a very good criterion for denture design, but undoubtedly it is the most important one from the patient's point of view. We suspect that when a denture is uncomfortable it is likely to be damaging to the tissues, but we must be aware that

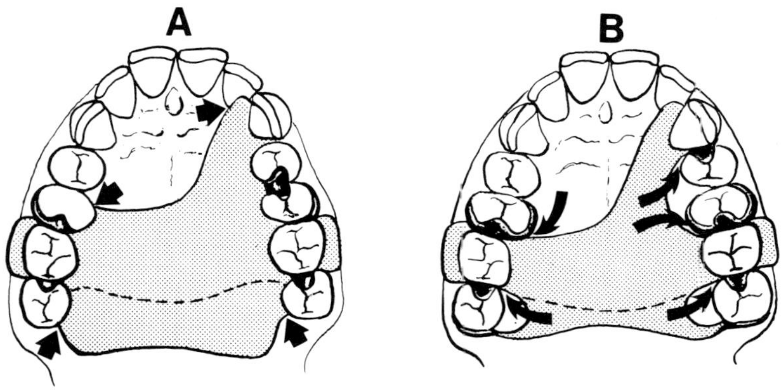

Fig. 9.1. **A**, Where the denture base crosses the gingival margins the angles (*arrowed*) between the edge of the denture and the gingival margins should be obtuse. **B**, Acute angles allow food-trapping and cause inflammation. The designs of both '**A**' and '**B**' would be improved by removing the denture base behind the interrupted line. Design '**A**' is stronger and more easily tolerated than design '**B**' which, although it avoids the gingival margins, requires lingual clasp arms to reciprocate the forces of the buccal arms. These lingual arms would irritate the tongue.

continuing and severe tissue damage can occur without the patient experiencing discomfort. The factors upon which comfort depends are likely to be related to the adaptive demands placed on the periodontium and this in turn is related to the rigidity of the denture base and the rigidity of the clasp connectors, particularly when the saddles are mucosa-borne.

Hygiene

We put a high priority on hygiene and feel that a very important part of partial denture design is to ensure that the gingival margins are not covered by the denture. However, it is virtually impossible to design a removable denture that does not cross the gingival margins somewhere, and at these positions the margins are most at risk, especially if the edges of the denture cross the gingival margins at an acute angle. The angle between the denture and the gingival margin should not be less than 90° and should preferably be quite obtuse to make it self-cleansing (*Fig.* 9.1). Acute angles between the denture periphery and the gingival margins tend to trap food and sometimes occur when the periphery is cut back from single teeth. In such designs the periphery of the denture may become unduly extended. Avoidance of gingival coverage can sometimes be taken too far and consequently in some denture designs small areas of gingivae are left uncovered. This is sometimes detrimental to the gingival mucosa, which tends to proliferate into these small areas.

In general, the shorter the denture periphery and the simpler the design, the easier it is for the patient to wear the denture and keep it clean. A fairly simple rule for designing a denture to maximize oral hygiene is that if the denture is tooth-borne it is not usually worth while complicating the shape of the lingual or palatal plate by keeping it away from the gingival margin of a single standing tooth. There should be at least two adjacent natural teeth to make the cut-away space sufficiently self-cleansing.

Support Classification

The factors associated with support of partial dentures have been fully discussed in Chapters 3 and 4. Partial dentures should be designed to distribute the masticatory and occlusal loads to the remaining teeth and/or residual alveolar ridges, so that these structures are not damaged. Maximum use should be made of the supporting tissues because a support deficit exists in every partially edentulous mouth. In this chapter we use a support classification of partial dentures as a basis for their design. Many methods of classifying partial dentures have been devised and are summarized in Appendix IV, but the classification we use for

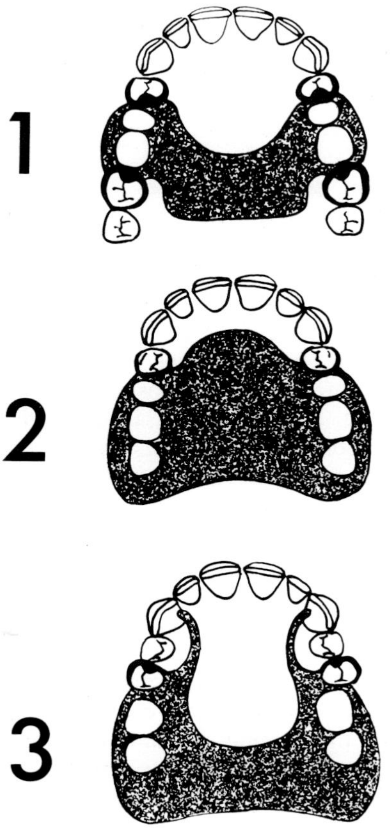

Fig. 9.2. Support classification of partial dentures: **1**, Tooth-borne. **2**, Mucosa-borne. **3**, Tooth-and-mucosa-borne.

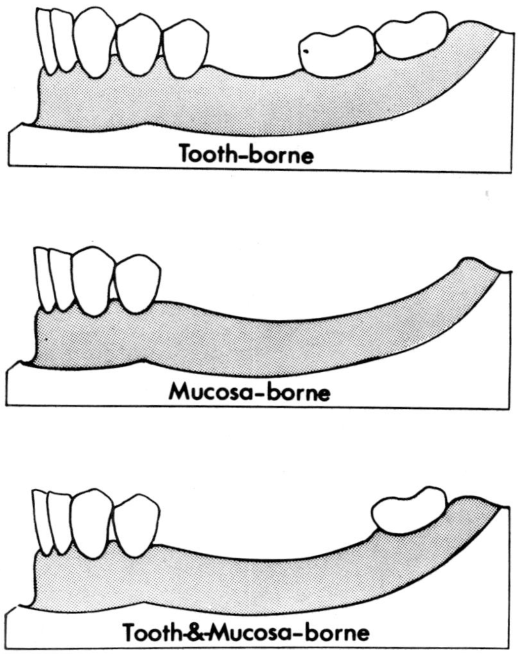

Fig. 9.3. Types of saddle areas.

the systematic designing of partial dentures is as follows (*Fig.* 9.2):

Tooth-borne partial dentures:
All the support for the partial denture comes from the teeth.

Mucosa-borne partial dentures:
The denture is entirely supported by the mucosa and underlying alveolar ridge.

Tooth-and-mucosa-borne partial dentures:
Some parts of the denture are supported by the teeth and some by the mucosa.

Which of the three means of support is used for a partial denture depends on the health of the teeth, the quality of the mucosa, the bone density, and on the age, general health and oral hygiene of the patient, but most of all on the type of saddle area. There are three types of saddle area (*Fig.* 9.3):

Short bounded saddle areas are caused by the loss of one or two teeth and have abutment teeth at both ends. Dentures fitting these gaps should be tooth-supported, provided the R/L ratio is more than 0·70 and the periodontal tissues are healthy.

Free-end saddle areas have abutment teeth at only one end. The type of support for the saddles depends on the type of connector used. If two free-end saddles are connected to each other with no connection with the tooth-borne part of the denture, they are entirely mucosa-borne. The amount of support from the teeth is related to the stiffness of the connector to the tooth-borne part of the denture. The different methods of connection are discussed in Chapters 8 and 10.

Long bounded saddle areas have three or more teeth missing. This indicates tooth support if the R/L ratio is about 0·70 or above and the periodontal prognosis is favourable. Mucosa-support or tooth-and-mucosa-support is indicated if the R/L ratio is less than 0·70 and the periodontal health is poor.

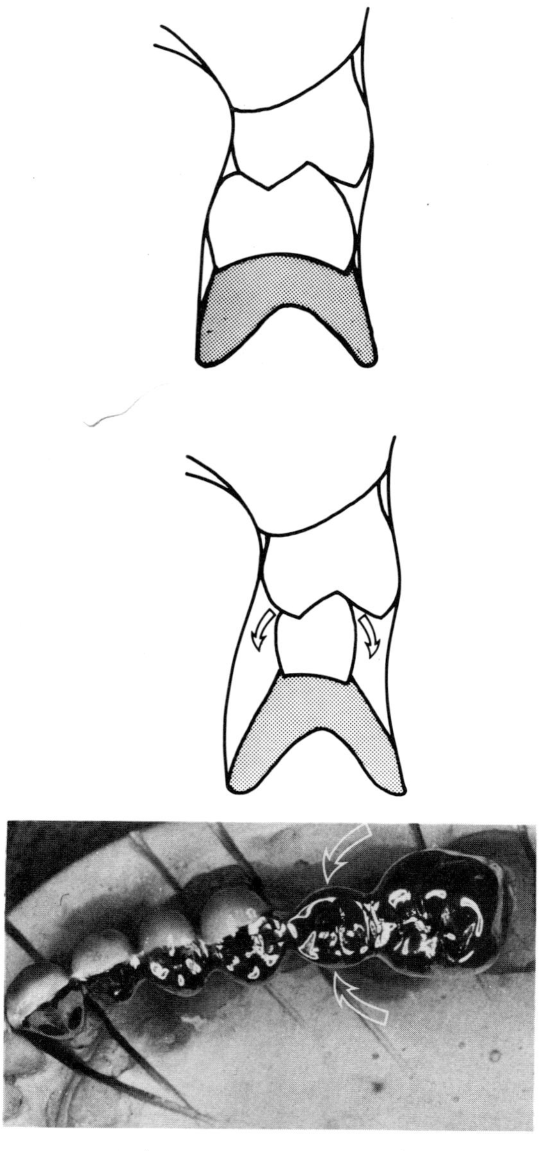

Fig. 9.4. Artificial teeth on tooth-borne dentures should be the same size as the natural teeth they replace, as they fill the denture space and are more comfortable for the patient. Narrow artificial teeth on tooth-borne dentures encourage food-packing in the buccal and lingual sulci (*arrows*).

Occlusion

The occlusion of a partial denture does not usually present much of a design problem, provided the occlusion of the natural teeth has been adjusted and stabilized before the partial denture is made (*see* Chapter 1 and Appendix II). However, it might be worth while asking the question 'Should the posterior teeth of partial dentures be the same size as natural teeth or should they be smaller?' It is generally accepted that by placing teeth with smaller occlusal surfaces on tooth-borne saddles of partial dentures, the masticatory load on the abutment teeth and supporting tissues is reduced, but when we examine this more carefully we find that the possible advantage of narrow teeth on tooth-borne saddles is outweighed by their disadvantages (*Fig.* 9.4). For instance, when a narrow artificial lower tooth opposes a broad upper molar, the bolus of food is divided by the narrow tooth and is thrust into the lower buccal and lingual sulci and is difficult to remove from there, especially if the denture flanges are too thick. With narrow teeth the mastication of food is less efficient and the occlusion of the narrow artificial tooth against the broad natural tooth is such that food particles are left sticking to the natural teeth. On the other hand, a broad artificial tooth produces a self-cleansing occlusion and feels better to the patient since it is in alignment with the rest of the dental arch. Its broad occlusal surface and high cusps provide better intercuspation and if the natural teeth are rotated or displaced, as commonly occurs, the cusps can be adjusted easily to provide self-cleansing contacts with the natural teeth. The management of the occlusion of partial dentures with displaced natural teeth is discussed in Chapter 1 and Appendix II.

Now let us look again at the only apparent advantage of placing narrow teeth on artificial dentures: the limitation of masticatory load. It has been assumed that the masticatory load should be limited to avoid overloading of the abutment teeth, but the normal protective mechanisms of our bodies ensure that we will not knowingly damage our bodily structures. The control mechanisms are arranged so that the muscles will not exert damaging forces except in dilemma situations in which such forces cannot be avoided. Thus, overloading the teeth is avoided by a reduction in the force exerted by the masticatory muscles. You can test this quite easily for yourself by attempting to crack a nut between your teeth. There comes a point when you will be unwilling to exert a greater force because of the possibility of damaging a tooth, and yet your masticatory muscles would be quite capable of exerting sufficient force to crack the nut.

There are some circumstances in which we may produce trauma in order to relieve a slight irritation. Scratching an itch is an example of this. Small occlusal interferences can also cause mild irritation that might be relieved by clenching or grinding habits. Minor periodontal irritations caused by infection or calculus can be considered as 'periodontal itches' and may also precipitate clenching or grinding habits, although Yemm (1979) believes that these are more likely to have a central origin. By their movement on the mucosa, some partial and complete dentures can produce series of light touches that may cause clenching. We are all familiar with patients whose speech is interrupted by sudden clenching of the jaws or contractions of the lips in response to slight displacement of their dentures. The merest suspicion of movement is often followed by a reassuring clench. What we have said about the use of broad teeth on tooth-borne saddles is not applicable to mucosa-borne saddles, because the mucosa is less able than the teeth to support masticatory loads. It is therefore better to place narrow teeth on mucosa-borne saddles as less force is required to penetrate the bolus when narrow teeth are used (*see Fig.* 7.11). Matsumoto (1984) has studied the effects of changing the size and shape of the artificial occlusal surfaces on masticatory movements and pressures. When the saddle is mucosa-borne the mucosal receptors appear to take second place to the periodontal receptors and the occlusal force is not limited as in tooth-borne saddles. Thus, the mucosa may be traumatised (*see* Chapter 4 and *Fig.* 4.8).

Cost and Technical Resources

Cost and technical resources must always be considered when designing partial dentures. Many insurance schemes only meet certain costs and the patient may be unable or unwilling to pay for what might be considered to be ideal treatment. In some parts of the world technical resources for carrying out the work may not be available, although payment is possible, and simpler designs must then be used. Cost often greatly influences the choice of clinical and laboratory materials from which the denture is made and this in turn affects the design. Written prescriptions from clinicians do not always result in accurate, well-made partial dentures. Clinical errors, faults in the laboratory services and misunderstandings can lead to difficulties that can be avoided if all persons involved in the treatment of the patient are aware of these possibilities.

Types of Partial Dentures

Partial dentures may be grouped into four main categories:

- Fixed partial dentures
- Acrylic removable partial dentures
- Metallic removable partial dentures
- Complex partial dentures

Fixed Partial Dentures

When few teeth are missing and the saddle areas are bounded, fixed partial dentures should always be considered first (*Fig.* 9.5) as they do not require connectors crossing the palate or passing behind the lower anterior teeth. In many ways they are the acme of streamlining as they occupy only the denture space and have no extra-anatomical parts, so are easily tolerated. Thus, provided the patient maintains a high level of oral hygiene and is willing to have the teeth prepared, fixed partial dentures of a high technical standard are the best type of appliance for many partially edentulous mouths.

Dentists often prescribe tooth-borne removable partial dentures in cases where they feel that the prognosis of the abutment teeth is not good enough for making a bridge or fixed partial denture. This course is unwise for three reasons:

1. A tooth-borne removable partial denture obtains no support from the mucosa and therefore the abutment teeth are subjected to just as large loads as those from a fixed partial denture.

2. Wolff (1884, 1891, 1892, 1899) described the 'biologic plasticity' of bone. Teeth might therefore be regarded as being embedded in a plastic material subject to movement when loaded. When a tooth-borne removable partial denture is loaded, the forces

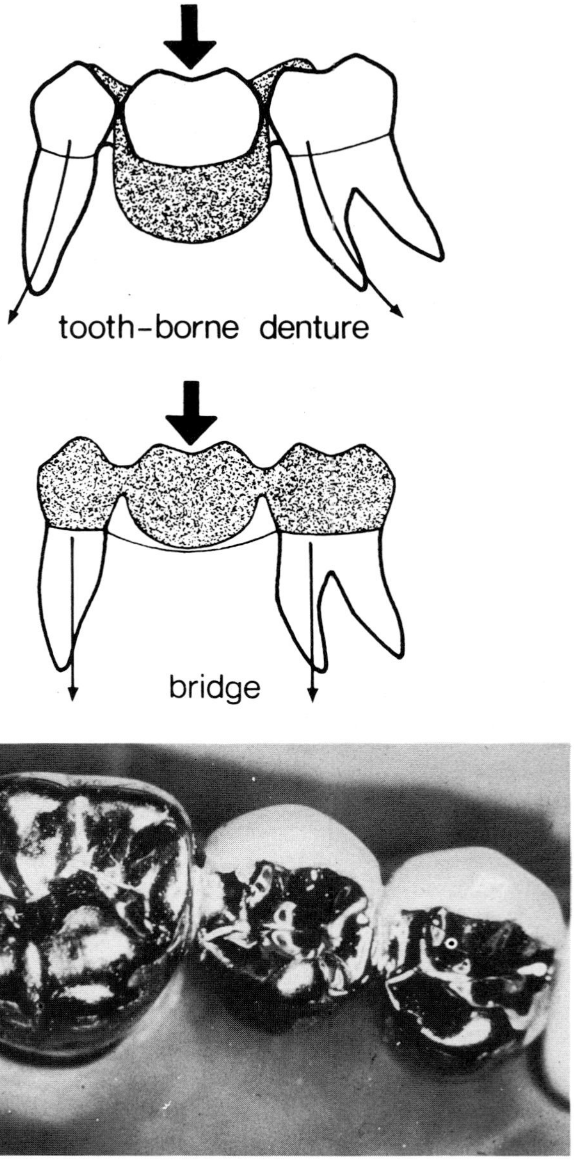

Fig. 9.5. Removable tooth-borne partial dentures (*upper*) do not obtain any support from the mucosa and it is unwise to fit such appliances when the teeth are of poor prognosis, as the loading of the periodontium is less favourable than if a bridge is fitted (*middle* and *lower* illustrations). Imagine the teeth embedded in a plastic material (Wolff described the biological plasticity of bone). The *heavy arrows* indicate the load and the *thin arrows* the movement of the teeth.

on the teeth tend to tip them towards each other and move the roots in the bone away from each other (*Fig.* 9.5). In contrast, with a bridge or fixed partial denture the occlusal loads are transmitted to the roots more favourably and therefore the teeth are less likely to be traumatised by this type of appliance (Glantz and Nyman, 1982).

3. Removable partial dentures are usually removed at night and thus forces on the abutment teeth are changed while the denture is out. A fixed partial denture remains in place

all the time and the forces on the teeth are reasonably constant, so that the periodontium does not have to adapt and re-adapt to changing forces.

Lundgren et al. (1975) reported a functional analysis of loads in a group of 18 patients with reduced periodontal support and concluded that fixed bridges are superior to removable partial dentures.

Acrylic Removable Partial Dentures

When large numbers of teeth are missing and long saddles remain, mucosa-borne acrylic partial dentures may provide the best solution, particularly if opposed by a complete denture that reduces the masticatory load on the partial denture. The simple acrylic 'gum-stripper' with no clasps or rests is probably the commonest type of removable partial denture. Although these appliances are damaging (*see* Chapter 4), they nevertheless retain their popularity because of their simplicity and low cost and because the patients are not aware of the dentures rocking on occlusal rests or tugging teeth that have retainers placed on them. They should be considered the most temporary and damaging of all partial dentures and should not be expected to assist in any way with preservation of the remaining teeth. They are more likely to be successful in the upper jaw than in the lower because of the greater area of mucosal support available. Gingival margin coverage should be avoided wherever possible (*see Fig.* 9.8). Careful surveying and blocking out, together with a meticulous laboratory technique, help to avoid damage and failure. A certain amount of rocking on a soft-tissue fulcrum is bound to occur as the patient chews, compressing first one saddle area, then the other. This rocking is likely to cause mucosal damage and papillary hyperplasia of the palate. Polishing the fitting surface of the denture can reduce the trauma (*see Fig.* 4.16). This may be achieved by the use of thin tin foil on the cast before the denture is processed.

Metallic Removable Partial Dentures

Partial dentures with alloy bases and acrylic saddles are best for patients with tooth-borne and mucosa-borne components distributed widely in the mouth. The strength of the alloy enables light designs to be made that cover as little of the oral tissues as possible. This generally improves the comfort of the patient. However, some patients complain about the rigidity of alloys, and major connectors crossing the anterior part of the palate are occasionally unacceptable.

There is little excuse for making alloy dentures that are entirely supported by mucosa and cover gingival margins. These are every bit as damaging as the so-called acrylic 'gum-strippers'. For example, metallic lingual plate connectors for bilateral free-end saddles are often well-tolerated, but traumatize the gingivae because a gap appears between the anterior plate and the lingual surfaces of the incisors as the denture sinks into the saddle areas under occlusal load. This gap acts rather like a cheese grater, enabling food to pack between the denture and the gingivae.

The main advantage of using alloys is the great variety of designs that can be made with these materials. Various components, such as rests, retainers, connectors, hinges and so on, can be incorporated into partial dentures made of metal alloys.

Complex Partial Dentures

We use the term 'complex partial dentures' to describe dentures that have some fixed parts and some removable parts. They are discussed in Chapter 13 and should be used when the least possible encroachment beyond the denture space is required, but where the post-extraction tissue loss cannot be restored by a fixed appliance or where cross-arch bracing is necessary because so few teeth remain. The complexity of these restorations makes them expensive. They must be designed very carefully to avoid encroachment beyond the denture space. The patients must be well motivated and must accept the responsibility for plaque control, which requires great care. Regular visits to the dentist should be arranged to ensure that a high level of oral cleanliness is maintained because without it complex restorations fail.

Choice of Design

In the last section we listed the types of partial dentures and some of the features that

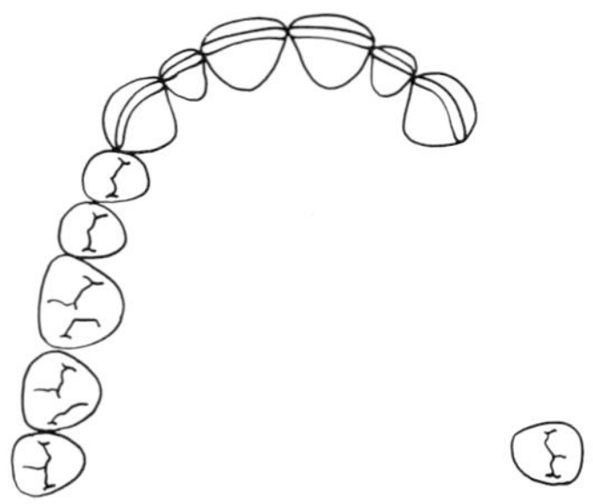

Fig. 9.6. Diagram of maxillary dental arch with the premolars and first two molars missing on the left. The designs of various appliances to replace the missing teeth are discussed in the text.

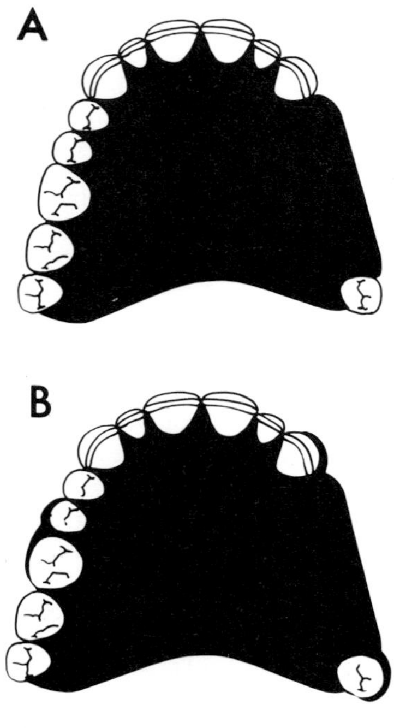

Fig. 9.7. **A**, Acrylic denture with no clasps or rests. **B**, Acrylic denture with clasps, but no rests.

influence the choice of a denture most suitable for a patient. Let us now consider the alternative designs for a partial upper denture to replace the left posterior teeth, as illustrated in *Fig.* 9.6. The simplest possible design, shown in *Fig.* 9.7**A**, is an acrylic denture with neither clasps nor rests. Lateral thrusts on this denture are transmitted to all the anterior teeth as well as to the posterior teeth. The ridges accept vertical thrusts during mastication, but little in the way of lateral thrusts. This design provides lateral bracing, but has many disadvantages. It damages the gingival margins round all the remaining teeth and the masticatory loads are sustained only by the mucosa and ridges. The lack of reciprocal action by clasp arms to the lateral thrusts on the base plate inevitably causes movement of the natural teeth and damage to the periodontium and gingival margins.

Now consider the effects of placing clasp arms on the abutment teeth (*Fig.* 9.7**B**). These clasp arms have two effects:

1. They provide reciprocation and thus movement of the clasped teeth is less likely to occur.

2. They provide retention on the opposite side of the arch to the side of mastication and the masticatory load is therefore spread over a larger area of mucosa (*see Fig.* 4.18).

The disadvantage of the clasp on the canine is that it shows when the patient smiles. The patient may complain that the clasps tug the teeth on chewing and the appliance feels bulky because it covers the rugal area of the palate.

Removal of the anterior part of the palate (*Fig.* 9.8**A**) undoubtedly improves the patient's comfort, but reduces the bracing from the anterior teeth. However, it might be argued that an improvement in periodontal health accrues from not covering the gingival margins. If this concept is pursued still further (*Fig.* 9.8**B**), less bracing against lateral loads is provided as fewer teeth are contacted by the denture base. Retention is by wrought clasp arms on buccal surfaces of the teeth. This arrangement produces the type of periodontal adaptive response described in Chapter 3 (*see Fig.* 3.5). The lateral thrusts of masticatory forces on the denture are much more severe in the buccal direction than in a lingual direction, since the rigid plate contacts the lingual sides of the teeth, but flexible clasp arms transmit smaller lingually-directed forces. This requires a lesser adaptive response from the lingual periodontium. If we now place occlusal rests on the canines and molars, the long bounded saddle becomes tooth-borne and the abutments are likely to be overloaded during chewing (*Fig.* 9.8**C**). The mucosa of the saddle accepts

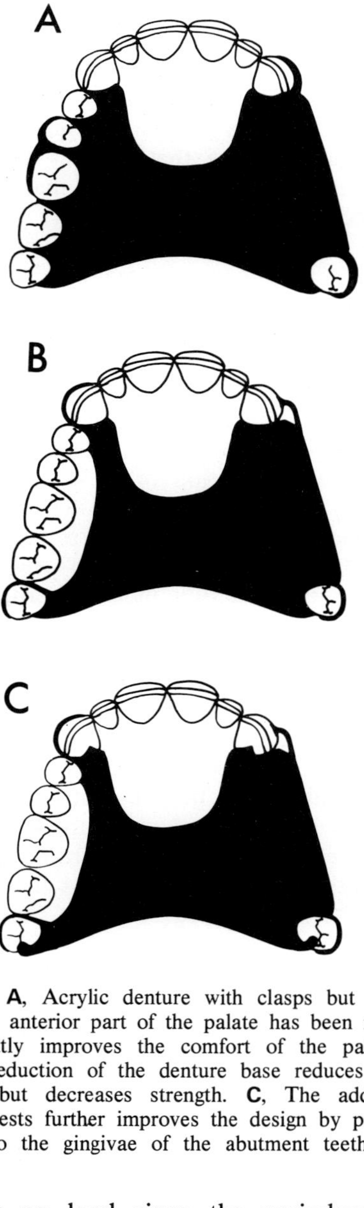

Fig. 9.8. **A**, Acrylic denture with clasps but no rests where the anterior part of the palate has been removed. This greatly improves the comfort of the patient. **B**, Further reduction of the denture base reduces gingival damage, but decreases strength. **C**, The addition of occlusal rests further improves the design by preventing damage to the gingivae of the abutment teeth.

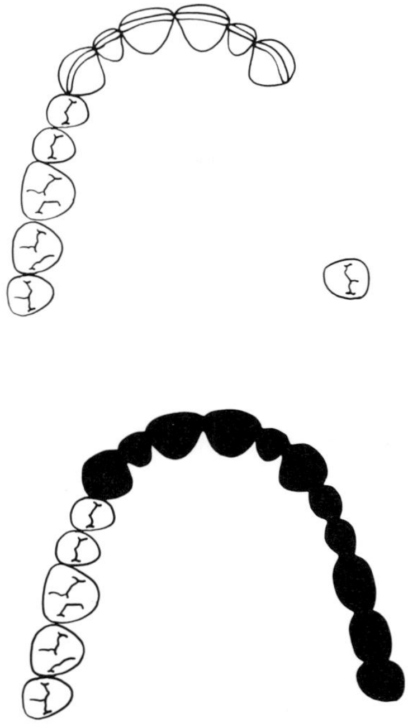

Fig. 9.9. A fixed partial denture to replace such a large tooth loss should include the anterior teeth as abutments to provide an element of cross-arch bracing against lateral loads. Six anteriors would only be used if they already had restorations that required replacement, but at least the left central lateral and canine should be used.

little or no load since the periodontium is much less compressible than the mucosa. The idea of 'overloading' teeth in a vertical direction may be more theoretical than real, as the load is likely to be limited by the ability of the periodontium to resist it. If the load exceeds a certain threshold, it is reasonable to suppose that the muscle activity will be diminished. Nevertheless, few would be prepared to place fixed partial dentures between canines and third molars and, if a fixed partial denture was contemplated, we would feel happier if all the anterior teeth were crowned to provide the necessary support (*Fig.* 9.9) and bracing against lateral loads. This extensive coverage would only be used if they already had restorations that required replacement. That indeed is the best design for the patient as it occupies only the denture space and leaves the palate uncovered, but it is obviously expensive and time-consuming to make an 11-unit bridge and the patient might object to having so many teeth prepared.

An alternative is to make a cast alloy removable partial denture. The properties of metal alloys make it possible to make many different designs. However, the general principle is to achieve maximum support for both vertical and lateral loads and to keep the anterior part of the palate free of connectors so as to improve the comfort of the patient and the health of the periodontium. A split bar

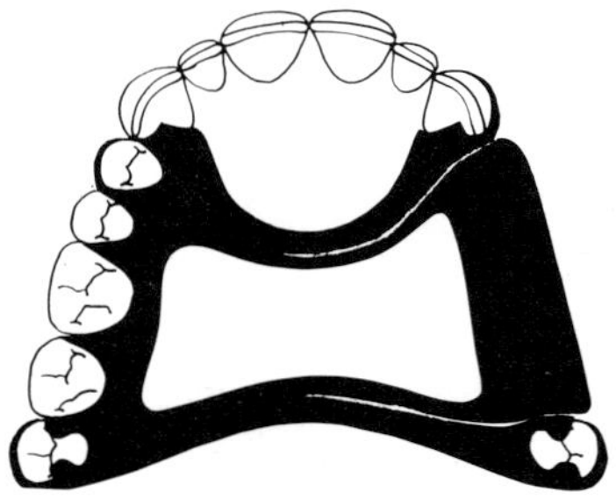

Fig. 9.10. A split bar stress-broken design divides the load between the teeth and the mucosa (*see also Fig.* 8.11).

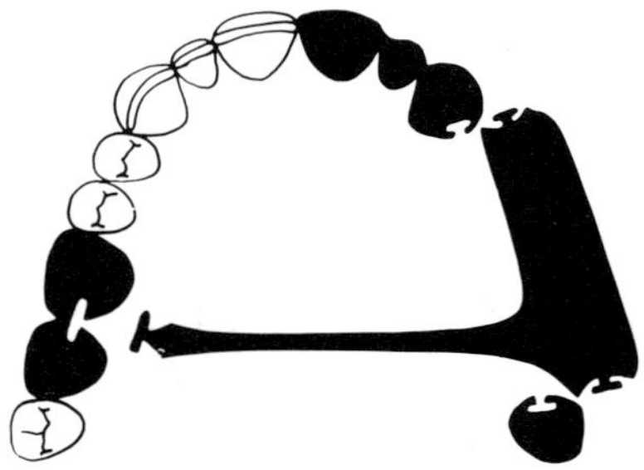

Fig. 9.11. A complex partial denture, with some fixed parts and some removable parts retained by precision attachments, provides a good solution to the design problem.

stress-broken design (*Fig.* 9.10) divides the load between the teeth and the mucosa and in this respect fulfils many of the criteria required, but the patient's tongue is likely to fiddle with the anterior bar. This design has already been discussed in Chapter 8 (*see Fig.* 8.11).

A complex partial denture (*Fig.* 9.11) provides a very good solution to the design problem posed by this case. Three anterior teeth are crowned to give the anterior tooth support and full veneer crowns are placed on the third molar on the left and on the first and second molars on the right. Flexible precision retainers on the canines and molars provide support and retention for the removable part of the complex partial denture, which replaces lost soft tissue. Cross-arch bracing provided by the palatal bar on the removable part of the denture is more efficient than that provided by the anterior teeth on a fixed restoration. In addition, the removable part makes it easier to remove plaque from the abutment teeth. The discussion of alternative designs for this case on a simple two-dimensional view of the arch does not take into account the many other factors that operate when designing a partial denture, but we hope that it gives an insight into at least some of the factors that must be considered.

We will now discuss alternative denture designs for a patient with mandibular second premolars and first molars missing (*Fig.* 9.12). Let us assume that the maxillary arch is intact and the oral hygiene is good. It seems clear that fixed partial dentures (bridges) are best for restoring function without encroaching beyond the denture space. This treatment involves the preparation of at least four (or, more likely, six) abutment teeth. There may be good reasons in some cases for considering simpler designs. At the bottom end of the spectrum is an all-acrylic mucosa-borne design with the connector in the form of a lingual plate. This is a destructive and inefficient denture because of the support deficit and the small area of coverage by the saddles. The denture may be made less damaging by using a lingual bar connector, but the clasped teeth are more likely to be traumatised because there is no bracing of the denture around the anterior teeth. The first premolars and second molars should be used to support the saddles because the saddle areas between these teeth are small and mucosal support is inefficient. Occlusal rests placed mesially on the premolars and molars must be made of cast alloy in order to be accurate and strong. Thus little extra work would be required to cast the whole denture base in cobalt-chromium alloy (*Fig.* 9.13). The rests can then be made to fit accurately and can be suitably placed on the abutment teeth. Connectors with little bulk but of sufficient rigidity can also be made. Cast or wrought clasps give adequate retention for this denture. Unfortunately such a design is not completely streamlined, as there are many extra-anatomical components.

A complex partial denture (*Fig.* 9.14) with full veneer crowns and internal channel attachments for retention and support provides better streamlining than the cobalt-chromium alloy denture in *Fig.* 9.13, but the cost and technical requirements are greater than those

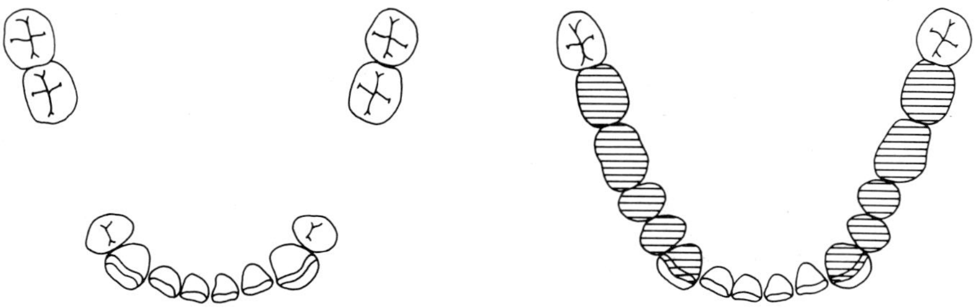

Fig. 9.12. Where mandibular second premolars and first molars are missing, fixed partial dentures (bridges) provide the best restoration. A suitable removable partial denture is illustrated in *Fig.* 9.13.

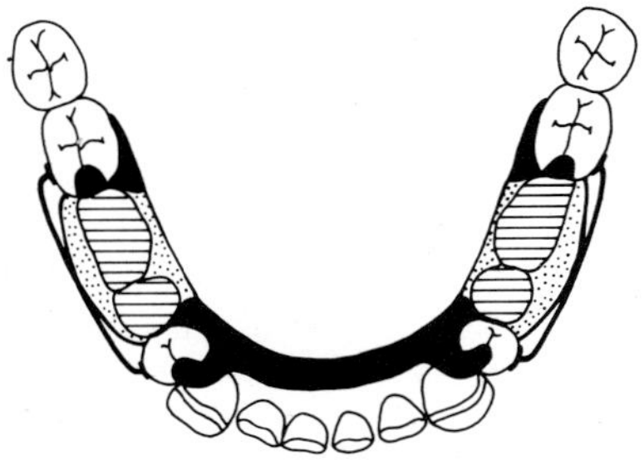

Fig. 9.13. The cast occlusal rests on this cobalt-chromium alloy base make the denture tooth-borne. Retention is provided by gingivally-approaching clasps. The lingual bar connector avoids the gingival margins of the natural teeth. This is a hygienic and efficient removable partial denture and would be our second choice in this case.

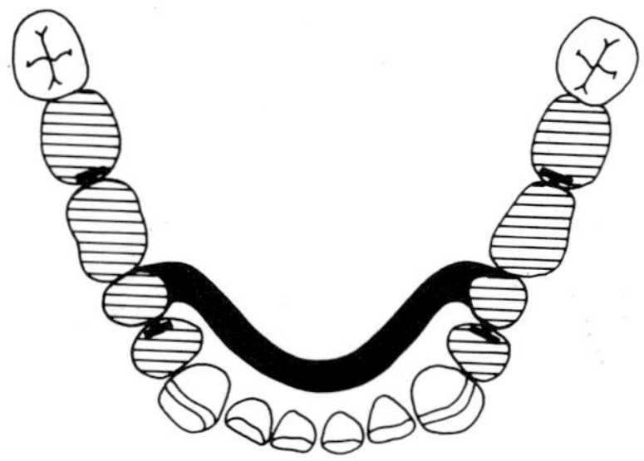

Fig. 9.14. A complex partial denture with internal channel attachments in full veneer crowns is more streamlined than the cobalt-chromium alloy denture in *Fig.* 9.13. The bar of the complex denture provides cross-arch bracing, but is an extra-anatomical encumbrance and, as the denture requires much tooth preparation, technical skill and additional expense, it has no advantage over fixed bridges.

necessary for fixed bridges and there is no advantage to the patient.

General Procedure for designing and making Partial Dentures

Every patient who is about to have a partial denture should be free of caries. The oral hygiene must be good and there must be no uncontrolled periodontal disease. There are two groups of partially edentulous patients:

1. Those who have sufficient teeth to indicate the stable intercuspal position of occlusion.

2. Those with so many teeth missing that the intercuspal position of occlusion is not indicated.

The procedure for making partial dentures varies a little for the two groups, and from one patient to another, but is generally as follows:

First Clinical Stage

Select upper and lower impression trays. In all cases the upper tray should be adapted by an addition of impression compound at the junction of the hard and soft palates, and elsewhere if necessary (for example, free-end saddle areas). Make first impressions in alginate and make a facebow record. The stem of the facebow fork should be on the right of the patient, but the orbital rod (indicating the anterior reference mark of the Frankfurt plane) may be dispensed with as it provides little added accuracy to the mounting.

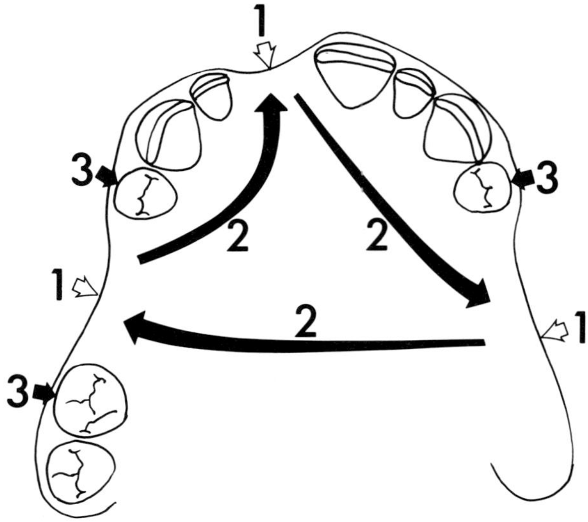

Fig. 9.15. The three main steps in designing: **1**, Plan the support. **2**, Plan the connectors. **3**, Plan the retention.

When a sufficient number of teeth is present, record the intercuspal position with a thin, D-shaped wafer of wax adapted to the maxillary teeth, making sure that the natural teeth perforate it and contact each other. If necessary the wafer may be reinforced with registration paste. When many teeth are missing, register the retruded contact position with wax or plaster with as much accuracy as possible. If wax is used, cool it in the mouth with a blast of air or a jet of cold water. Make sure the wax occlusal record does not become distorted. In some cases a retruded contact position record cannot be made and registration must be delayed until record blocks have been made on the casts.

First Laboratory Stage

1. Box and pour the impressions in dental stone. Survey the casts in relation to the path of displacement (black carbon) and in relation to the path of insertion and removal (red marker).

2. Make an individual acrylic tray (*see Figs.* 2.13, 2.14).

3. Mount the upper cast on an articulator by means of the facebow and, when the orbital rod has not been used, adjust the occlusal plane to lie at approximately 10° to the horizontal. Mount the lower cast with the occlusal record.

4. Make record blocks when there are insufficient teeth to indicate the retruded contact position.

Before the Second Clinical Stage

Examine the occlusion in the intercuspal and eccentric positions and decide what occlusal (or other) modifications may be necessary (*see* Chapter 1 and Appendix II) before proceeding with the three main steps in designing the denture (*Fig.* 9.15).

1. *Plan the Support of the Denture* (*see* Chapters 3, 4 and Appendix II)

Decide the position and outline of occlusal and incisal rests and outline the saddles. In taking this first step you decide which oral structures will support the forces of mastication on the denture. Later, when the retention is planned, check the occlusal rest positions to ensure that they provide indirect retention. That is, they should resist rotation of the saddles, away from the mucosa, round the fulcrum axes through the clasp arm tips (*Fig.* 9.16).

2. *Plan the Saddle Connectors*

The principles governing the choice of connectors are discussed in Chapter 8. In general, like saddles should be connected rigidly and unlike saddles may be connected

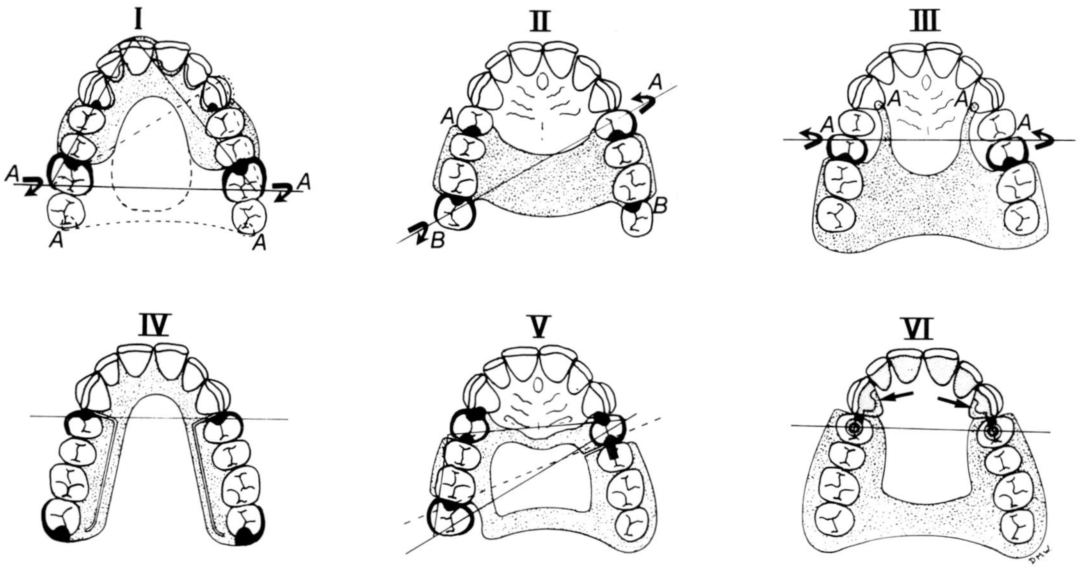

Fig. 9.16. Designs of removable partial upper dentures to illustrate various types of connectors and to show the placement of clasps and rests. **I, II, III,** Anterior, middle and posterior rigid saddle connectors. **IV, V, VI,** Stress-broken designs. *See* text for discussion.

flexibly. Some rigid and flexible connectors for removable partial upper dentures are shown in *Fig.* 9.16. Designs I, II and III are rigid anterior, middle and posterior palatal connectors. In the complex denture VI a rigid posterior connector joins the like mucosa-borne saddles, which are then connected flexibly by means of CEKA attachments to the tooth-borne parts of the prosthesis, comprising soldered porcelain-fused-to-gold crowns on the central and lateral incisors and canine teeth on both sides. In designs IV and V split plates provide flexible connectors to the mucosa-borne saddles. Various rigid connectors for mandibular dentures with bilateral free-end saddles are shown in *Fig.* 9.17. 'A' is a conventional lingual bar. It is hygienic and reasonably comfortable, but could be improved by thinning its upper edge to make its cross-section more pear-shaped. 'B' is a sublingual bar which is very comfortable if correctly formed and positioned, but can be very damaging to the tissues if placed too low. Neither 'A' nor 'B' provides indirect retention for the appliance. 'C' is a continuous clasp (Kennedy bar) in conjunction with a lingual bar. This provides indirect retention, but is uncomfortable for the patient. 'D', a thin lingual plate, provides indirect retention and is comfortable for the patient but, by covering the gingival margins, it is unhygienic. 'E', a lingual plate that lies only on the teeth and avoids the gingival margins, is hygienic and provides indirect retention, but because it is much narrower than the conventional lingual plate ('D') it must be made thicker to give it sufficient strength. The thickness and position of this plate may make it uncomfortable for some patients. 'F', a labial bar, is used where lingual undercuts or lingually inclined teeth preclude the use of a lingual bar. It is hygienic, but as a rule it is not as easily tolerated as a lingual bar. It does not provide indirect retention. 'G': Thin buccal and lingual bars are sometimes used in mucosa-borne dentures, but although thin they are no more comfortable than lingual or sublingual bars. 'H': The swing-lock system usually combines a thin lingual plate or a continuous clasp and lingual bar as a connector. The swing-lock retainer in the labial sulcus tends to trap food and is uncomfortable for the patient. Thus, the comfort and hygiene rating for this appliance

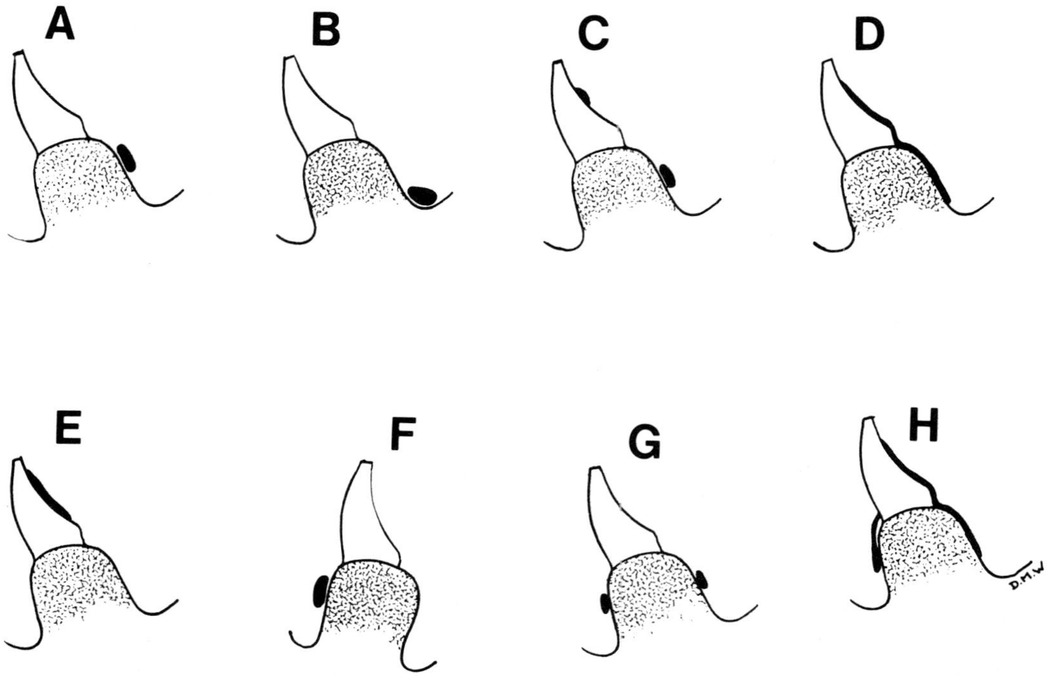

Fig. 9.17. Sections of various types of rigid connectors for mandibular dentures with bilateral free-end saddles. **A**, Lingual bar. **B**, Sublingual bar. **C**, Continuous clasp and lingual bar. **D**, Lingual plate covering gingival margins. **E**, Lingual plate on teeth only. **F**, Labial bar. **G**, Labial and lingual bars. **H**, Lingual plate and swing-lock retainer.

is usually low, but this may be offset by the improved retention. It is obviously important to assess both the patient's oral hygiene and ability to tolerate an appliance before deciding which connector to use. In general, lingual or sublingual bars are best, but provision for indirect retention must be made by means of suitably placed occlusal rests or Cummer arms.

3. *Plan the Retention*

The type and positions of retainers must be decided. If precision retainers are to be used they should provide stress-breaking if placed at the ends of mucosa-borne saddles (*Fig.* 9.16, VI), but may be rigid if used for retaining tooth-borne dentures. In general, one retainer on each side of the mouth is sufficient to retain a tooth-borne denture provided the line joining them bisects the denture. The occlusal rests then resist rotation of the saddles away from the mucosa round the axis through the retainers. In *Fig.* 9.16,II, rotation in the direction of arrow 'A' is resisted by occlusal rest 'A' and, similarly, rotation in the direction 'B' is resisted by rest 'B'. The retention systems shown in *Fig.* 9.16, III and VI would be unsatisfactory without the provision of indirect retainers to stop rotation about the axis through the direct retainers. In III rotation in the direction of the arrows 'A' is resisted by the Cummer arms 'A.A' resting on the canines. In VI the short extensions of the denture (arrowed) which lie in prepared recesses in the canines provide indirect retention and bracing for the denture. The retention system in *Fig.* 9.16, I is essentially triangular. The centre of the triangle lies about the middle of the denture. The labial flange of the saddle carrying the right central incisor enters the mesiolabial undercuts on the abutment teeth and provides retention against forces in the common path of displacement. Thus the clasps which form the other corners of the triangle can be kept out of sight on the molars. In this way the appearance is not marred. However, should there be no appropriate undercuts on the left central or right lateral incisors, it would be necessary to clasp the left canine to preserve the triangular retentive system. This might spoil the appearance. A spring-loaded retainer (e.g. Ipsoclip) on the distal surface of the canine might be used instead. Another option would be to extend the denture to form a 'ring' design and place occlusal rests at 'A.A' to resist rotation in the direction of the arrows round the clasp axis and thus provide indirect retention for the anterior part of the denture. This option has little to recommend it as it makes the denture unnecessarily cumbersome.

Thus, wherever possible, retention by extra-coronal clasps should be assisted by rigid parts of the denture base lying in undercuts in relation to the common path of displacement. Where the black and red survey lines are at different positions, flexible tips of clasp arms should be in appropriate undercuts in relation to both lines.

Where designs incorporate flexible saddle connectors, three or even four retainers are necessary to hold the tooth-borne parts of the dentures in position when the mucosa-borne saddles are loaded and the connectors bend. A four-clasp system is used in *Fig.* 9.16, IV. When the anterior teeth are used for biting, the denture tends to rotate towards the mucosa round an axis through the occlusal rests on the premolars. This rotation is prevented by the clasps on the second molars which provide 'indirect support', but the direct support comes partly from the mucosa of the anterior saddle and partly from the first premolars.

In V a three-clasp system is used. When the mucosa-borne saddle on the left is loaded, the L-shaped posterior connector bends. The fin projecting from the clasp on the left premolar lies in the slot in the artificial premolar and allows vertical movement of the saddle. On eating, the denture would tend to rock towards the mucosa round an axis (interrupted line) through the occlusal rests nearest the mucosa-borne saddle. This is prevented by the clasp on the right first premolar which provides 'indirect support'. Rotation of the free-end saddle away from the mucosa takes place through the axis of the clasp arm tips nearest the saddle (solid line) and is resisted by the occlusal rests on the right canine and premolar, which provide indirect retention. The effectiveness of the indirect retention depends chiefly on the direct retention of the clasps, but also on the distance of the occlusal rest from the axis of rotation. Thus, although the occlusal rest positions are decided early in the designing procedure, these positions should be reviewed later when indirect retention is being looked at in the overall assessment of the design.

When the planning is completed the exact design is drawn on the laboratory card and the material to be used is recorded, together with the dimensions and types of the various components (clasps, rests and connectors). In cases in which the occlusion is not indicated, the design should only be tentative until the occlusal relationship has been verified.

Second Clinlcal Stage

1. Rehabilitation of the mucosa, occlusal surface correction, restorations, guide plane and rest seat preparations must be completed before the master impressions are made.

2. Make master impressions in alginate or other appropriate elastic material and have them poured as soon as possible.

3. Make an accurate occlusal record in the stabilized intercuspal position, or when this is not indicated, register the jaw relationship in the retruded contact position with the record blocks, which must have rigid bases.

4. Make a facebow registration.

5. Note the shade and mould and any unusual characteristic of the teeth. Complete the instructions on the laboratory card.

6. In those cases where the design has only been tentative up to this stage, mount the primary casts on the articulator by means of record blocks in the retruded contact position before confirming the design.

Second Laboratory Stage

1. Mix dental stone under vacuum and vibrate it into the master impressions. When set, base the casts with plaster. Treat the casts with the utmost care as they must not be rubbed or damaged in any way.

2. Survey and prepare the master casts. Block out the undercuts that are not required

for retention in relation to the path of insertion and removal. Prepare shelves round the abutment teeth to indicate the positions of the clasp arms. Relieve the ridge areas that will lie under the cast alloy framework. Prepare shallow border seal lines.

3. Duplicate the master casts in refractory material.

4. When the occlusion is indicated, mount the master casts on an articulator by means of the facebow and occlusal record. Make sure remounting keys have been cut on the bases of the casts. Proceed with making the cast alloy base.

5. When the occlusion is not indicated, make record blocks on the master casts with the relieving tin foil attached to the blocks. When a shellac base (or other hard material) is used, great care is necessary to avoid the slightest abrasion or damage to the stone surface of the casts.

Third Clinical Stage

The trial of the cast alloy base is made in the mouth, usually without teeth added. We prefer to verify the accuracy of the base with indicating paste without the encumbrance of teeth and wax. The teeth are then added at the chairside or in the laboratory and checked in the mouth for position, appearance and occlusion. If the whole is satisfactory, decide the colour and type of matrix acrylic and instruct the laboratory to finish the denture. If the occlusion is not indicated, register the jaw relationship in the retruded contact position. Mount the upper cast on an articulator by means of a facebow and use the record block to mount the lower cast. Confirm the accuracy of your articulator mounting and at the patient's next visit verify the cast alloy base as above.

Subsequent Stages

The prepared master casts, which have been accurately blocked out with wax around the abutment teeth and soft tissues, should now be duplicated in artificial stone. Use the duplicate casts for processing the dentures. After deflasking and polishing, fit the dentures to the master casts on the articulator. Correct any minor faults in the occlusion that may have arisen during processing before delivery of the dentures on the articulator to the chairside.

It should be unnecessary to have to make any adjustments or alterations at the chairside, although the various time lapses between recording master impressions, verifying occlusal relationships, checking alloy bases in the mouth, and finishing the dentures, may readily account for minor errors due to small but uncontrollable changes in the mouth. In addition to a meticulous clinical and laboratory technique, the time between the start and completion of a partial denture should therefore be as short as possible.

Wide labial flanges may be used when replacing anterior teeth and adjacent lost tissue. Fit these flanges most carefully in the mouth to obtain the best appearance. Modify the edges of the flanges with carborundum stones at the chairside and lightly polish them before final delivery to the patient.

At this point instruct the patient in the care of the denture and re-emphasize the importance of oral hygiene. Make a recall appointment for one week ahead.

Chapter 10

Partial dentures with free-end saddles

In the previous chapter we have discussed alternative designs for maxillary and mandibular partial dentures with bounded saddles and have sketched the general procedure for designing and making them. In this and the following chapters we discuss in more detail the designs of various kinds of dentures.

We may consider partial dentures plus the natural teeth as one hard object, and the alveolar bone and residual ridges as a second hard object, and between these two hard objects there is a continuous layer of soft tissue, comprising the mucous membrane and the periodontal membrane (*Fig.* 10.1). One part of this layer of soft tissue, the mucous membrane, is very much more compressible than the other part, the periodontal membrane. The comfort of the patient depends on how effectively the load is distributed through this soft-tissue layer. The average mucosa-borne denture is reasonably comfortable because the loads are limited to the thick part of the soft-tissue layer, and the average tooth-borne denture is also comfortable because the loads are limited to the thin part of the soft-tissue layer (the periodontium). It is when the denture is both mucosa-borne and tooth-borne that trouble starts. If the abutment teeth hurt, it is because the periodontium is being traumatised by torsional and lateral forces transmitted to them through the denture. If the mucosa is painful, it is usually because loads shared with the teeth are concentrated on comparatively small areas of mucosa because of the difference in compressibility of periodontium and mucosa.

Dentures for saddle areas that have abutment teeth at only one end are called free-end saddle dentures or distal extension dentures. Kennedy (1928) classified them as Class I dentures when the saddles were bilateral and Class II when the saddle was unilateral. These dentures present special design problems because of the different properties of tooth support and mucosa support. A tooth can be intruded into its alveolus by about 20 μm, whereas the mucosa

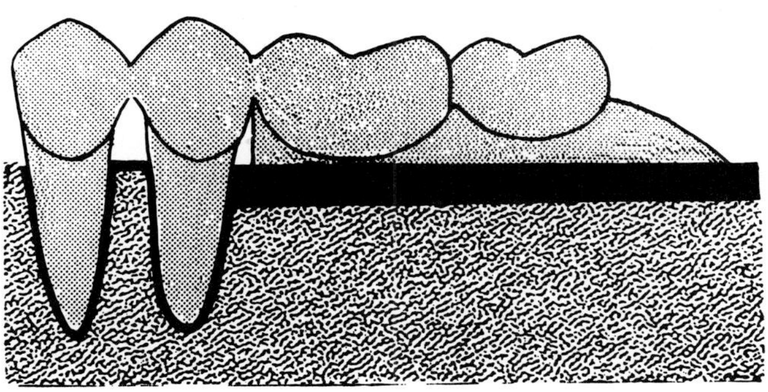

Fig. 10.1. The periodontal membrane and mucoperiosteum represent a continuous layer (black) of soft tissue of unequal compressibility lying between two hard objects: the alveolar bone on one side and the teeth and partial denture on the other. The comfort of the patient depends on how effectively the masticatory loads are distributed in this soft-tissue layer.

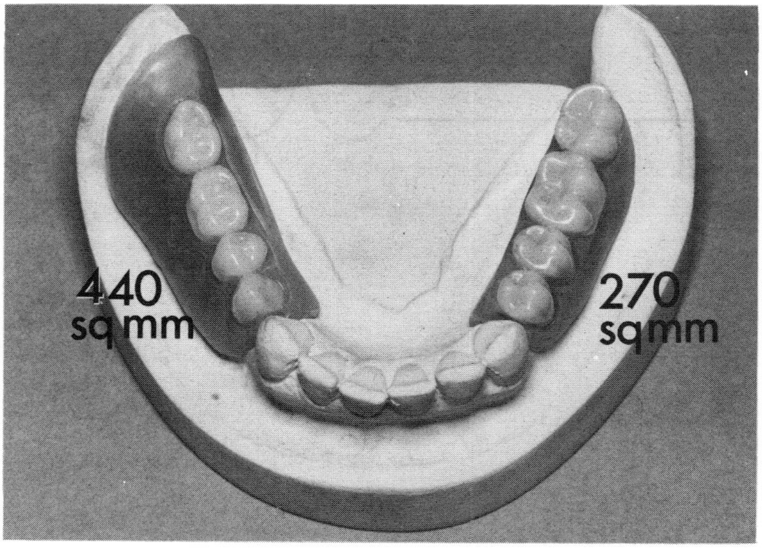

Fig. 10.2. Correctly extended and under-extended saddles. A 4-kg load on the saddle on the patient's right side would load the mucosa 9 g/sq mm, but a similar load of 4 kg on the under-extended saddle would be transmitted to the mucosa as 15 g/sq mm. Note that the narrower teeth on the larger saddle on the patient's right side reduce the masticatory load.

can be displaced as much as 500 μm (*see Fig.* 3.4). The support deficit resulting from the loss of the molar and premolar teeth also causes difficulties in designing free-end saddle dentures. When teeth are lost, the supporting periodontal membrane is also lost and the surface area of mucosa that remains amounts to about 25 per cent of the original area of periodontium. Thus, in all mandibular free-end saddles there is a support deficit of about 75 per cent (*see Table* 3.2).

The supporting tissues that remain are of two distinct types. Anteriorly, the teeth and periodontal tissues may be considered rigid and immovable unless subjected to abnormal forces. Posteriorly, on each side the free-end saddle areas are covered by mucosa of varying thickness and of varying compressibility. Thus, any part of the denture resting on the saddle area moves when subjected to load.

When designing a free-end saddle denture it must first be decided whether the denture is going to be a rigid rocker or if the connectors between the tooth-borne and mucosa-borne parts are to be sufficiently flexible to enable the tooth-borne part to remain in position while the saddles sink. The decision is chiefly influenced by the number of the remaining teeth and their health. If only the six lower anterior teeth remain and are of poor prognosis, it might be decided to make a very simple mucosa-borne denture. If the patient has no maxillary teeth, this denture might act as a temporary training appliance before the patient is rendered edentulous, but if it is possible to retain one or two teeth and to place an overdenture, this is generally a more satisfactory solution. Overdentures are further discussed in Chapter 14.

One of the principles in saddle design is to cover as large an area as possible. In *Fig.* 10.2 one saddle is under-extended and covers only 270 sq mm; the other saddle is correctly extended and covers an area of 440 sq mm. If equal loads of 4 kg are applied to both these saddles, the mucosa under the correctly extended saddle is subjected to less load per unit area (9 g/sq mm) than the mucosa under the under-extended saddle (15 g/sq mm). Narrow teeth on the correctly extended saddle penetrate the food more easily than the broad teeth on the under-extended saddle and thus reduce the load on the underlying mucosa during mastication. An additional benefit from using narrow teeth is that the tongue and cheek can control the saddle more easily than

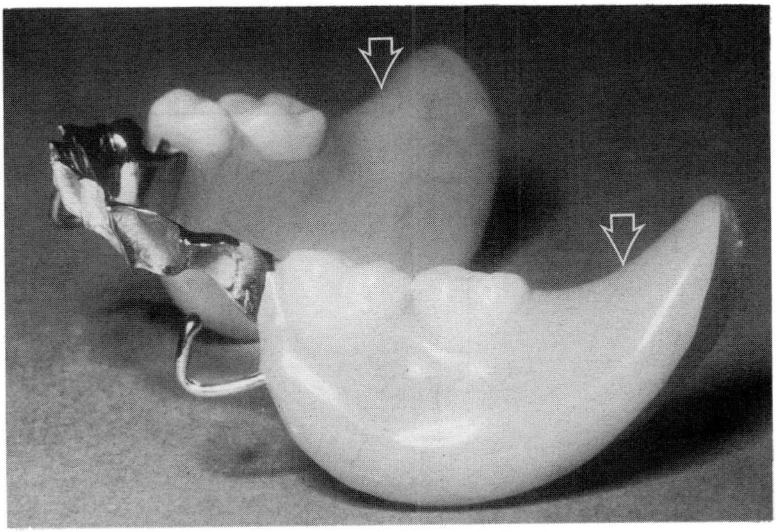

Fig. 10.3. Posterior shelves (*arrows*) provide more space for the tongue and help tongue and cheek to control the denture. In addition, the absence of artificial teeth opposite the steeply sloping parts of the residual ridge reduces displacing forces during mastication.

when the teeth are broad. A posterior shelf behind the last molar (*Fig.* 10.3) is a further aid to control of the denture in the mouth, because the shelf enables the tongue to spread on to the saddle. This is similar to the design of complete lower dentures (Watt and MacGregor, 1976). The advantages of using narrow teeth on mucosa-borne saddles outweigh the disadvantages. However, on tooth-borne bounded saddles the use of natural-sized teeth has much to recommend it (*see* discussion in Chapter 9).

Much has been written about free-end saddle dentures (MacGregor, 1960; Hekneby, 1969; Fish, 1970; Osborne and Lammie, 1974; Zarb et al., 1978; Johnson and Stratton, 1980; Henderson and Steffel, 1981; Taylor et al., 1982; Lofberg et al., 1982; Matsumoto, 1984). The majority think that a rigid connector is desirable between the tooth-borne part and the mucosa-borne part, since it simplifies the design. Some believe that it is possible to compress the mucosa sufficiently to give a relatively stable denture, but the weight of evidence is in favour of the contrary view that in time a rigid tooth-and-mucosa-borne denture rocks round a fulcrum axis through the occlusal rests nearest the saddles (Watt et al., 1958; Wills and Manderson, 1977; Picton and Wills, 1978; Kydd and Daly, 1982).

Thus, there are two main types of saddle connectors used in these designs: rigid and flexible. The flexibility can be achieved by the inherent property of the material or by mechanical stress-breakers, such as hinged joints between the tooth-borne and mucosa-borne parts. Alternatively, disjunct dentures can be designed with complete disjunction between the tooth-borne and mucosa-borne parts of the dentures (*see* Chapter 11).

Rigid Designs

Two simple rigid designs for bilateral free-end dentures are shown in *Fig.* 10.4. These designs are minimal and unsatisfactory. Both are entirely mucosa-borne and the remaining natural teeth play no part in the support of the dentures. Rigid connectors are used in both cases. In one the saddles are connected by a lingual bar and there is nothing to stop backward movement of the denture when the mandible is moved forwards, or to stop forward movement when the mandible is moved backwards. The denture also pivots and moves from side to side with nothing to resist

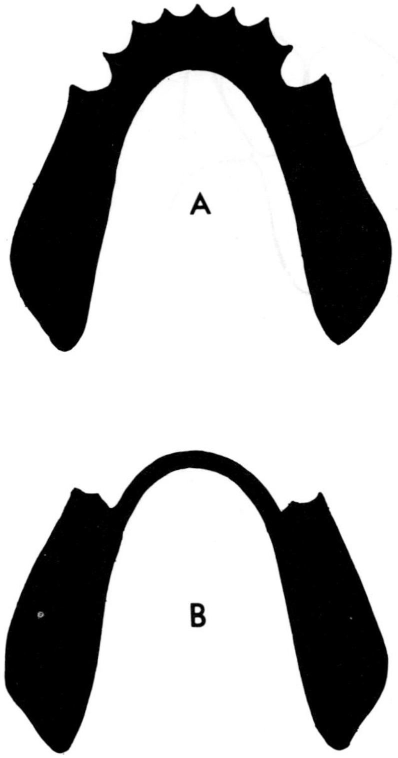

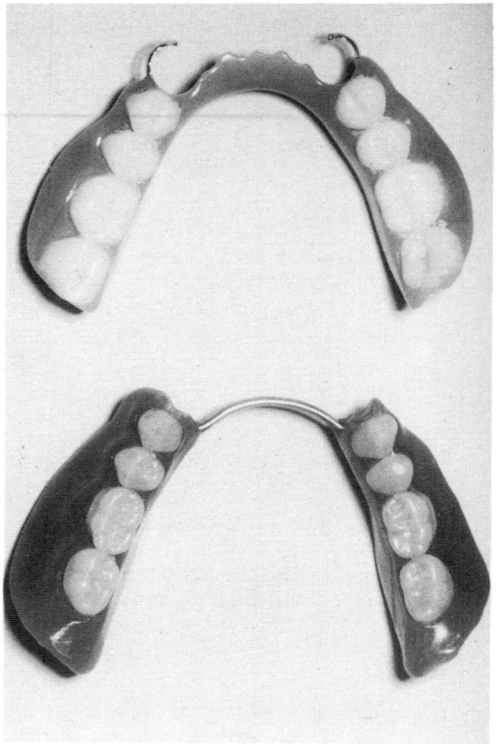

Fig. 10.4. Silhouettes and photographs of simple designs for free-end saddle lower dentures. These designs are *unsatisfactory* and are discussed in the text. **A**, All acrylic. **B**, Acrylic with lingual bar.

this movement except the residual alveolar ridge, which is damaged by it. In the other design in *Fig.* 10.4 the saddles are connected by a lingual plate made of acrylic. This denture does not move as much as the lingual bar denture because the acrylic lingual plate contacts the teeth, but this plate damages the gingival margins and mucosa. Simple clasps made of 0·8 or 0·9 mm stainless steel, placed on the canines, stop the backward movement of the denture when the mandible moves forwards.

It is a popular misconception that the acrylic on the lingual surfaces of the standing teeth contributes some support for vertical loads (*Fig.* II.1). The lingual surfaces of the lower incisors are almost vertical and tooth support cannot be obtained by this means when clasps are absent. This is further discussed in Appendix II. The acrylic connector behind the incisors provides some indirect retention if clasps are present, and some bracing against lateral forces, but it usually damages the gingivae in the process. The saddles of these dentures sink into the mucosa after a short time and play no part in accepting clenched loads against the opposing teeth, although they may assist in mastication. The main criticism is that they damage the remaining hard and soft tissues and this is sufficient reason to avoid these designs. The damage is particularly severe if the patient's oral hygiene is poor. More acceptable designs for free-end saddle lower dentures are shown in *Fig.* 10.9 and are discussed in detail later.

When the occlusal rests are placed mesially on the premolars and the clasp arms engage the distal undercuts, the denture can rock towards the mucosa, freely round the fulcrum axis passing through the occlusal rests. This puts minimum stress on the abutment teeth. When both premolars are present on each side, occlusal rests may be placed between the

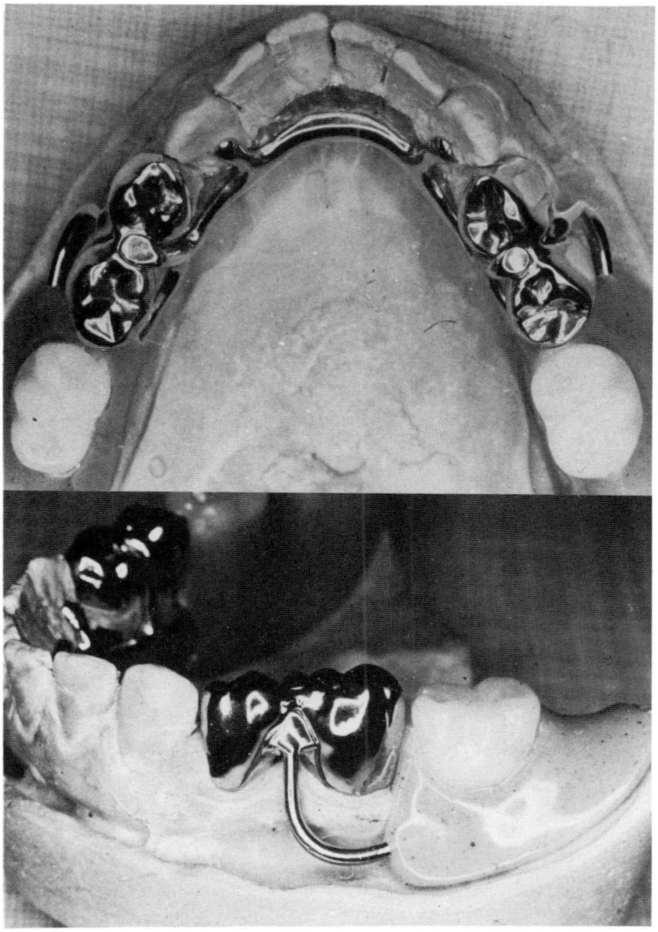

Fig. 10.5. Full veneer crowns soldered together on the premolars provide double abutments for this partial denture. The occlusal rests are in the occlusal embrasures and the clasp arm tips in the buccal embrasures near the fulcrum axis of the denture. Thus the stresses on the teeth are minimized. This denture continues to give good service after 15 years.

premolars. The retention is provided by gingivally-approaching clasp arms engaging buccal undercuts in the same coronal plane as the rests (*Fig.* 10.5). Thus, when the partial denture rotates towards the tissues, the axis of rotation through the occlusal rests is near the tips of the clasp arms. This minimizes the stresses on the teeth, particularly if soldered crowns are placed on them to provide strong double abutments. This design is especially useful when the form of the anterior natural teeth is such that posterior displacement of the denture base is difficult to control. Under these circumstances clasp arms that engage distal undercuts are useless, as they lose contact with the teeth when the denture moves distally.

When the saddles are loaded the movement of lingual bars is closely related to the position of the occlusal rests on the abutment teeth. In bilateral free-end saddles rotation of the denture is usually round an axis through the occlusal rests (*Fig.* 10.6). If the occlusal rests are on the distal marginal ridges of the second premolars, movement of the saddles towards the mucosa makes the lingual bar rise on an arc with its centre at the occlusal rests. When the occlusal rests are placed on the canines or

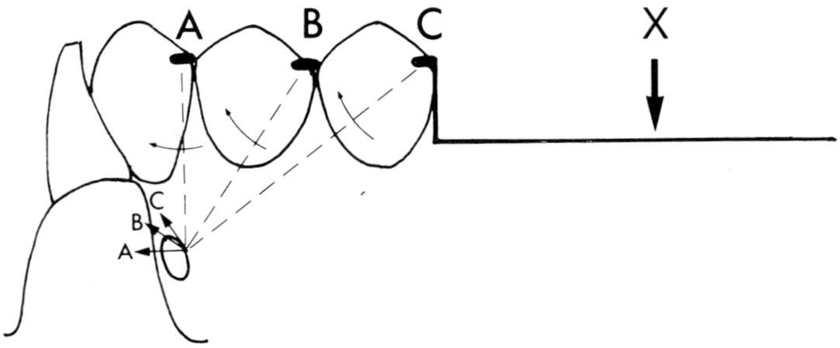

Fig. 10.6. Diagram to illustrate how the position of an occlusal rest on a free-end saddle partial lower denture affects the movement of the lingual bar when the saddle is loaded. When the occlusal rest is at 'A', the lingual bar moves forwards in the direction shown by the arrow marked 'A'. An occlusal rest at 'B' causes the movement of the bar to be forwards and upwards. At 'C' the lingual bar may move more or less parallel to the lingual mucosal surface. The movement of the bar depends on the compressibility of the tissues of the free-end saddle and the proportion of AA to AX, BB to BX, and CC to CX. Thus the smallest movement is the forward one at 'A' and the largest is the upward movenent at 'C'.

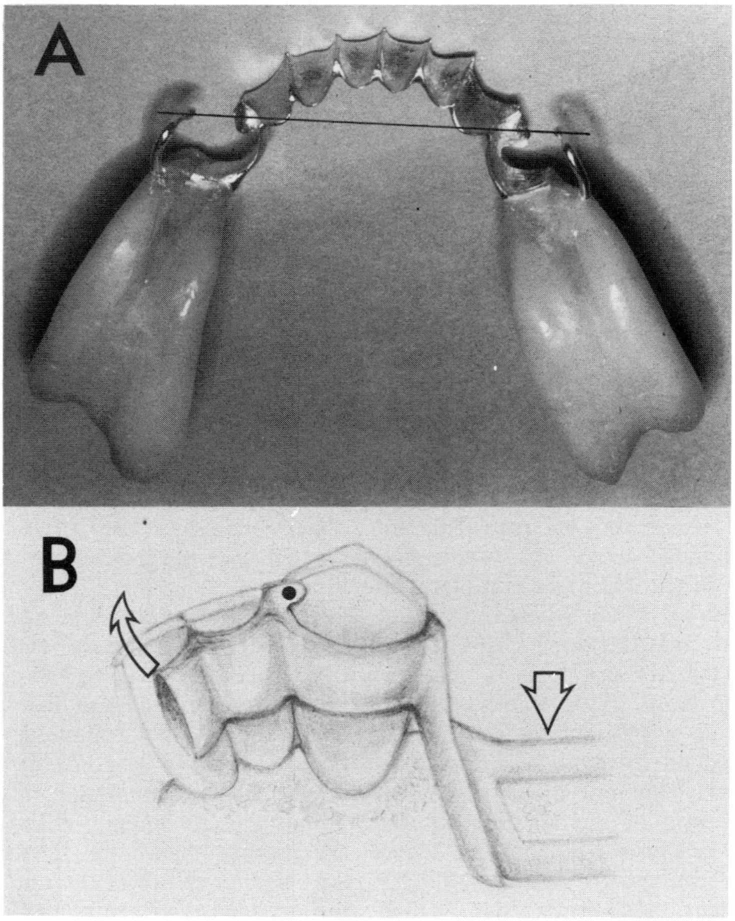

on the mesial marginal ridges of the first premolars, the movement of the lingual bar is forwards towards the lingual gingival tissues when the saddles are loaded. The forward movement of the bar may be as much as half the downward movement of the saddle. Thus, for safety, a 0·5 mm spacer of foil or wax must be placed on the cast before the lingual bar is fabricated. If this is not done the tissues are traumatised by the lingual bar. The greater the vertical distance between occlusal rest and lingual bar, the greater the forward movement, and consequently the more relief is required.

Where only six lower front teeth remain, the occlusal rests are placed on the canine teeth. In these cases the fulcrum axis may be in front of the lingual bar, which then moves downwards and forwards when the saddles are loaded (*Fig.* 10.6) and adequate relief is essential. In some cases the dangers of lingual bar trauma can be avoided by making the primary connector a heavy continuous clasp or lingual plate that lies on the lingual surfaces of the anterior teeth, but does not cover the gingival margins. By bringing the connector nearer the fulcrum axis, this arrangement reduces the chance of trauma since it tends to rise on the lingual surfaces of the teeth when the saddles are loaded (*Fig.* 10.7).

A labial swinglock system may be used to improve the retention of distal extension dentures. *Fig.* 6.24 and 6.25 show the retentive system in detail. The labial bar swings from one side, rather like a door hinge, and clips into the other. The contact of the

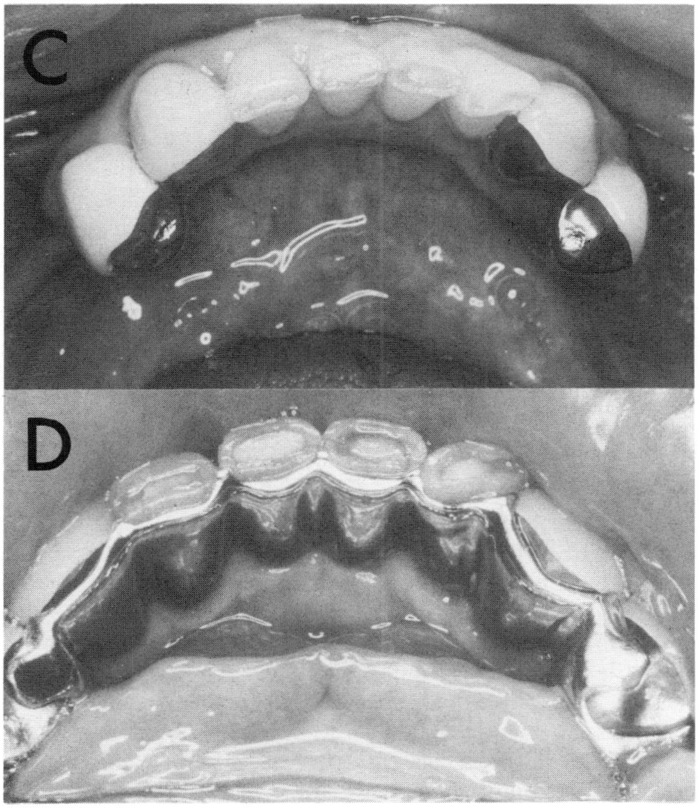

Fig. 10.7. **A**, A heavy continuous clasp should be used as a primary connector when occlusal rests are placed on or near the canines. Note that in this case the fulcrum axis through the occlusal rests lies close to the tips of the clasps. **B**, This arrangement brings the connector near the fulcrum axis and avoids trauma. **C**, Full veneer crowns on the abutment teeth. **D**, The denture in place.

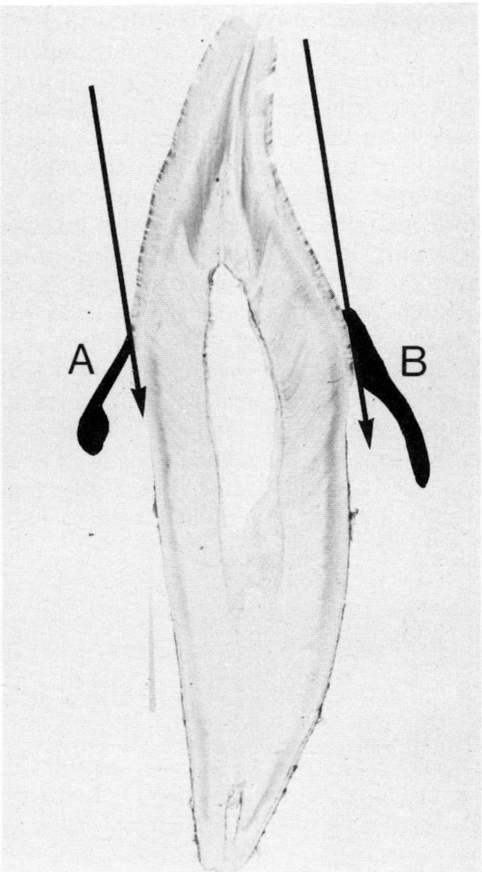

Fig. 10.8. Sagittal section through lower central incisor with diagrammatic section of badly designed swing-lock superimposed. If the labial spur (A) or the lingual plate (B) are not placed sufficiently high on the tooth, the tooth support of the appliance may be endangered and serious damage to the gingivae can occur.

denture against the teeth resists downward movement of the anterior part of the denture in most cases, but if the lingual plate and labial spurs are short and badly positioned, downward movement of the appliance may be possible (*Fig.* 10.8) and labial gingival trauma can occur when sticky food displaces the posterior saddles (Gomes et al., 1981).

In *Fig.* 10.9 are shown four different designs for alloy denture bases for patients who have lost all their posterior teeth, except for the first premolars, and have six lower anterior teeth still in position.

Design 'A' has a cobalt-chromium lingual plate with occlusal rests on the mesial marginal ridges of the first premolars. Gingivally-approaching embrasure clasps provide retention and are positioned as near as possible to the fulcrum axis of the denture. The criticism of this design is that it covers gingival margins and therefore does not promote good oral hygiene, but on the other hand the lingual plate is relatively easily tolerated by the patient as it presents a smooth surface to the tongue. Forward movements of the mandible may cause backward movements of the denture that are resisted by the embrasure clasps and the occlusal rests. Bracing against lateral forces is provided by the lingual plate that transmits these forces to the anterior teeth.

Design 'B' leaves the gingival margins uncovered as much as possible. The distally facing lingual arms of the occlusally-approaching clasps dip further into the undercuts when the saddles are loaded and the denture rotates round the fulcrum axis through the occlusal rests. Similarly, the gingivally-approaching arms of the De Van clasps (De Van, 1935) also move more deeply into the undercuts when the saddles are loaded, thus protecting the abutment teeth from tilting stresses. The two small arms resting on the lateral incisors provide indirect retention for the appliance. While this design leaves some gingival margins uncovered and in this respect may promote their health, its fussiness is likely to cause the patient discomfort as the tongue may fiddle with the lingual clasp arms and indirect retainers. In addition, the design might not provide enough resistance to distal movement which, if it takes place, makes the retainers ineffective. Further modification using the rest, plate and I-bar (RPI) system of retention (Kratochvil, 1963; Krol, 1973a, b; 1981; Kurrasch, 1983) does little to reduce the peripheral length of the base (*see Fig.* 6.20).

In design 'C' some of the fussiness has been eliminated by placing a single indirect retainer in the midline and by replacing the lingual arms of the clasps by a plate that provides reciprocation for the buccal arms. The buccal arms in this case have been made occlusally-approaching since they are less likely to trap food, but the appearance of the denture suffers

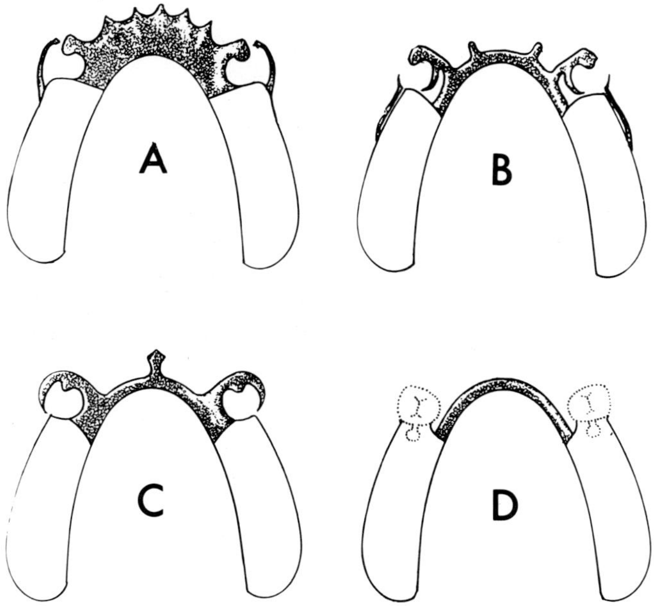

Fig. 10.9. Rigid designs for free-end saddle dentures. **A**, Mesial occlusal rests on the first premolars with gingivally-approaching clasp arms in the mesial embrasures. These arms engage the teeth in the fulcrum axis of the denture and cause little trauma. The thin lingual plate is easily tolerated by the patient, but may traumatise the gingival margins. **B**, The trauma to the gingival margins is reduced by this design, except where the two indirect retainers and minor connectors cross the margins. The clasp arm tips engage distal undercuts and thus allow free rotation of the denture without trauma to the teeth when the saddles are loaded. The lingual clasp arms might traumatise the tongue. **C**, Further simplification of the design reduces the chance of trauma to the tongue, but possibly increases the risk of gingival trauma. The clasps are likely to be ugly. **D**, The Dalbo attachments on full veneer crowns on the first premolars further streamline the design and improve the comfort, hygiene and appearance of the denture. The attachment prevents rotation of the denture away from the tissues and thus rests to provide indirect retention are unnecessary.

badly since these clasp arms are likely to be fairly obvious at the corners of the mouth. This design can easily be modified by substituting De Van clasp arms for the occlusally-approaching arms that have been drawn.

Design 'D' is a complex partial denture with Dalbo attachments fixed to crowns on the abutment teeth. As these attachments provide indirect retention, considerable streamlining of the removable denture base is possible and the only extra-anatomical part is the lingual bar, which can easily be tolerated. Although only single abutments are shown in this case, it is wiser to include the canine teeth as abutments since the tooth support from the appliance is distal to the first premolars and this puts unfavourable stresses on the abutment teeth. For this reason double abutments are better.

As already mentioned, in designs 'A', 'B' and 'C' it is necessary to relieve the lingual bars and plate connector as forward movement is likely to occur when the saddles are loaded. The amount of forward movement also depends on the shape of the dental arch. If it is of wide radius the rests are relatively further forward and it may be necessary to use a strong continuous clasp as a primary connector (*see Figs.* 10.3 and 10.7) to avoid trauma to the soft tissues.

Designing removable partial dentures for patients who have only six anterior teeth in the maxillary arch presents problems. Although retainers are placed on the canines, the posterior part of the denture drops as there is usually insufficient indirect retention, especially if the labial arch is flat. In order to improve the indirect retention the denture is sometimes

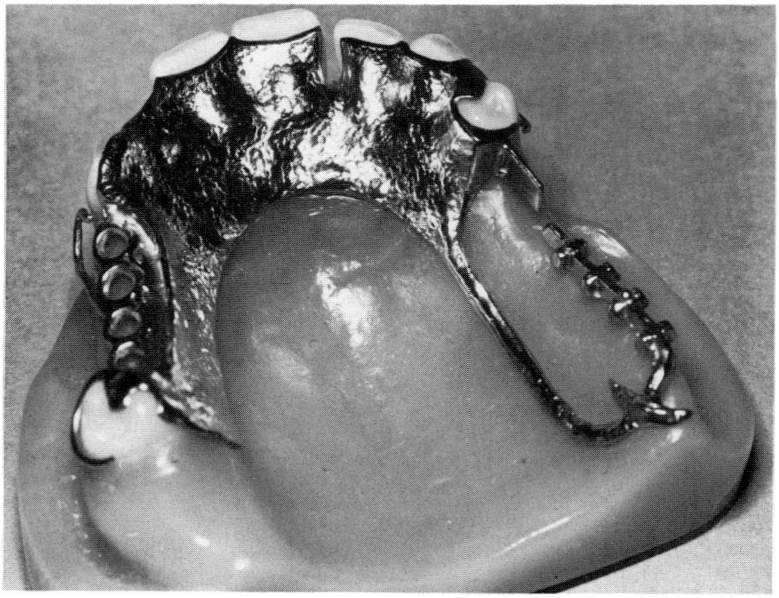

Fig. 10.10. This 'stress-broken' denture is likely to act like a rigid design because the palatal stress-breaking bar would have to bend edgewise and the tooth-borne part is likely to be displaced. However, when the distal end of the free-end saddle is fully compressed the anterior end of the saddle could be loaded by virtue of the torsional elasticity of the L-shaped stress-breaker.

made to cover the gingival margins of the anterior teeth. This causes gingivitis and is uncomfortable for the patient because the rugal area of the palate is covered. An alternative simple design leaves the anterior part of the palate uncovered, and the indirect retention for the posterior part is obtained by simple extension of the denture to the labial part of the gingivae (*see Figs.* 6.22 and 6.23). The effectiveness of this design can be further improved by cutting tiny horizontal notches on the distal surfaces of the canine teeth near their incisal edges. The notches should be designed so that the denture can spring into them, using the elasticity of the gingival tissue, but should not be so deep that the mucosa is traumatised. This simple design, made in acrylic, can be very effective, but some patients find that the labial extensions are uncomfortable.

Removable partial dentures made of cobalt-chromium alloys and retained by clasps are not always successful because the patients object to the clasps showing. Alternative designs that use prefabricated attachments to provide retention are usually more acceptable to patients.

Flexible Designs

The designs of flexible connectors that depend on the elasticity of the material have been fully discussed in Chapter 8 and the necessity of having adequate retainers on dentures with these connectors has been emphasized. For instance, the supposedly stress-broken denture in *Fig.* 8.12 acts in the same manner as a rigid design. It rocks round the fulcrum axis through the occlusal rests because the clasps are not sufficiently retentive to keep the tooth-borne part in place when a masticatory load falls on the saddles. The force required to bend the 'stress-breaker' is greater than the retentive force of the clasps. The fins projecting from the distal surfaces of the tooth-borne part prevent buccal twisting of the saddles when loaded, but are also an unnecessary embellishment of this design. A similar criticism can be levelled against the design shown in *Fig.* 10.10. The palatal stress-

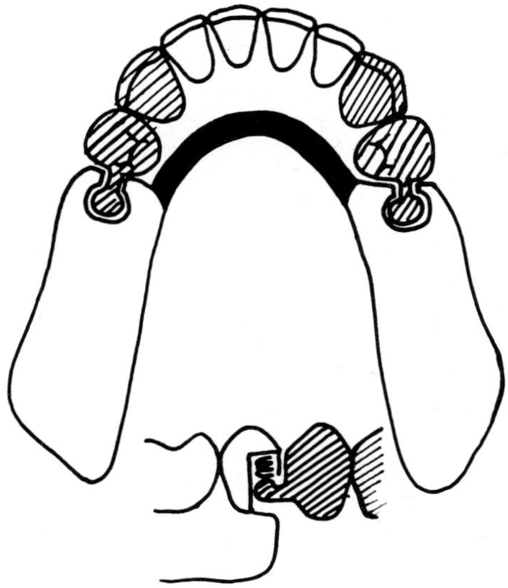

Fig. 10.11. Denture with male Dalbo attachments soldered to full veneer crowns providing double abutments for removable partial free-end saddle lower denture. By using these attachments the denture design can be streamlined, as indirect retainers on the anterior teeth are not required.

breaking bar is unlikely to bend when the saddle is loaded, although its L-shaped form may help to distribute the load at the anterior end of the free-end saddle when the posterior end is fully compressed. The fin projecting from the distal surface of the premolar prevents buccal rotation. The clasping in this case is slightly more favourable since the gingivally-approaching clasp arm on the right canine tooth and the clasp on the molar might prevent tilting of the appliance. Stress-broken designs that depend upon the elasticity of the material are generally not satisfactory because extracting forces are placed on the clasped teeth and this in itself is undesirable. Mechanical stress-breakers do not have this disadvantage.

Mechanical Stress-broken Designs

Various types of mechanical stress-breakers have been discussed in the chapter on prefabricated attachments (Chapter 7) and only general applications of these attachments to free-end saddles are discussed here.

Mechanical stress-breakers should be used when mandibular anterior teeth are not sufficiently strong to support a free-end saddle denture of rigid design. Where two abutment teeth on each side can be crowned and fixed together to provide support, Dalbo No. 63.02.2, CEKA 6.96/KS or similar attachments should be placed distally. These attachments provide both stress distribution and retention (*see Figs.* 7.8, 8.10, 10.11). The springs in these attachments ensure that some of the load is transmitted to the teeth, but it is important that the saddles are relined frequently to avoid the spring reaching maximum compression when the attachment would act as a simple hinge. A simple lingual bar connector behind the anterior teeth completes the design since the attachments provide indirect as well as direct retention. Thus a streamlined denture is produced with the minimum number of extra-anatomical parts.

If the abutment teeth at the ends of free-end saddles require to be root-filled, stud retainers can be used with a lingual bar saddle connector. This design is also streamlined and is inconspicuous (*Fig.* 10.12). Flexible stud retainers that provide stress distribution have been designed by Gerber, Dalla Bona, Battesti and others.

Removing the crowns of teeth and placing studs for retention improves the prognosis by greatly reducing the crown/root ratio of the teeth (*Fig.* 10.13). Where there has been much bone loss round abutment teeth it is worth carrying out this procedure and root-filling the teeth, even if the pulps are vital. However, where there has been much attrition, the crowns of some of these teeth can be radically reduced without the necessity of root-filling as much secondary dentine has been deposited in the pulp chamber.

Hinged Designs

Simple hinges of various types can be used as saddle connectors (*Fig.* 10.14), but they have the disadvantage, already mentioned, that they deliver 50 per cent of the load to the abutment tooth and about 50 per cent to the distal end of the saddle, the amount of load diminishing to zero immediately distal to the abutment tooth. The Frey joint (*Fig.* 10.15) distributes more load to the saddle by means of a

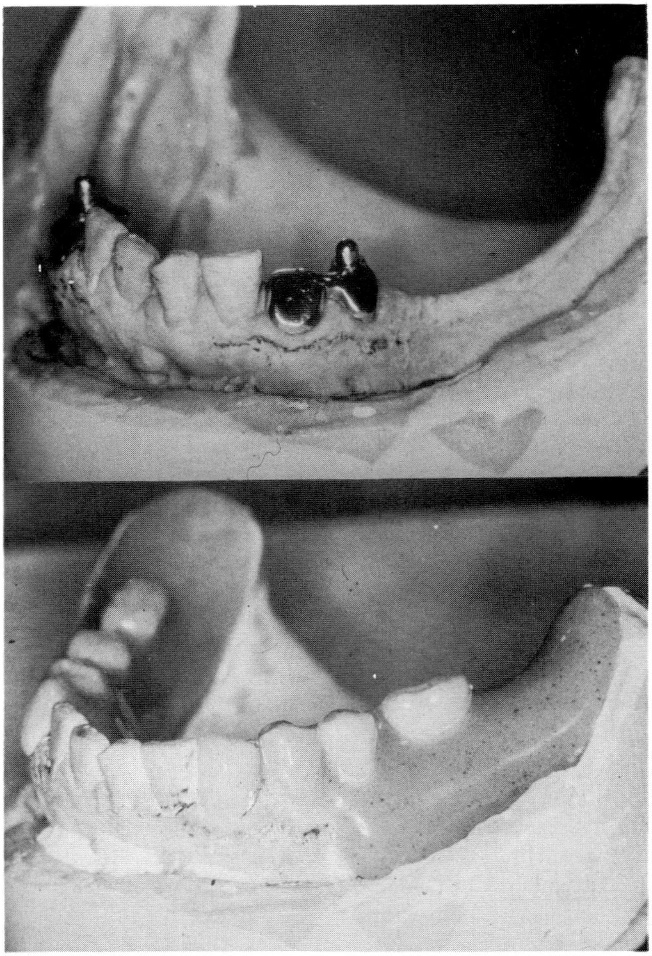

Fig. 10.12. Caps on the canines and stud retainers on the first premolars provide support and retention for a streamlined partial lower denture.

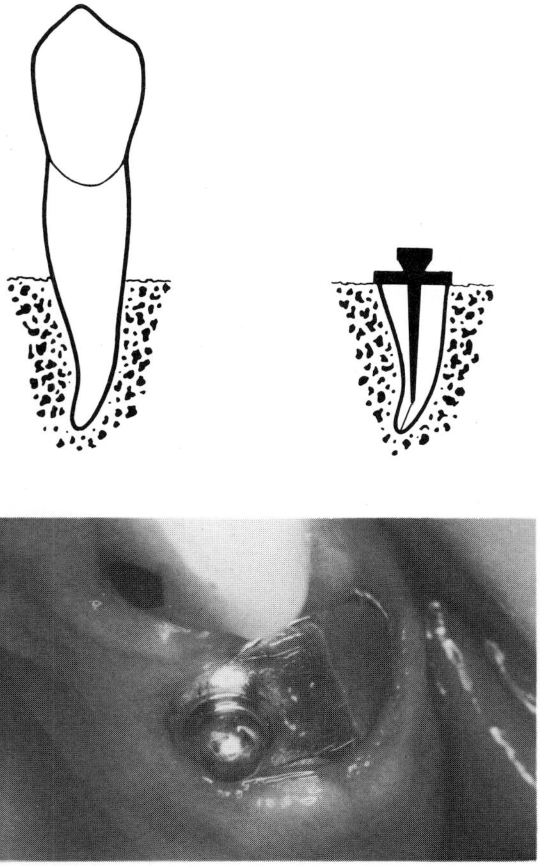

Fig. 10.13. The prognosis of an abutment tooth with an unfavourable crown/root ratio can be greatly improved by cutting it down and placing a stud retainer on the root face. The photograph shows a Bona Ball-Anchor.

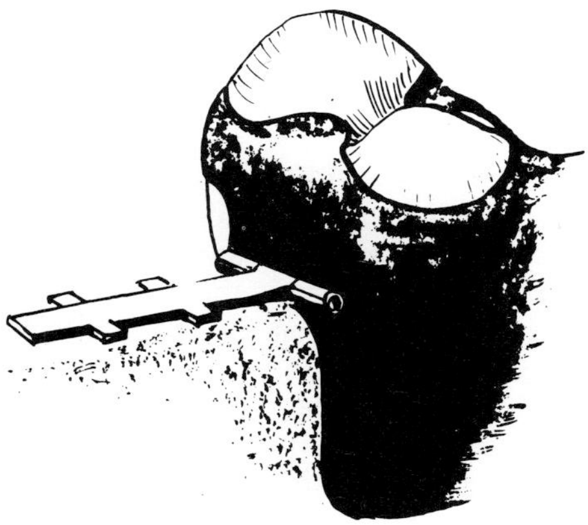

Fig. 10.14. Simple hinge connecting a free-end saddle to tooth-borne part of the denture.

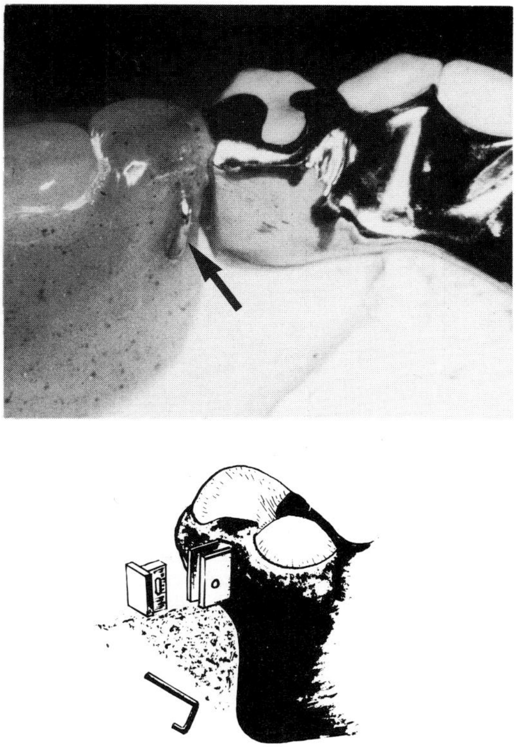

Fig. 10.15. The Frey joint for a free-end saddle has a pin (*arrow*) which can be withdrawn from the lingual side of the denture to permit easy relining of the saddle and replacement when the pin wears. The pin, entering a slot in the patrix, enables more even distribution of the load to the mucosa of the saddle area.

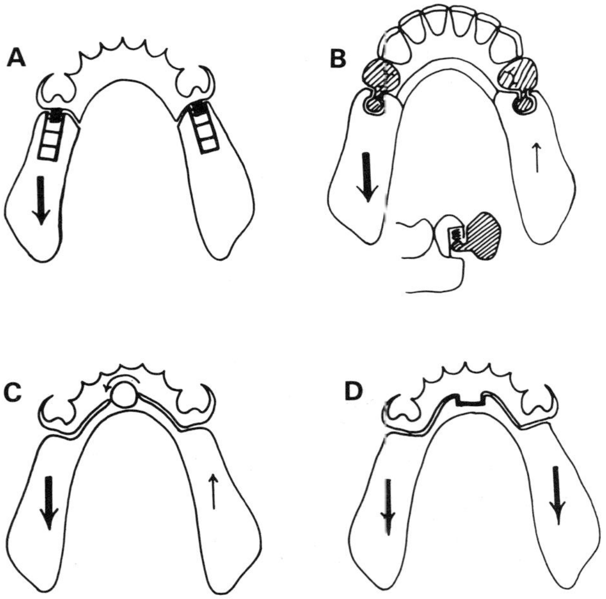

Fig. 10.16. Comparison of load distribution to free-end saddles when different hinge connectors are used. *Heavy arrows* indicate downward movement towards the mucosa when load falls on saddle. *Light arrows* indicate secondary movement of the contralateral saddle away from mucosa. **A**, Hader hinge; the load on one saddle does not affect the other. **B**, Dalbo attachments connected by lingual bar; saddle opposite the loaded saddle tends to rise. **C**, Button hinge; opposite saddle tends to rise. **D**, Dimple hinge; load shared by both saddles and standing teeth.

removable pin that passes through a slot in the patrix and is set in the lingual surface of the free-end saddle. The pin can be withdrawn so that the saddle can be removed for re-lining or adjustment. Some of these appliances tend to develop lateral 'wobble' when the pin wears, but a fresh pin can be inserted. However, when the holes in the hinge wear, it is not so easy to cure the 'wobble'. When it is possible to place a hinge some distance anterior to free-end saddles, there is a better distribution of load on the mucosa of the saddles and proportionately less load goes on the abutment teeth (*Fig.* 10.16). The midline button hinge allows rotation and hinged movement, so that when one free-end saddle is loaded the other tends to rise from the mucosa.

Dimple-hinge Attachments

The dimple hinge has a rigid transverse axis, so that when one side is loaded the other side is also depressed into the mucosa and, provided the retention on the tooth-borne part is adequate, both saddles are loaded during unilateral chewing. The additional advantage of the dimple hinge is that the load is applied at the lower edge of the tooth-borne segment and thus all the anterior teeth are loaded during mastication. This arrangement gives an efficient distribution of load to the remaining

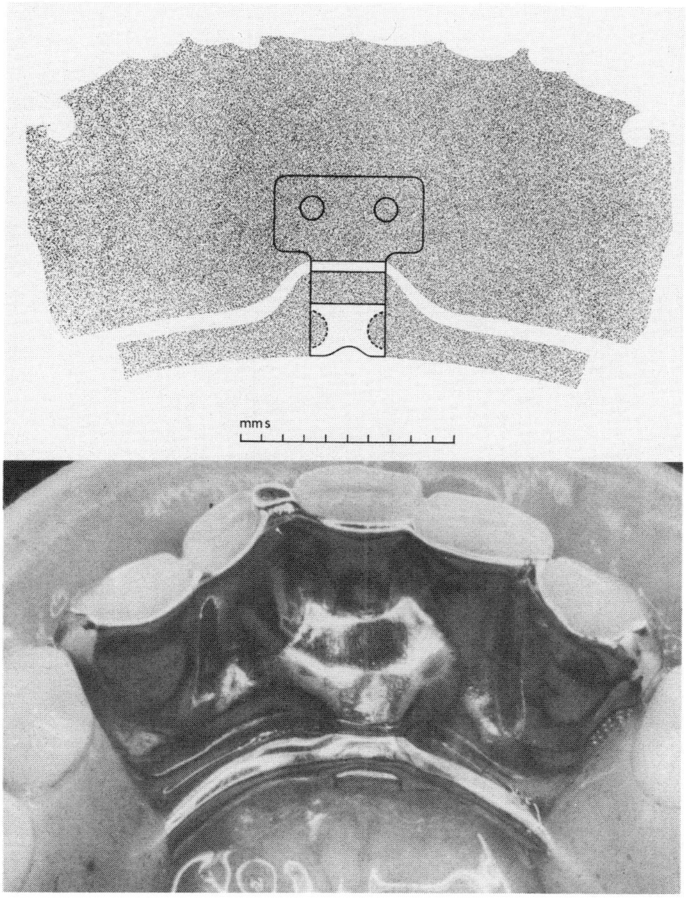

Fig. 10.17. *Upper,* Diagram of a double dimple attachment in the midline between the lingual plate and lingual bar of a Kennedy Class I partial lower denture. *Lower,* The finished appliance.

structures in bilateral free-end saddle lower dentures. The load transmitted to all the remaining teeth is about 50 per cent of the masticatory load at the anterior end of the saddle, but the actual proportion on each tooth depends on the number of remaining teeth and the distance of the saddles from the hinge. Dimple hinges are cheap and easily fabricated attachments that can be used in most types of tooth-and-mucosa-borne dentures where stress relief is required. They are simple cobalt-chromium alloy castings that can be made in batches and used as required (Watt, 1972). The melting range of the alloy used for the attachments must be higher than that used to cast the dentures to which they are attached. There are two types of dimple hinge attachments: double and paired. The cast cobalt-chromium double dimple-hinge attachment is incorporated in the wax pattern between the lingual plate and the lingual bar portion of a Kennedy Class I denture (*Fig.* 10.17). When the denture is cast the cobalt-chromium ridge on the attachment prevents the molten metal in the lingual plate portion from joining that in the lingual bar. As the metal flows in the lingual bar portion of the casting, it enters the dimples in the cylindrical part of the attachment and thus forms a hinge.

Paired dimple hinges comprise two 2-mm

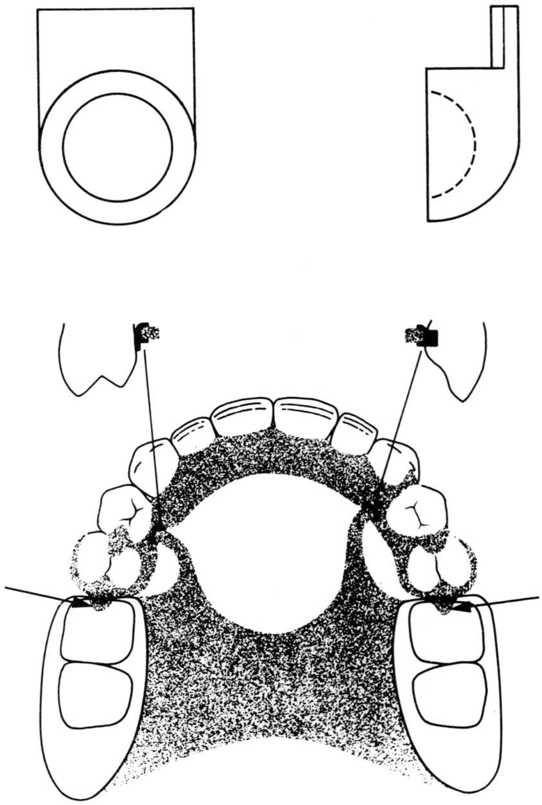

Fig. 10.18. *Upper,* Front and side view of a dimple hinge attachment. These are used in pairs to provide a hinge between the tooth-borne and mucosa-borne parts of a partial denture. *Lower,* Diagram of a bilateral free-end saddle upper denture with a pair of dimple hinges. Note the extensions (*arrows*) on to the first artificial molars prevent the saddles losing contact with the mucosa.

diameter dimples made of cobalt-chromium alloy. These are placed on opposite sides of a partial denture (*Fig.* 10.18) and provide a hinge between the mucosa-borne and tooth-borne parts of the denture. Thus, the position of the fulcrum line can be decided without regard to the position of the clasps or rests.

Disjunct Dentures

When the remaining teeth are of poor prognosis, and it is felt that they should not be used to provide support but should be splinted, a disjunct design can be used. With this design (*Fig.* 10.19) there is a complete disjunction between the tooth-borne part and the mucosa-borne part; the tooth-borne part provides splinting of the anterior teeth and only retention for the mucosa-borne part. The mucosa-borne part is connected to the tooth-borne part by means of disjunct bars that carry pins sliding in slots placed at the mid-points of the mucosa-borne saddles (*see* Chapter 11). When one side of a disjunct denture is loaded, the other side tends to rise as the loaded

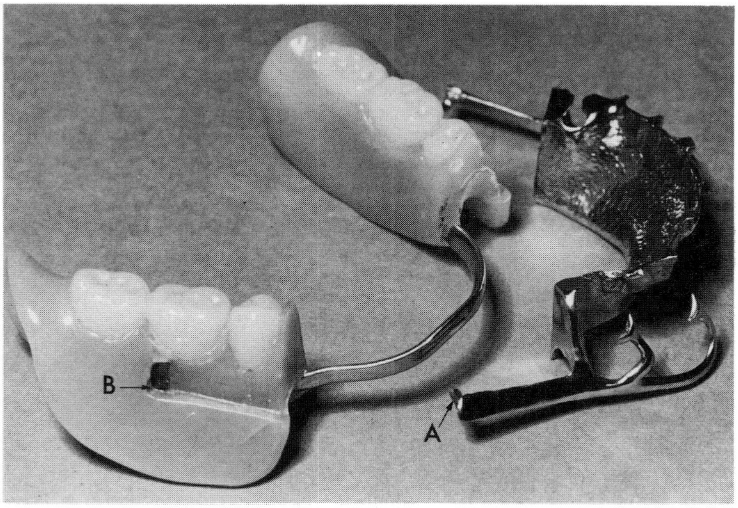

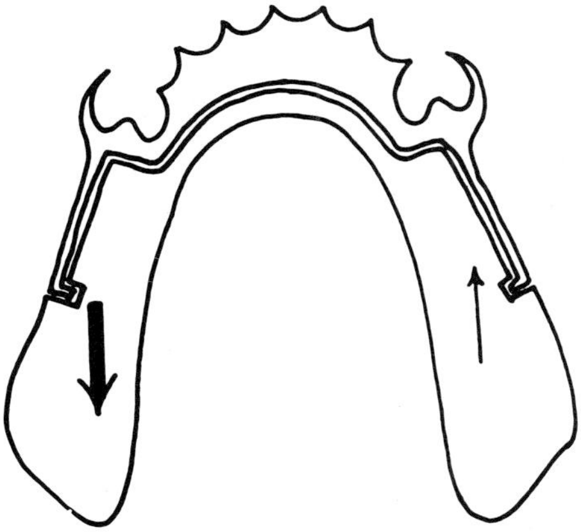

Fig. 10.19. *Upper,* Disjunct partial denture before assembly. The cast metal tooth-borne part splints the anterior teeth and provides retention for the mucosa-borne part. *Lower,* When one saddle is loaded (*heavy arrow*) the other saddle tends to rise, but is prevented by the pin on the disjunct bar (A) resting on the bottom of the slot (B).

saddle rotates round a soft-tissue fulcrum. However, the saddle on the contralateral side cannot lose contact with the mucosal surface as the pin rests at the bottom of the slot and maintains it in light contact with the mucosa. Thus the disjunct denture is particularly suitable when it is wished to put no additional occlusal load on the remaining teeth.

These dentures are further discussed in Chapter 11.

Chapter 11

Disjunct dentures

The idea of 'disjoining' tooth-borne and mucosa-borne parts of partial dentures is not new. Nally (1961) classified some types of prefabricated precision attachments as 'disjunctors'.

Disjunct dentures may be used when the remaining teeth are of poor prognosis. The disjunct principle of denture design (Geissler and Watt 1965; Geissler 1968, 1973) is that the tooth-borne and mucosa-borne parts of the denture are disjoined, the tooth-borne part providing splinting of the remaining teeth and only retention for the mucosa-borne part. All the support for the saddles comes from the mucosa. This principle of denture design has many applications and the following guidelines will help to produce the most suitable design.

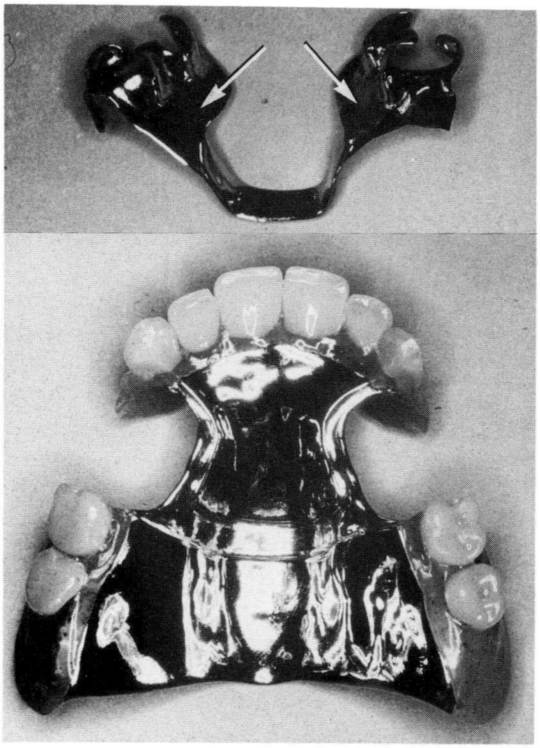

Fig. 11.1. Separate parts of a disjunct denture for a strong young man with an intact mandibular arch and only premolars remaining in the maxilla. *Upper,* The cobalt-chromium tooth-borne part with gingival skirts (*arrows*). *Lower,* The mucosa-borne part, usually made of acrylic, was made in cobalt-chromium alloy to avoid fracture in this case.

Guidelines to Designing

1. The tooth-borne part should be rigid and carry all the retainers of the denture. It should be constructed to provide gingival 'skirts' that cover the gingival margins round the abutment teeth and prevent the mucosa-borne part from pressing on the gingival margins (*Fig.* 11.1).

2. A step should be formed along the margins of the gingival skirt to provide retention for the mucosa-borne portion of the denture. The skirt should be in close contact with the underlying mucosa, except where the step is formed at its margins (*Fig.* 11.2).

3. In the case of bilateral free-end saddle lower dentures, the gingival skirt should be formed distal to the abutment teeth (*Fig.* 11.3) by thickening that portion of the denture. If possible, the undercut in this area should not be blocked out, but a path of insertion should be chosen so that the tooth-borne part of the denture can closely engage the distal undercut and contact the gingival margin. In some cases the gingival skirt can be extended by attaching the first artificial tooth to the tooth-borne part of the denture. However, this may make the tooth-borne part rock round a fulcrum axis through the occlusal rests.

4. In the case of maxillary disjunct dentures with premolar abutment teeth on each side of the arch, care should be taken with the design

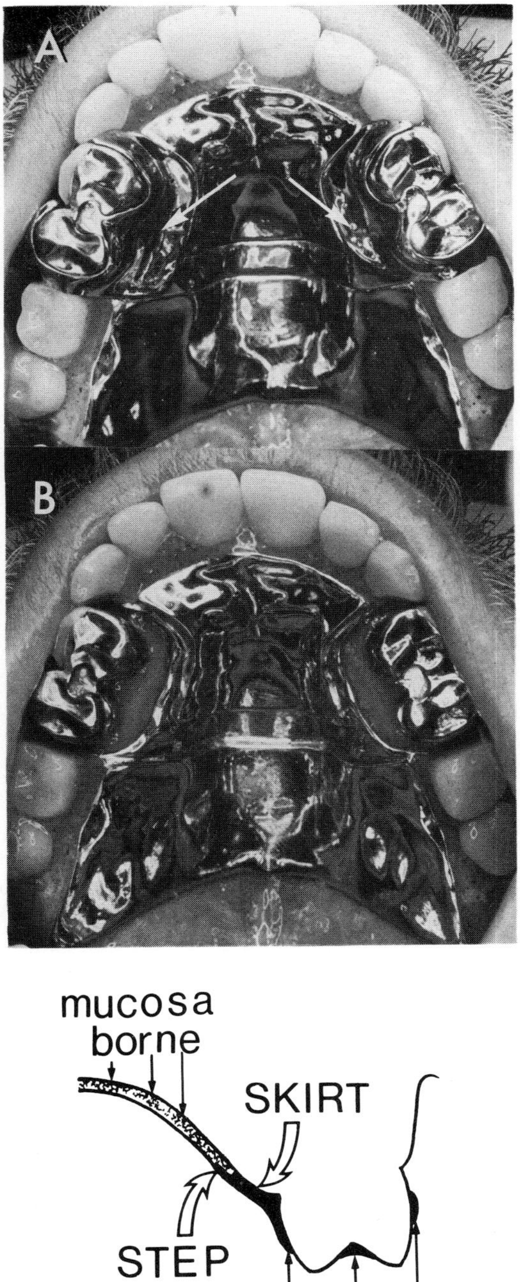

Fig. 11.2. **A**, Disjunct denture in mouth, showing gingival skirts (*arrows*). **B**, Tooth-borne part of disjunct denture removed to show how the mucosa-borne part is kept clear of the gingival margins. Diagram of cross-section of gingival skirt on partial upper disjunct denture, showing step.

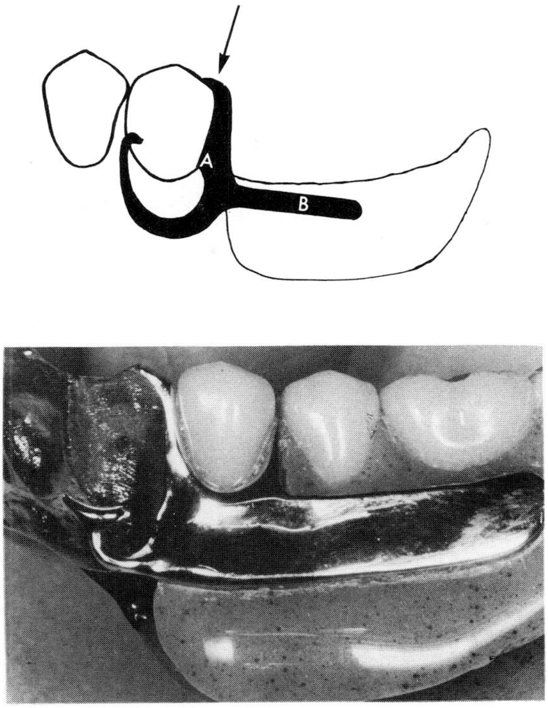

Fig. 11.3. *Upper,* Diagram of a partial lower disjunct denture, showing the usual design of a gingival skirt (A) and the disjunct bar (B); the arrow indicates the path of insertion. *Lower,* A partial lower disjunct denture with an extended gingival skirt produced by attaching an artificial tooth to the tooth-borne part.

of the bar connecting the two halves of the tooth-borne part. A bar crossing the anterior part of the palate often leads to fracture of the mucosa-borne part of the denture behind the anterior teeth (*see Fig.* 11.1) and in addition may obstruct the tongue. If possible, therefore, the connector should be formed as shown in *Fig.* 11.4 to reduce the danger of a fracture and to improve the comfort of the patient. When the upper anterior teeth are present and the patient has bilateral free-end saddles, a disjunct denture design can be used (*Fig.* 11.5), but this design has the disadvantage that it covers the anterior part of the palate. The patient is usually more comfortable with a fixed splint placed on the anterior teeth and a denture designed like that shown in *Fig.* 11.6, being attached to distal abutments by Dalbo or other precision attachments.

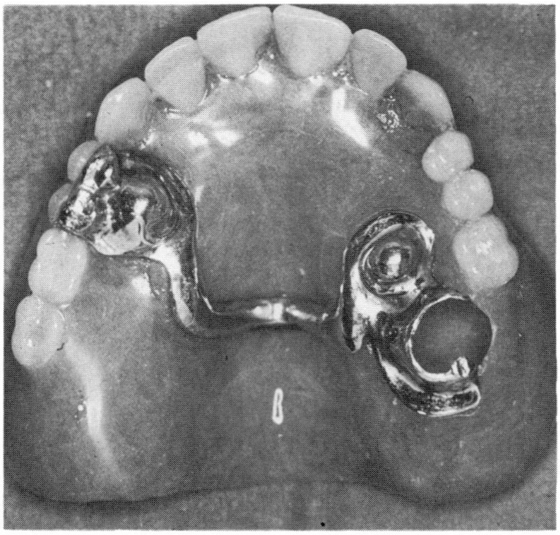

Fig. 11.4. The tooth-borne connector of this disjunct denture for a patient with a cleft palate crosses the middle part of the palate to avoid obstructing the tongue and to prevent a line of weakness near the front of the mucosa-borne part.

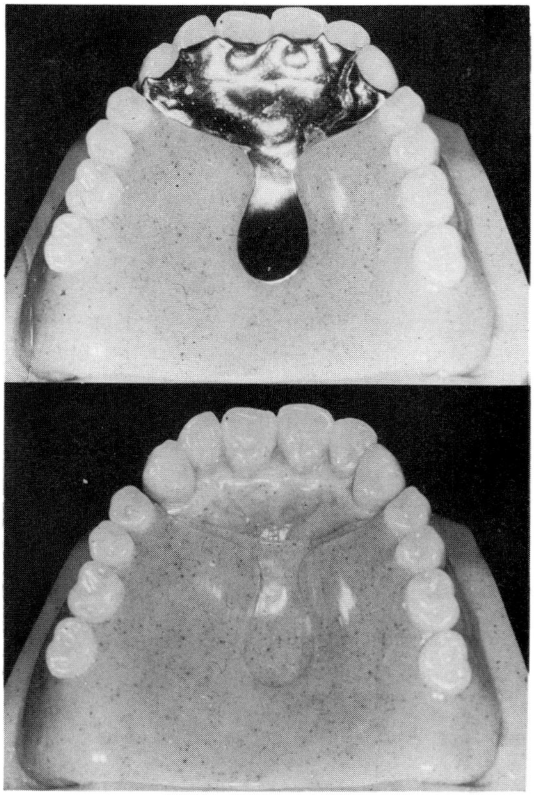

Fig. 11.5. *Upper,* Disjunct denture design for a patient with six maxillary anterior teeth remaining. *Lower,* The same denture without the tooth-borne part.

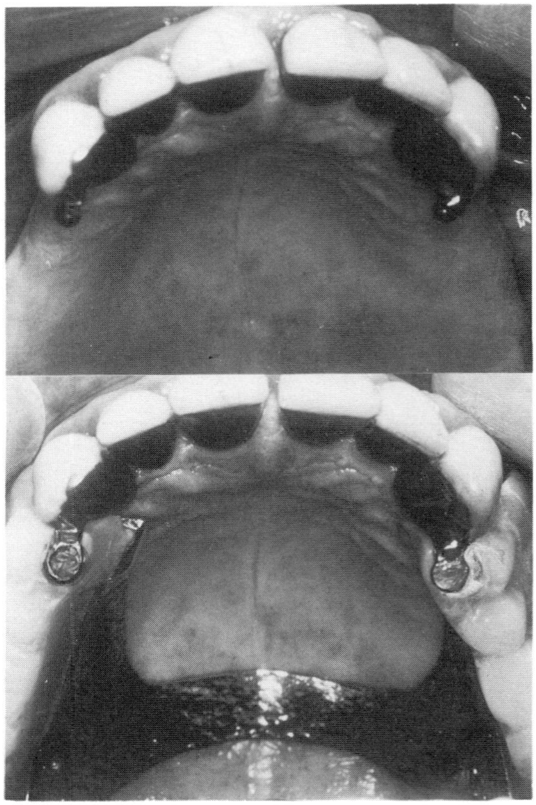

Fig. 11.6. When anterior teeth of poor prognosis are present, soldered full veneer crowns may be used and the denture retained by prefabricated retainers. This design leaves the anterior part of the palate uncovered and improves the patient's comfort and gingival health.

Advantages of Disjunct Dentures

The disjunct principle of denture design has the advantage that it provides cross-arch splinting for mobile teeth. The saddles of the dentures are entirely mucosa-borne and require no tooth support. The designs can be made as simple or as complex as you wish and many variations can be made to suit the needs of individual patients (MacGregor and Miller, 1974). When very few teeth are left in the mouth, it is sometimes advisable to place thimble crowns on the remaining abutment teeth and attach caps to the tooth-borne part of the disjunct denture. This gives much more precise splinting than placing ordinary clasps on the abutments (*Fig.* 11.7). Disjunct dentures are particularly useful for cleft palate

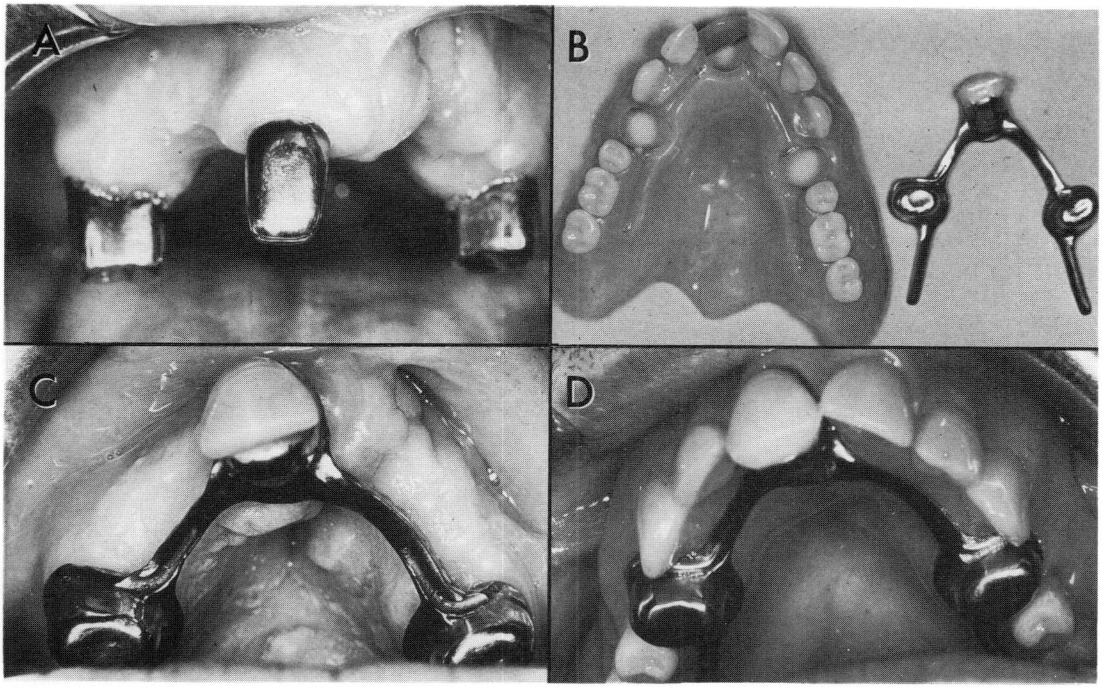

Fig. 11.7. **A**, Thimble veneer crowns on abutment teeth of cleft palate patient. **B**, Disjunct denture (parts separated). **C**, Tooth-borne part of disjunct denture in place. The tooth-borne part provides cross-arch splinting for the abutment teeth and retention for the mucosa-borne part. **D**, Both parts in place in the mouth.

patients whose few remaining teeth are vital for the retention of the obturator, but are awkwardly placed and quite inadequate to support it. Various designs that can be used for these difficult cases are shown in *Fig.* 11.4, 11.7, 11.8 and 11.9.

Mandibular Disjunct Dentures

Mandibular disjunct dentures usually have an anterior tooth-borne part that splints the remaining anterior teeth and a posterior mucosa-borne part that carries two free-end saddles connected by a rigid lingual bar. The connection between the tooth-borne and the mucosa-borne parts is made by pins at the end of the disjunct bars (*Fig.* 11.10) which slide in slots on the mucosa-borne part. When the denture is placed in the mouth, the pins rest at the bottom of the slots and hold the free-end saddles against the mucosa. When these saddles are loaded they can be displaced into the mucosa without putting stresses on the anterior teeth. Many patients with teeth of poor prognosis have lost so much supporting bone that there is little room for a lingual bar between the gingival margins and the floor of the mouth. In such cases the lingual bar can lie on the polished surface of the lingual plate of the tooth-borne part of the denture that protects the gingival margins. Where more space is available, the bar can lie in a groove at the lower edge of the lingual plate. An alternative disjunct denture design that eliminates the disjunct bars is shown in *Fig.* 11.11. The connection between tooth-borne

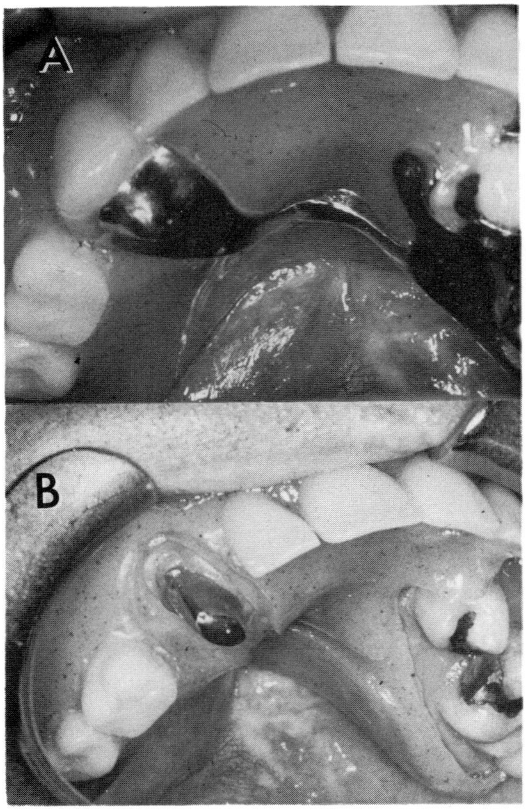

Fig. 11.8. **A**, Disjunct denture for cleft palate patient. Note that the tooth-borne part carries an artificial facing on the buccal side of the right canine, extending the gingival skirt so that the mucosa-borne part (**B**) does not damage the gingival margin of the abutment tooth.

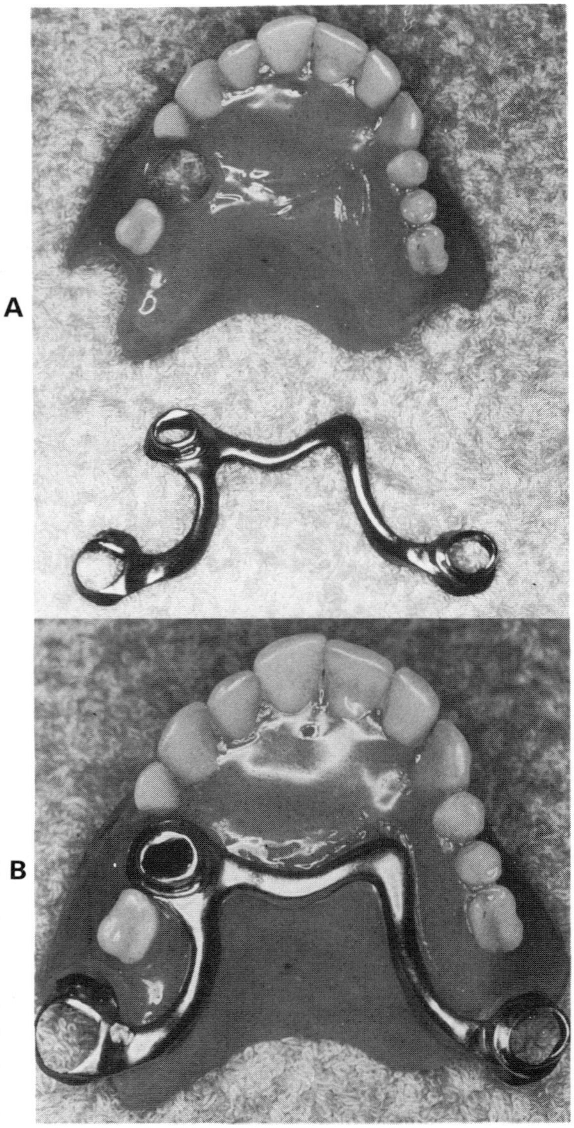

Fig. 11.9. Disjunct denture for cleft palate patient. **A**, Separated. **B**, Assembled.

and mucosa-borne parts is made by downward facing tubes on each side in which slide vertical rods attached to the first artificial teeth of the free-end saddles. A little play between the rod and the tube is necessary to allow movement of the saddles, but the closed end of the tube must contact the rod so that the saddle is held against the mucosa when the mucosa is not compressed. Alternatively, to simplify fabrication the rod may be attached to the cast tooth-borne part and the tube to the mucosa-borne part.

Although disjunct dentures may appear to be rather complicated, their main clinical advantage is the comfort they give to the patient. As there is complete disjunction between the mucosa-borne parts and the tooth-borne parts, patients are not conscious of stress on the teeth when eating. Many patients who are unable to wear other types of bilateral free-end saddle dentures find comfort with disjunct dentures.

Three-dimensional photo-elastic stress analysis has been used to examine the stresses on disjunct partial dentures. MacGregor et al. (1978) showed that more stress was distributed to the abutment teeth when the pin/

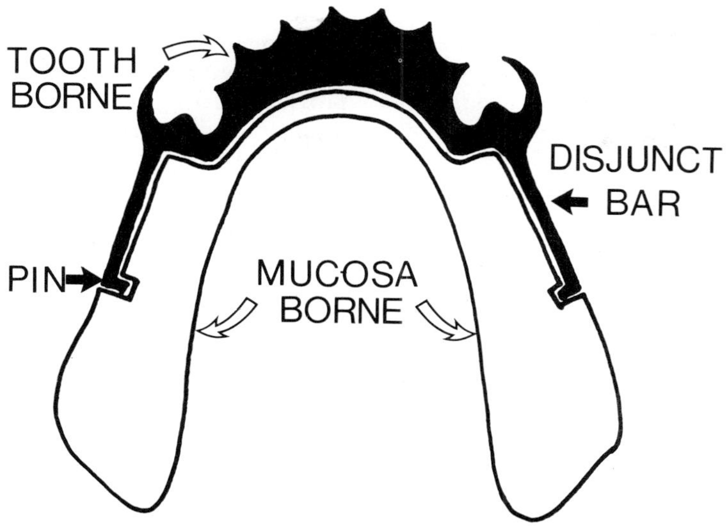

Fig. 11.10. Diagram of mandibular disjunct denture for bilateral free-end saddles. The disjunct bars carry pins that lie at the bottom of slots and hold the mucosa-borne part of the denture against the surface of the mucosa when the denture is inserted. When a masticatory load falls on the mucosa-borne part of the denture, it sinks into the tissues.

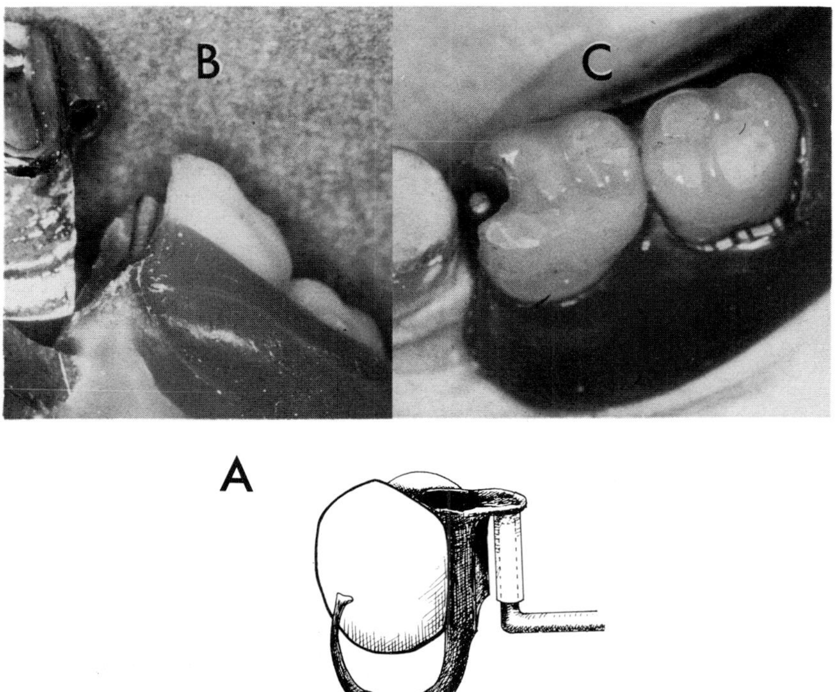

Fig. 11.11. An alternative method of connecting the tooth-borne part to the mucosa-borne part of a disjunct denture. **A**, Diagram showing connector. **B**, The two parts separated, showing how the tube on the tooth-borne part engages the rod on the mucosa-borne part. **C**, The wax mucosa-borne saddle with the rod in place.

slot mechanism was rigidly fixed, converting the denture to a rigid design. When the pin/slot mechanism was freely moving, however, the stress was distributed to the saddle area and much less stress was distributed to the teeth. It is essential that wearers of disjunct dentures maintain a very high level of oral hygiene as the gingival margins are covered by these dentures, but since the cover is tooth-borne gingival damage does not take place provided oral hygiene is good. Patients should be instructed in the hygiene of the mouth and should also be taught how to keep the denture clean (Appendix I).

Chapter 12

Sectional dentures

Sectional dentures (Lee, 1963, 1964; Pullen-Warner, 1964, 1965) have already been mentioned in Chapter 6, in which reference was made to the book by Pullen-Warner and L'Estrange (1978) which describes these appliances in detail.

In some partially edentulous mouths there may be undercuts that oppose each other (i.e. mesial and distal or buccal and lingual). The choice of blocking out one or other of these opposed undercuts has then to be made. This leaves an unsatisfactory space that may trap food when the denture is in the mouth. By using a sectional denture, both undercuts can be used, as the sections of the denture are inserted in two different paths. This has the advantage of filling all undercut spaces and giving very positive retention. Such dentures comprise two parts. In some designs the two parts are separate, assembled by the patient in the mouth, and locked together by split pins, locking bolts, tubes and clips, or similar devices. In other designs the two parts are hinged and after being placed in the mouth they are locked together (hinge-flange design).

Indications for Sectional Dentures

1. When a patient is unwilling to have teeth prepared for a bridge, a small sectional denture can often satisfy the patient by occupying little space in the mouth and restoring the patient's appearance (*see Fig.* 2.7).

2. Where there has been much soft-tissue loss and the construction of a fixed bridge would fail to restore that loss, sectional dentures can often provide the best type of appliance.

3. Where a clasp on an anterior tooth would be necessary for retention, it can sometimes be replaced by a hinge-flange or sectional part of the denture (*see Fig.* 5.16).

Advantages of Sectional Dentures

1. Undercuts do not have to be blocked out and therefore there are no food-trapping spaces left between the denture and the abutment teeth.

2. They do not require extensive tooth preparation.

3. They can usually be constructed within the limits of the denture space and have very few extra-anatomical parts.

4. They can be removed for cleaning.

5. They restore both hard and soft tissues.

6. They can be used in many different situations in the mouth because many different kinds of design can be employed (*Fig.* 12.1).

Disadvantages of Sectional Dentures

1. After some time in the mouth the locking devices begin to wear and small lateral movements of the appliance can occur.

2. Skilled technicians are required to construct and maintain them.

3. Their use is dependent on appropriate undercuts being present around the teeth and saddle areas.

4. They must be carefully handled to avoid distortion and breakage by the patient.

5. They are expensive to produce.

Some may argue that Rochette and Maryland bridges (Rochette, 1973; Nathanson and Moin, 1980; Hopkins, 1981; Thompson et al., 1983), which are bonded by composite resin to acid-etched tooth surfaces, are easier to make and are just as satisfactory, but these

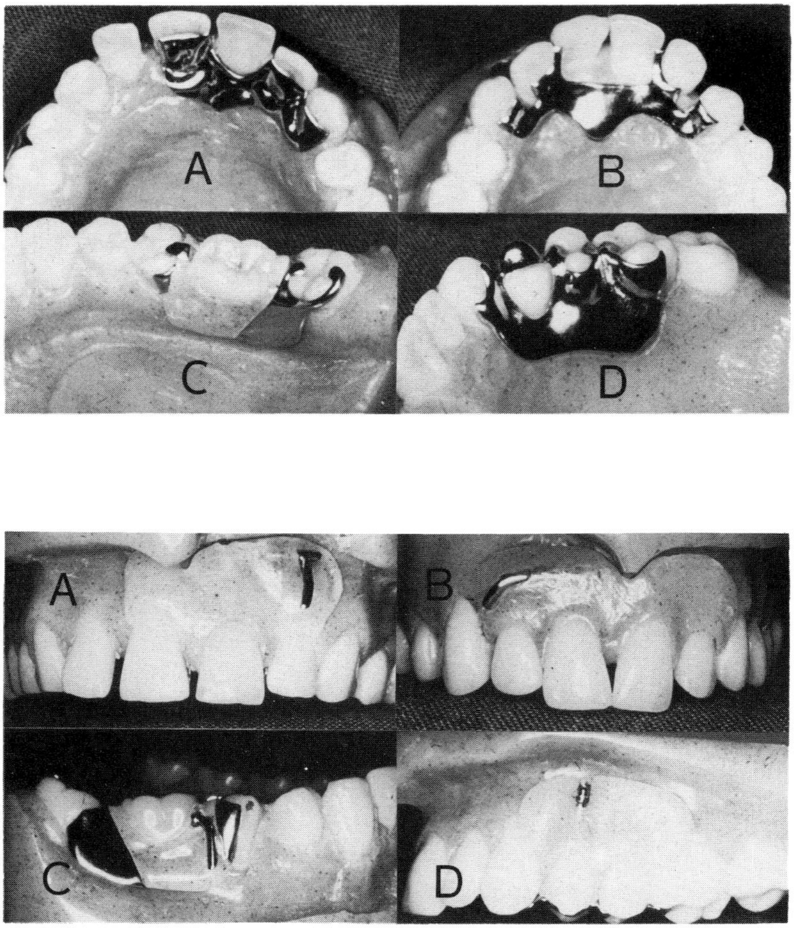

Fig. 12.1. Different types of sectional dentures. *Upper,* Lingual views. *Lower,* Buccal views. **A,** Buccal and lingual parts inserted separately and bolted together. **B,** Buccal and lingual parts hinged and bolted. **C,** Separate parts enter mesial and distal undercuts and are joined with a horizontal bolt (*see Fig.* 12.2). **D,** Separate parts enter buccal and lingual undercuts and are joined with a vertical bolt.

appliances, in common with most bridges, do not restore lost soft-tissue parts.

Types of Sectional Dentures

Sectional dentures for posterior gaps usually employ the mesial and distal undercuts in posterior teeth for their retention and are of two types, mesiodistal and linguobuccal.

With the mesiodistal type the distal portion is usually inserted first into the distal undercut, then the mesial portion is put into the mesial undercut and the two parts are locked together with a horizontal bolt (*Fig.* 12.2).

With the linguobuccal type the lingual portion of the denture engages the lingual part of both mesial and distal undercuts and the buccal portion of the denture engages the buccal part of both mesial and distal undercuts (*Fig.* 12.3). It is necessary to survey the ridge crest and mesial and distal parts of the teeth with the surveying lead parallel to the occlusal plane. This draws the line of demarcation between the buccal and lingual parts (*Fig.*

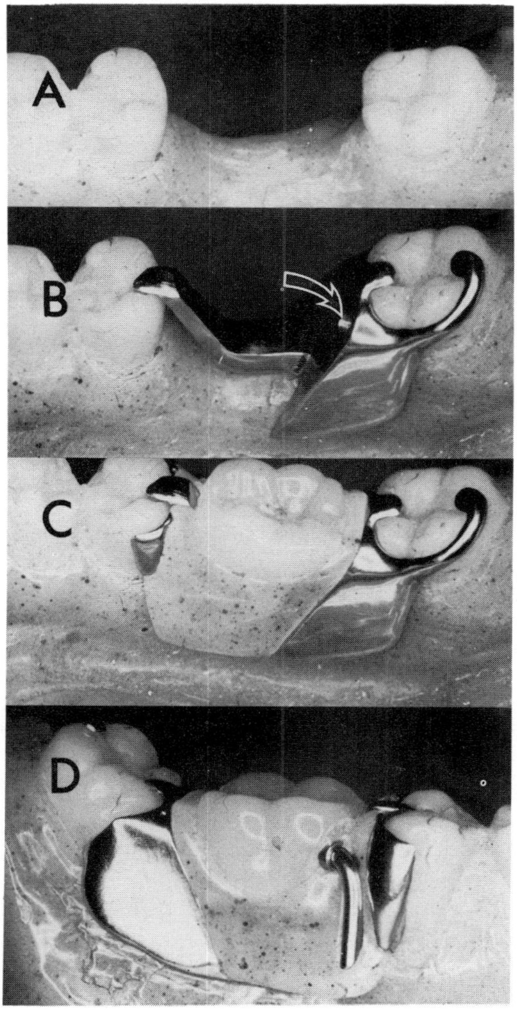

Fig. 12.2. **A,** Posterior saddle area suitable for mesio-distal type of sectional denture. **B,** Lingual view of distal part inserted first; note hole for bolt (*arrow*). **C,** Lingual view of assembled denture. **D,** Buccal view, showing horizontal bolt, the handle of which lies in a vertical recess.

12.4). The disadvantage of this type of appliance is that the division along the ridge crest may nip the mucosa and much stress is placed on the bolt. This can be avoided by carrying the lingual part of the denture across the ridge towards the buccal side without engaging the buccal part of the mesial and distal undercuts. The buccal portion placed upon the lingual extension is fixed with a horizontal bolt (*Fig.* 12.5). This is similar to the arrangement for replacing anterior teeth in which the lingual portion is placed first and the buccal portion locked on to it.

The buccal part can be located by means of a hinge, which allows it to swing into the buccal portion of the mesial and distal undercuts (*Fig.* 12.6).

An alternative arrangement for locating the

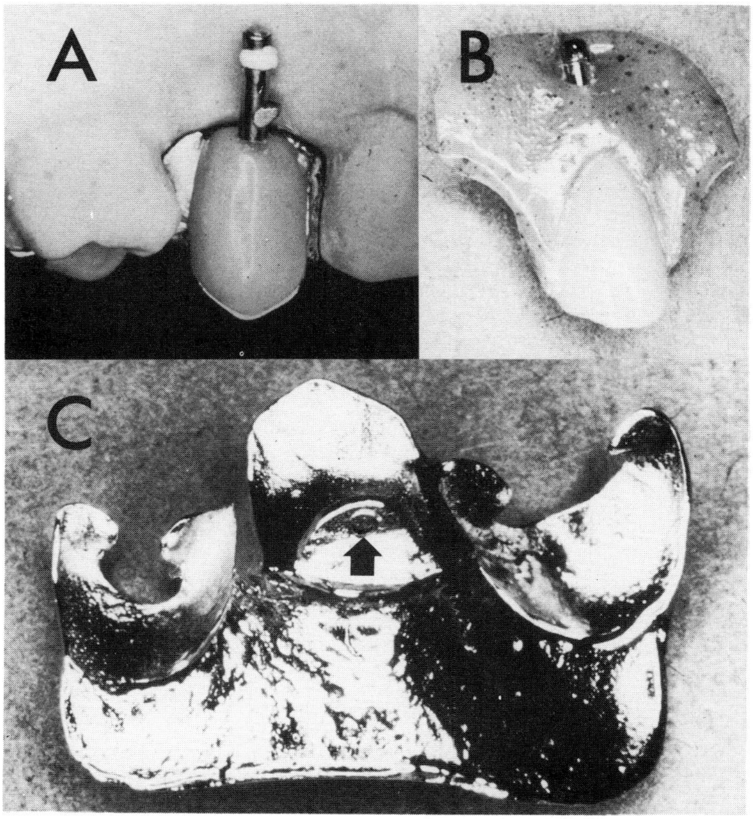

Fig. 12.3. Sectional denture with vertical bolt. **A,** Bolt before buccal flange is waxed up. **B,** Completed buccal flange. **C,** Fitting surface of cast base, showing horizontal plate which guides the buccal section into position. The *arrow* indicates the vertical hole through this plate that is engaged by the vertical bolt that locks the two parts together.

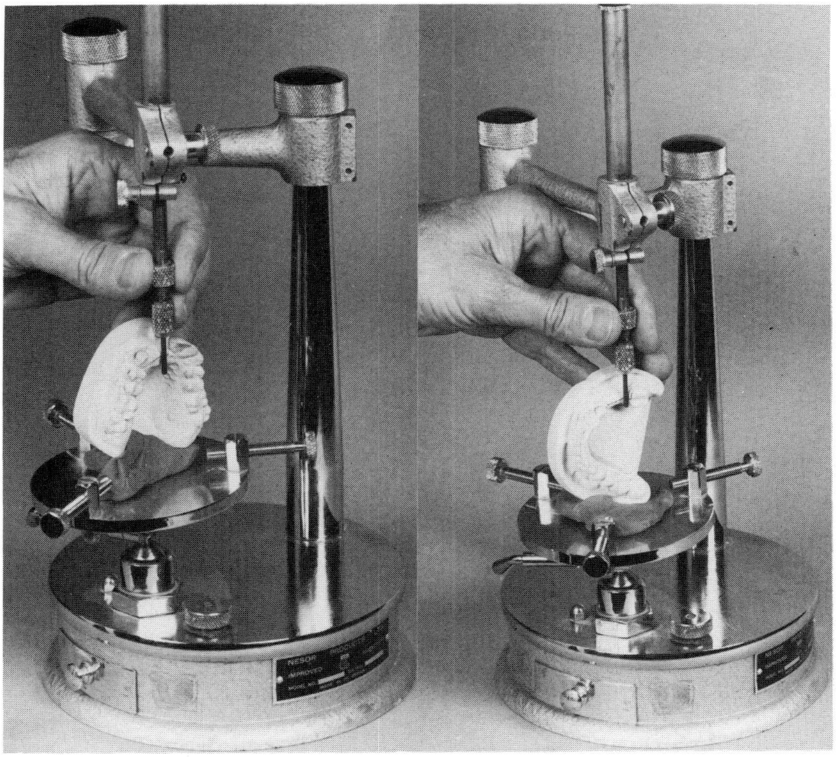

Fig. 12.4. Surveying the teeth and ridge crests of maxillary anterior and mandibular posterior saddle areas to indicate the dividing line between the buccal and lingual parts of sectional dentures.

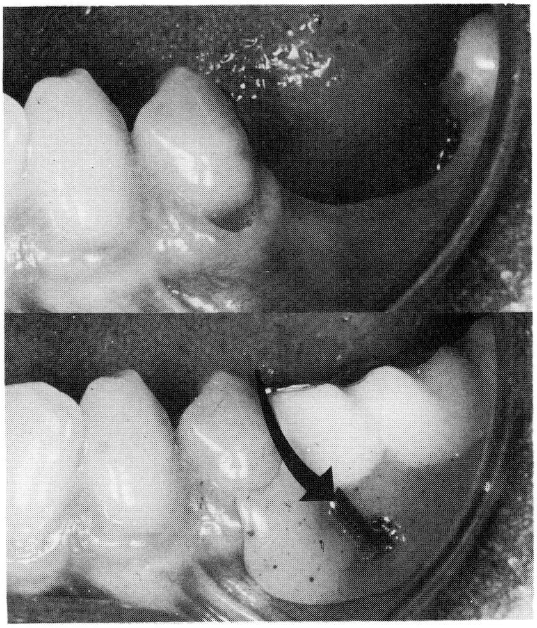

Fig. 12.5. Linguobuccal sectional denture for posterior saddle area. Part of the lingual portion is extended across the ridge without entering mesial or distal undercuts. The buccal portion is fixed to it with a horizontal bolt. The handle of the bolt (*arrow*) has been eased out of the recess that houses it.

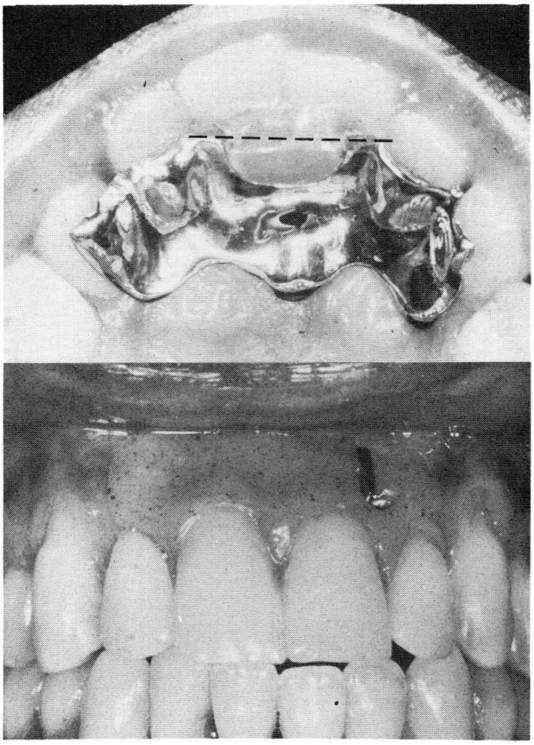

Fig. 12.6. Hinge-flange sectional denture replacing central incisors. Interrupted line indicates position of hinge.

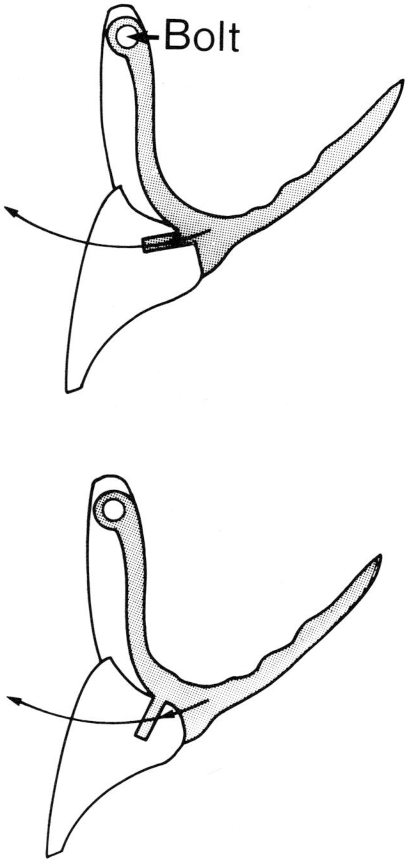

Fig. 12.7. *Upper,* When the guiding rod of a two-part denture is tangential to an arc centred on the bolt of the denture, the rod provides no resistance to displacement of the labial flange round the bolt. *Lower,* Correctly positioned guiding rod prevents rotation round the bolt that locks the labial flange in place.

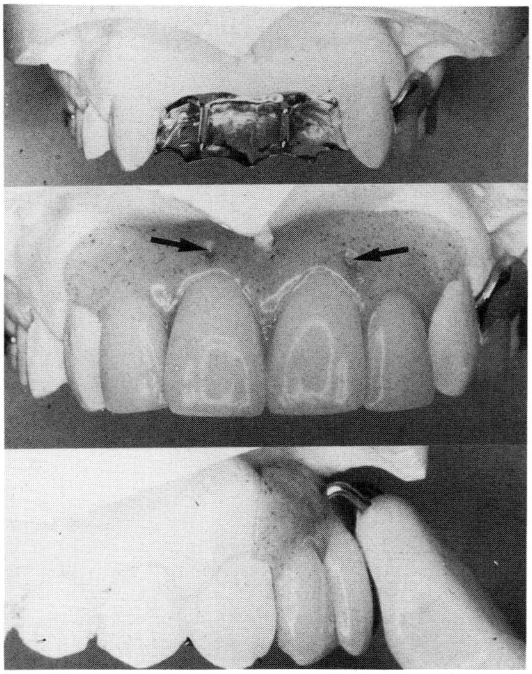

Fig. 12.8. Sectional denture retained by frictional attachment. Long guiding rods guide the labial part into position. Frictional sleeves in this part of the denture provide the retention. The depressions (*arrows*) enable the patient to remove the labial portions by means of a simple instrument (lower) which engages them.

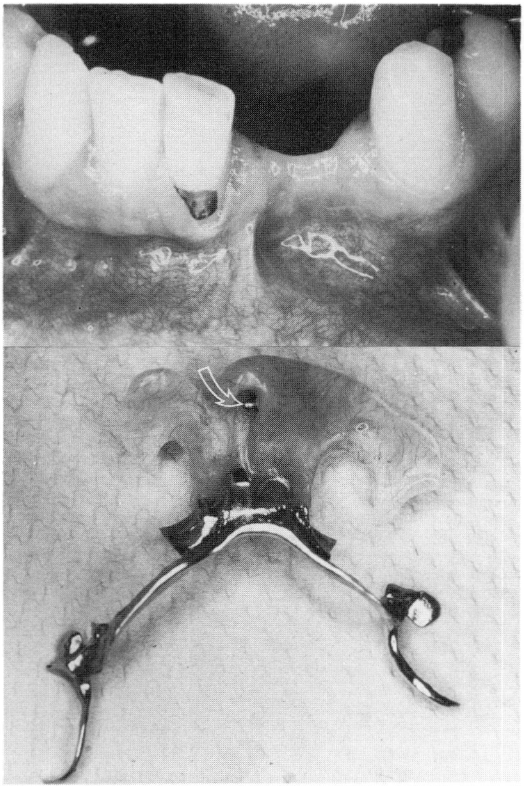

Fig. 12.9. Lower left central and lateral incisors replaced by a hinge-flange sectional denture. The fitting surface of the denture is shown with the flange open to show the plunger of the spring-loaded attachment (*arrowed*).

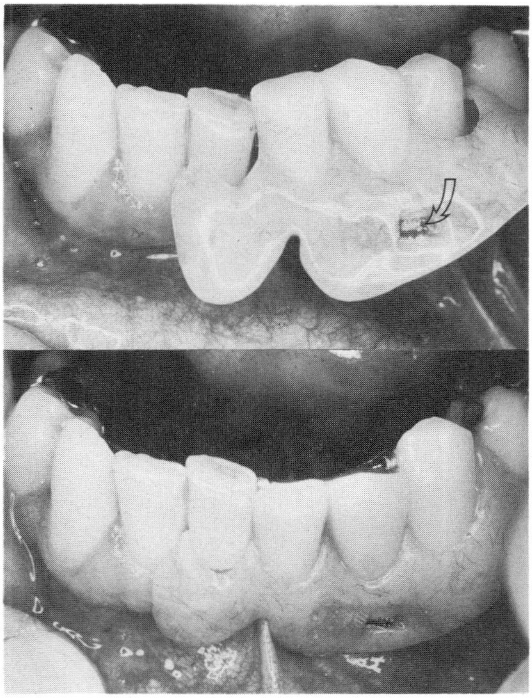

Fig. 12.10. The hinge-flange denture shown in *Fig.* 12.9 in position in the mouth. *Upper,* With the flange open. *Lower,* With the flange clipped shut. The *arrow* indicates the screw-housing of the spring-loaded attachment.

parts is by means of guiding rods, which must lie in the path of insertion of the buccal portion of the appliance and guide it into position in the undercuts (*Figs.* 5.16, 12.7). It is then locked into this position, usually by means of a bolt. The bolt may be either horizontal or vertical, depending on the space available and the position of the appliance in the mouth. Where a horizontal bolt is used the buccal portion of the appliance may swing outwards round the bolt like a hinge. It is therefore essential that the guiding rod is not tangential to the arc of rotation, because if it is the buccal flange will not be held firmly in position (*Fig.* 12.7). *Fig.* 12.3 shows a sectional denture fixed by a vertical bolt. Instead of a guiding rod, a short flat horizontal plate with a vertical hole in it carries out the double purpose of guiding and holding the buccal section in position.

In some cases the two parts may be held together by frictional sleeves on guiding rods. Such appliances usually require a little instrument to enable the patient to remove the buccal part (*Fig.* 12.8). Other means of holding the two parts together are magnetic retainers (Ling, 1982) and spring-loaded attachments. These are most appropriate on hinge-flange dentures since the hinge provides the strength between the two parts, while the magnetic retainer or spring-loaded attachment simply holds them together (*Figs.* 12.9, 12.10).

When constructing a hinge-flange denture which will be locked by a bolt, the hinge is usually designed to cross the gap from the contact point of one abutment tooth to the contact point on the other (*see Fig.* 12.6). The flange then swings towards the gingival margin to engage the mesial and distal undercuts. A

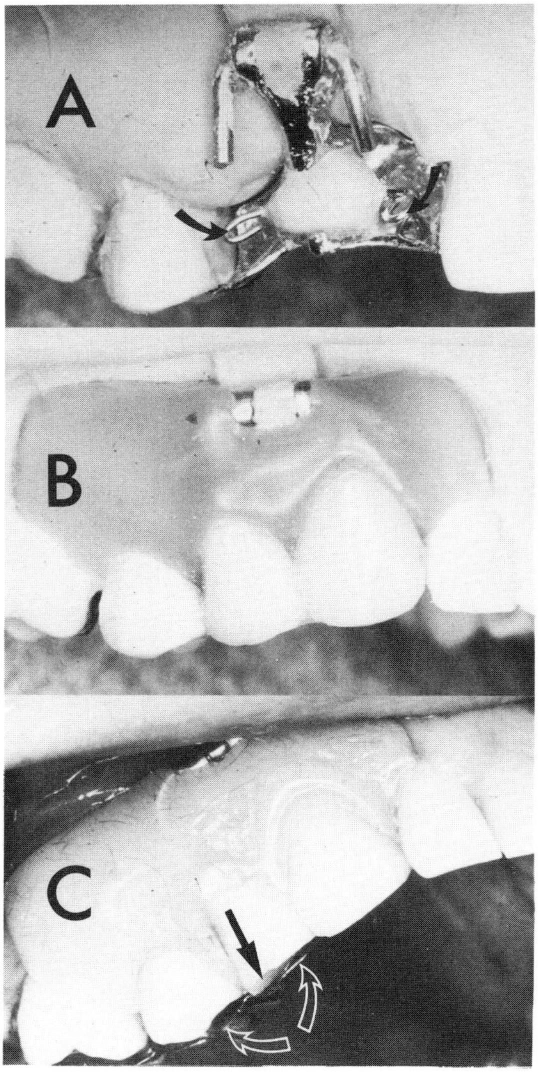

Fig. 12.11. Hinge-flange sectional denture with hinge in buccal sulcus. **A**, The hinge before waxing the buccal flange. The *arrows* indicate the ends of the stainless steel wire clip that holds the buccal flange against the cobalt-chromium lingual part. **B**, The appliance waxed up ready for flasking. **C**, The appliance in the mouth. The buccal flange was not pushed right home in order to show the small depression on the premolar (*black arrow*) into which the patient places an instrument to open the flange. The cobalt-chromium occlusal surface (*white arrows*) prevents the buccal flange being opened accidently when food is chewed.

less conventional way of hinging the flange is to place the hinge in the buccal sulcus (*Fig.* 12.11A, B). This enables the flange to engage

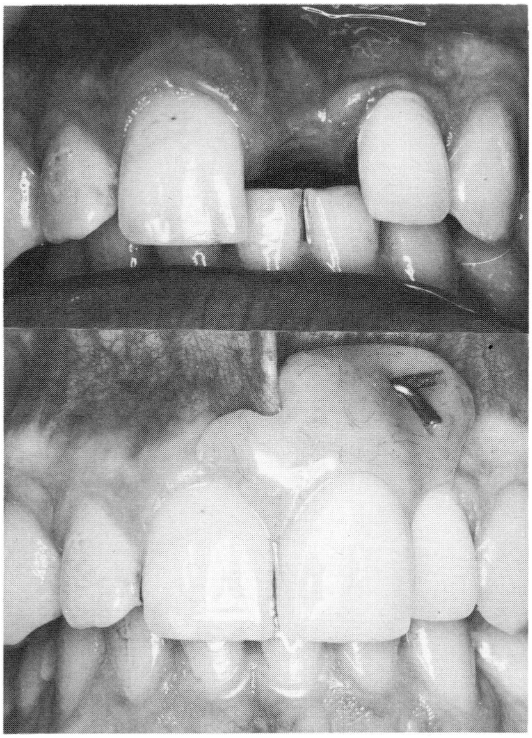

Fig. 12.12. Missing left central incisor replaced by a hinge-flange sectional denture.

the undercuts more easily and is easier for the patient to manipulate, but it has the disadvantage that it can spring out of position when the patient bites on the artificial tooth. To prevent this, the lingual portion of the denture must protect the incisal edge or occlusal surface of the tooth attached to the labial part (*Fig.* 12.11). The patient opens the two halves of the denture with a modified dental instrument placed in a little notch on the labial incisal edge of the tooth.

Although there are many different designs of sectional dentures and numerous methods can be used to fix the sections together, the main purpose of the design is to engage undercuts with rigid parts of the denture, using different paths of insertion. In this way good retention is provided for these small streamlined restorations which require little tooth preparation and replace all the missing parts (*Fig.* 12.12).

Chapter 13

Complex partial dentures

Complex partial dentures have some fixed parts (abutment pieces or bridges) and some removable parts (*Fig.* 13.1). The advantage over conventional removable partial dentures is that they can be kept within the limits of the denture space and are thus more streamlined.

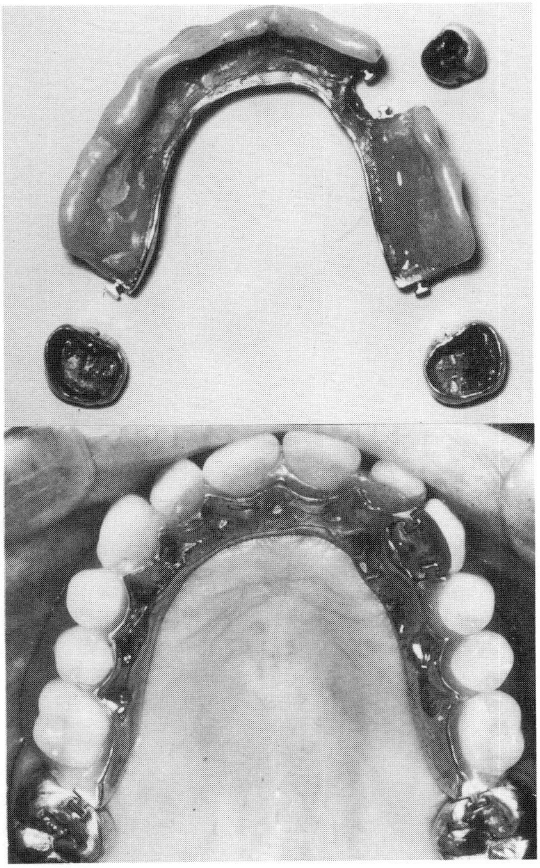

Fig. 13.1. Complex partial dentures have some fixed parts (the abutment pieces) and some removable parts. They are indicated when fixed partial dentures cannot replace all the lost tissues (the *lower* photograph is a mirror view).

Complex partial dentures are indicated when fixed partial dentures (bridges) cannot replace all the lost tissues. For instance, when there is considerable tissue loss following trauma (*Fig.* 13.2) or when an obturator is required (*see Figs.* 7.13, 7.14). These appliances are also indicated where cross-arch bracing is necessary (*Figs.* 13.3, 13.4) and where there are so few remaining teeth that mucosal support is required to supplement the tooth support (*see Fig.* 11.9). In some patients oral hygiene can be maintained more easily with a complex partial denture than with bridges. A complex partial denture should not be made unless the patient is fully aware of the need for careful maintenance of the appliance and is able to keep the mouth and teeth very clean.

An outline of the procedure for making a complex partial denture is as follows:

1. Treat any periodontal disease and ensure that the patient is able to maintain good oral hygiene.

2. Remove any caries and fill the teeth concerned.

3. Stabilize the occlusion. Investigate and treat muscle and temporomandibular joint pains before stabilizing the occlusion. When there are sufficient teeth present to indicate a precise intercuspal position, adjust the occlusal surfaces if necessary to ensure that this position coincides with the patient's muscle position. Do not prepare the teeth for abutment pieces until you have stabilized the occlusion. When there are too few teeth to indicate a stable occlusal position or when there is a gnathic dysfunction, construct a temporary acrylic appliance to stabilize the occlusion before further treatment.

4. Before proceeding with the design, make sure that there is adequate crown length for placing the attachments on the teeth.

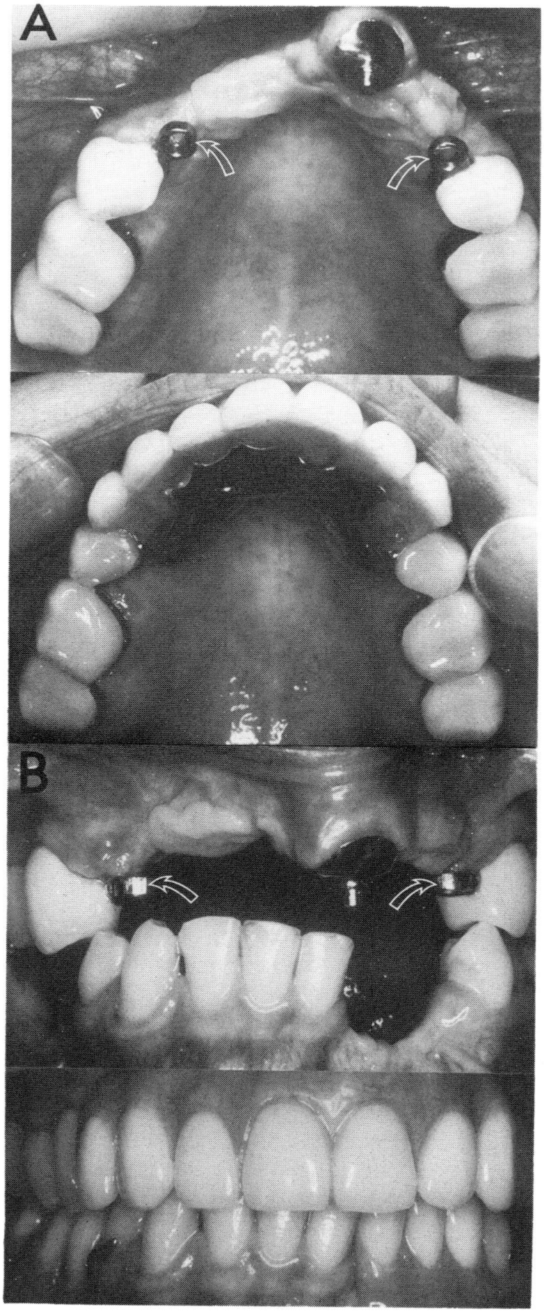

Fig. 13.2. Traumatic loss of anterior teeth following an accident has caused much tissue loss, which is restored by a complex partial denture. The attachments used are CEKA OL 444 rigid attachments (*arrows*) and a Baer cylindrical snap grip anchor (Cendres et Metaux 32.06.2 OSV) on the remaining central incisor. The posterior maxillary teeth are restored with full veneer bonded porcelain crowns. **A**, Occlusal view. **B**, anterior view.

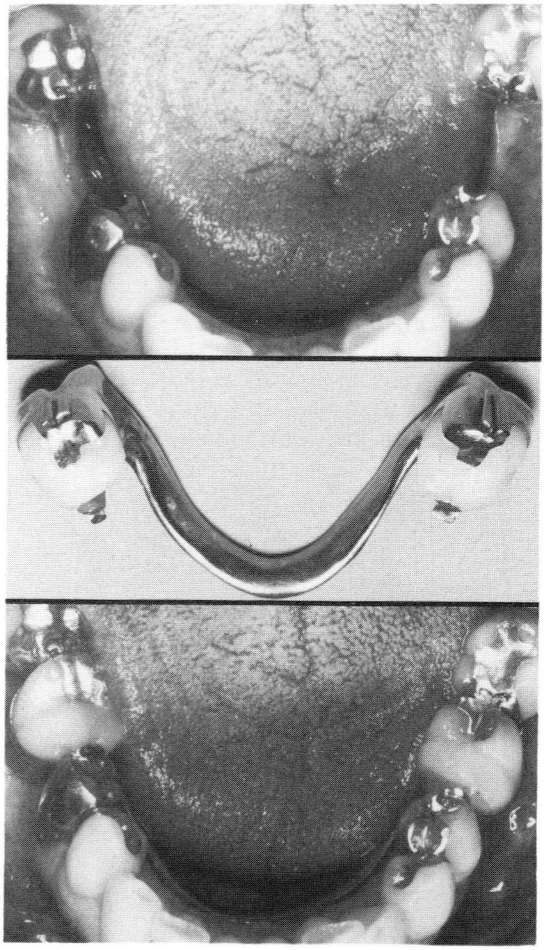

Fig. 13.3. A complex partial denture used to supply cross-arch bracing of 'weak' abutment teeth. This photograph was taken 30 years after the appliance was fitted. Fixed partial dentures are an obvious alternative in this case and would have been more streamlined, but would they have given such good service?

Occasionally, periodontal surgery may be necessary. If there is much attrition and the crown length is small, an overdenture might be indicated. These appliances are also classified as complex partial dentures, since they have some fixed parts and some removable parts. They are discussed separately in Chapter 14.

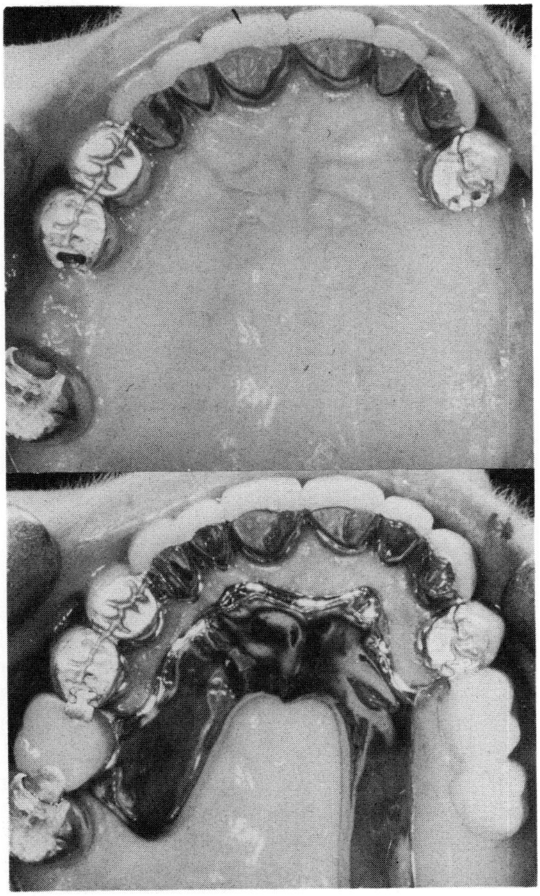

Fig. 13.4. Complex partial upper denture splints the remaining teeth and provides cross-arch bracing for the free-end saddle on the patient's left.

5. Take impressions and prepare study casts. Duplicate the casts and mount them on an articulator in the intercuspal position.

6. Survey the duplicate casts and with a milling cutter mounted on the parallelometer make minimal preparations of the plaster teeth (*see Fig.* III, 40). This is described in Appendix III.

7. To avoid undue cutting of tooth substance, identify groups of teeth on the cast with long axes that are nearly parallel to each other and decide on the types of locks that will be used between these groups. Arrange guide planes and formulate the general design as you survey the cast on the articulator, so that you can decide the type and distribution of the precision attachments for the removable part of the complex partial denture.

8. If some parts of the denture are mucosa-borne, decide the position and types of the stress-breaking attachments to the mucosa-borne saddles.

9. After completing minimal preparations with the milling cutter on the duplicate cast, construct temporary acrylic cover on the articulator to maintain the occlusion.

10. Next prepare the teeth in the mouth and take impressions of the preparations at the same visit. Also take an overall impression of all the preparations. In some cases adequate exposure of the gingival margins of the preparations is not obtained. If this presents a problem, place some retraction tape before the temporary cover is cemented and take the impressions at the next visit after removing the tape. There is a great advantage in doing all the preparations at the same time, but if this is not possible at least one quadrant should be prepared at each visit.

11. Correct and stabilize the occlusion on the temporary cover as soon as it is cemented. It is not good enough to 'hope that the occlusion will settle down'. The settling-down process may involve a change in the position of the mandible and hence a change in the occlusion of all the teeth and it is likely to cause a change in their position, which endangers the fit of the finished appliance (Watt, 1981).

12. Emphasize the need for maintaining gingival health while the temporary cover is in place.

13. Wax up the abutment pieces and with the appropriate tool on the surveyor carve or mill the wax surfaces adjacent to the removable partial denture. By means of a mandrel in the chuck of the surveyor, form recesses for the attachments or place plastic attachments. This ensures that they are parallel.

14. Cast the abutment pieces and where necessary mill them and solder the attachments before the patient's next visit.

15. Remove the temporary cover and fit each cast section in the mouth. Carefully adjust the occlusion before cementing the finished abutment pieces. Many practitioners

prefer to use a temporary cement at this stage to allow for 'settling down', but in our view it is better to stabilize the occlusion before cementing the crowns and then after cementing to check once again to ensure it is correct. If a temporary acrylic removable partial denture has been made, adjust it immediately after the crowns have been cemented so that the occlusion is maintained until the final appliance is ready.

16. After permanent cementation of the crowns, take an overall impression. The cast from this impression is used in the construction of the removable part of the appliance.

17. Complete the removable part of the denture and place it in the mouth. When precision retainers are used, do not tension them at this stage, but place them and attach them to the denture framework with self-curing resin, then remove and solder them.

18. Check the fit of the framework and then attach the teeth to it.

19. Instruct the patient in the care and maintenance of the appliance and again emphasize the importance of keeping the mouth exceptionally clean.

Advantages of Complex Partial Dentures

1. They are streamlined and can be kept within the limits of the denture space.
2. They are comfortable to wear and look good because no clasps show at the front of the mouth.
3. They last for many years provided a patient's oral hygiene is good.
4. The preparation and splinting of the abutment teeth ensures a favourable distribution of loads to these teeth.
5. The full veneer crowns, usually used as abutment pieces, protect the teeth against further caries attack.

Disadvantages of Complex Partial Dentures

1. They are expensive and time-consuming to construct.
2. If they break they are usually difficult to repair, unless special interchangeable attachments have been selected.
3. The high degree of clinical and technical precision that is necessary is not always available.
4. Gingival damage may occur because it is not always possible to make supragingival preparations for crowns used as abutment pieces.
5. Patients are not always sufficiently motivated to keep the appliance clean and it may fail because of this.

Summary

Complex partial dentures are sometimes considered to represent the acme of dental skills, bringing together the disciplines of periodontics, endodontics, prosthodontics and stomatognathic physiology to produce total mouth rehabilitation.

In the midst of prolonged treatment problems can arise when the patient tires and is unable or unwilling to 'take any more'. Treatment should therefore be planned to occupy as short a time as possible. It should be arranged so that completion of one stage at a time is possible and no great harm will come to the patient if a period of 'recovery time' is given before the next stage of treatment. This type of planning is welcomed by the patient, who pays for each section when it is completed. It is very important that the patient should fully understand the financial and therapeutic implications before treatment is started. The patient must also realize that regular visits for maintenance and plaque control are essential after the appliance has been fitted.

Chapter 14

Overdentures

Overdentures are made frequently nowadays because reliable endodontic treatment and good caries control techniques are available. Improved methods of oral hygiene and patient attitudes to tooth preservation also encourage this type of treatment.

As early as 1856 Ledger proposed a type of overdenture treatment when he wrote 'the remaining stumps I cut level with the gum. I then make a model of the jaw and a palate to fit. This will remain for years perhaps without the gums undergoing any material change.' Lukyn (1859) 'proposed removing the crowns and leaving the fangs, so as to prevent a loss of substance' and Atkinson in 1861 also recommended similar treatment. More recent publications have reviewed different aspects of treatment with overdentures and the types of attachments that can be used (Taylor et al., 1976; De Franco, 1977; Morrow, 1978; Brewer and Morrow, 1980; Jumber, 1981; Henking, 1982).

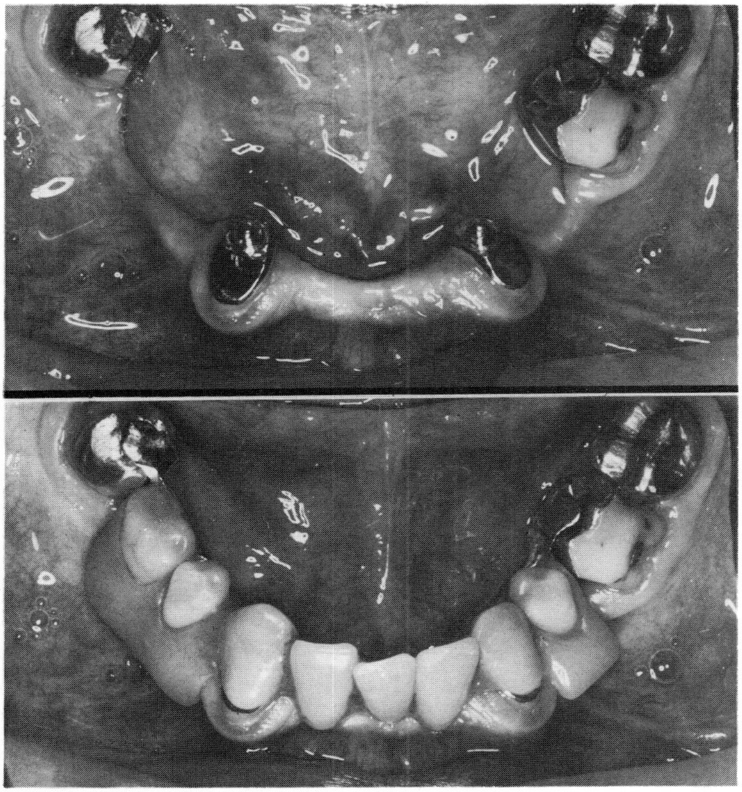

Fig. 14.1. Partial overdenture.

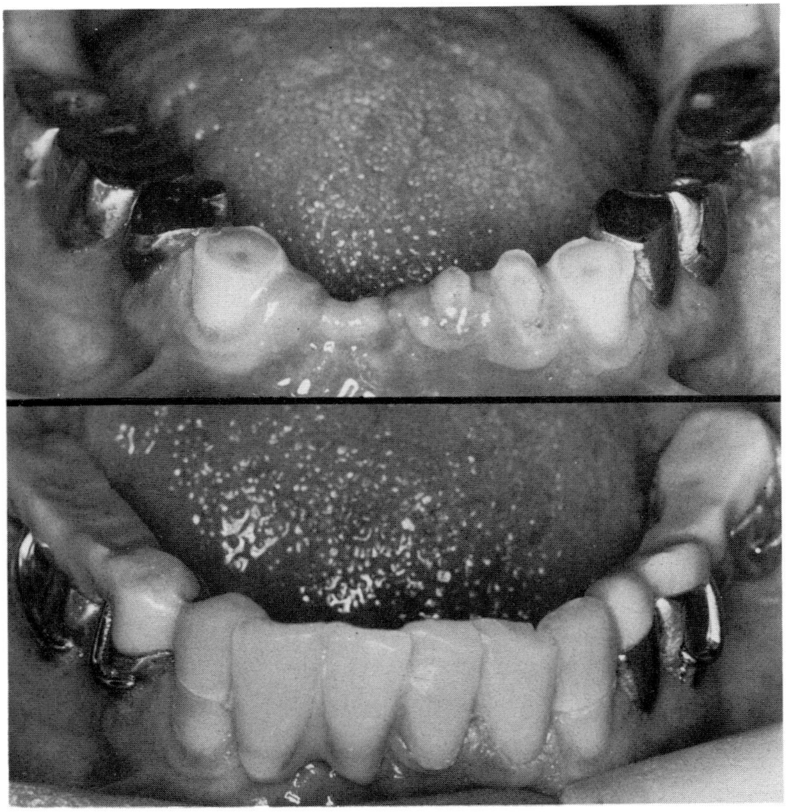

Fig. 14.2. An overlay partial denture.

Definitions

Overdentures may be defined as dentures that cover natural teeth or roots, but there is occasionally a confusion of terminology with regard to different types of overdentures and we use the following definitions:

A removable partial overdenture derives its support and retention from a combination of abutment teeth, retained roots, alveolar bone and mucosa. The design is similar to a partial denture except that some part or parts cover natural teeth that have been prepared or modified for that purpose (*Fig.* 14.1).

An overlay denture is a removable partial denture that has a metal casting or an acrylic extension on or over the occlusal or incisal surfaces of natural teeth (Heartwell and Rahn, 1974) (*Fig.* 14.2).

A hybrid denture (Brill, 1955) is a type of overdenture that looks like a complete denture but is retained and supported by natural teeth for which prefabricated or precision attachments have been made (*Fig.* 14.3).

Advantages of Overdentures

Preservation of Alveolar Bone

To a large extent alveolar bone depends for its existence on the presence of teeth. Treatment with an overdenture uses exposed tooth roots that in turn preserve the supporting alveolar bone (*Fig.* 14.4). However, MacEntee et al. (1982) urge caution in intentionally retaining submucosal roots to preserve the integrity of alveolar bone as exposure and sepsis with further loss of bone often occur.

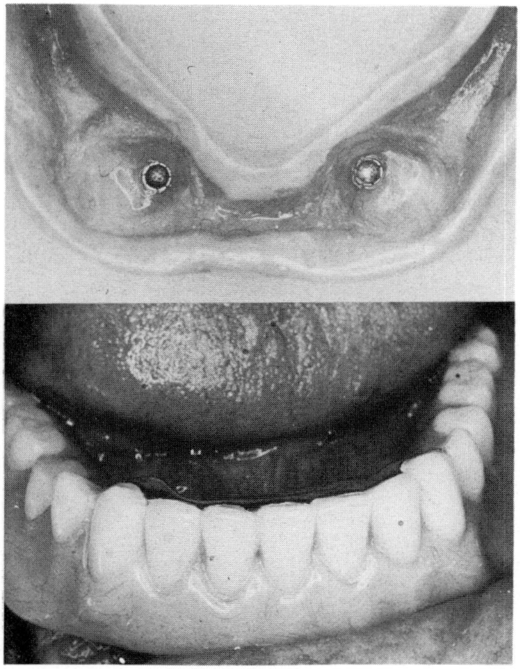

Fig. 14.3. Hybrid denture, as defined by Brill, looks like a complete denture but is retained by attachments on teeth covered by the denture. 'Overdenture' or 'stud-retained prosthesis' are other terms used for this type of prosthesis.

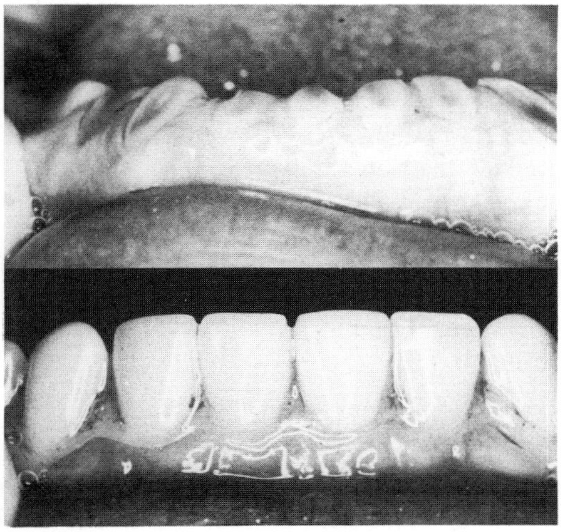

Fig. 14.4. Severely worn lower anterior teeth were rounded off and used to support an open-faced overdenture. The photographs were taken two years after the overdenture was fitted.

Support

In a patient with natural teeth the occlusal forces are sustained by the periodontal membrane. After the loss of teeth, the area of mucosa left for support is approximately one-quarter of the area of the periodontal membrane that originally supported the load (*see* Chapter 3). By retaining roots under an overdenture its support potential is increased. This leads to greater efficiency and comfort if the hygiene is good.

Retention

The retention obtained from clasps and the judicious use of undercuts is often sufficient for partial dentures, but the retention of overdentures is usually as good or better because of the accurate prefabricated attachments between the natural teeth and the denture. This makes the overdenture particularly suitable in cases where retention may be a problem, for example when the few teeth remaining have low crowns with no undercuts (*Fig.* 14.5).

Reaction of Patients

Losing teeth and wearing dentures may be thought of as a social stigma with psychological overtones of ageing. This is a complex problem with wide variations in attitude amongst different races and cultures. Partial overdentures provide a form of treatment that may be more acceptable than conventional partial or complete dentures. To some patients even one remaining natural tooth is sufficient to delay the helpless feeling of edentulousness.

However, the attitude of the patient towards preservation of teeth is important when considering the provision of an overdenture. It is worth remembering that the patient's neglect no doubt contributed to the loss of teeth, and the care of those teeth remaining may become a responsibility beyond their ability or interest.

Maxillo-facial Prostheses

Patients with congenital or acquired clefts, or defects arising from surgery or trauma, are often difficult to treat because of the deficiency of tissue and the subsequent problems of support and retention when designing

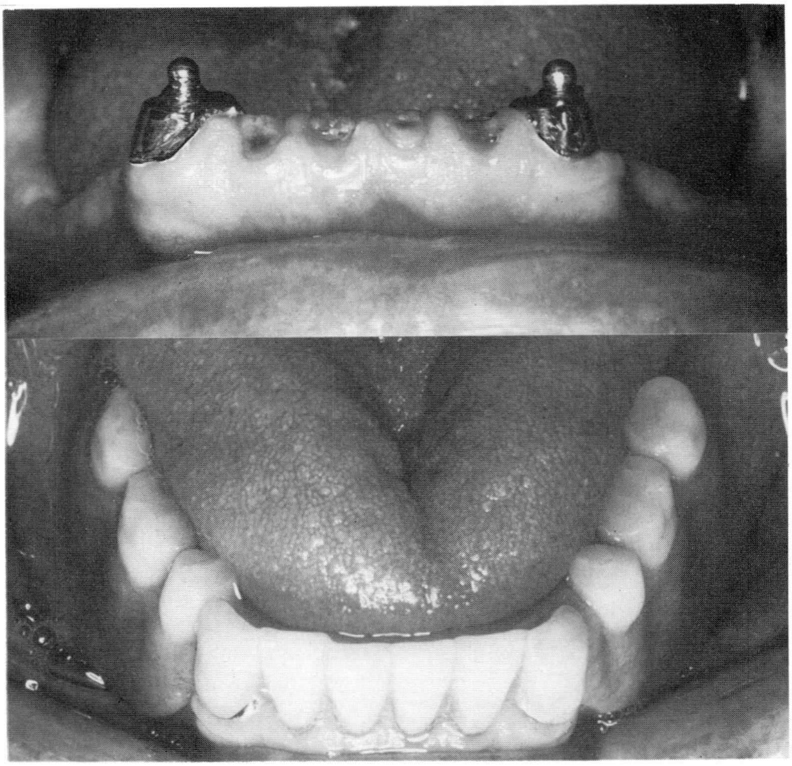

Fig. 14.5. Open-faced overdenture retained by Bona ball anchors on the mandibular canines. The photographs were taken four years after the prosthesis was supplied.

prostheses. In these cases partial overdentures, with the preservation of carefully selected abutment teeth, are a most useful form of treatment (*see Fig.* 7.14).

Some Indications for Overdenture Treatment

1. When there remain only a few natural teeth that are badly tilted or are unsuitably shaped to provide abutments for normal partial dentures.
2. When the prognosis of the few remaining teeth is poor, overdentures can often serve as transitional dentures prior to the loss of all the teeth.
3. When it is anticipated that the patient will have difficulty in adapting to complete dentures, especially elderly patients who have had little previous experience of wearing dentures.
4. When the mobility of the abutment teeth of a partial denture is increasing owing to an unfavourable crown/root ratio. Endodontic treatment should be given and the crown reduced in height and the overdenture provided to cover the abutment teeth. The reduction of the crown and the conversion to an overdenture improve the prognosis of the abutment teeth by reducing the crown/root ratio (*see Fig.* 10.13).
5. When patients have severe attrition of the teeth (*see Fig.* 14.4).

Patients with Severe Attrition

When a patient with severe attrition attends for treatment, the choice must be made between building up the worn teeth with restorations or grinding them down further and placing an overdenture (*see Fig.* 14.4). As a rule, the second alternative is easier, as making crowns or restorations on teeth with severe attrition presents many problems, not the least being finding root canals to retain the crowns. In addition, patients with severe attrition of anterior teeth frequently have missing posterior teeth that must be replaced with a removable appliance to prevent the patient damaging the new crowns by further attrition.

At this point the role of the periodontal and mucosal afferents in the control of the appliance replacing the posterior teeth must be considered. If the anterior teeth are restored by crowns and a mucosa-borne denture is placed behind them, it is likely that the denture will soon sink out of occlusion and the crowns will then have to take the greatest part of the occlusal load. Trauma to the teeth and breakage or displacement of the restorations or crowns may easily follow. Porcelain-fused-to-gold crowns are likely to last longest in this situation, but the crown/root ratio and the overbite of the restored teeth is likely to be greater than that of the worn teeth and the lateral forces on the crowned teeth are therefore increased.

On the other hand, with an overdenture the artificial anterior teeth are attached to the denture base itself, so that if the posterior part of the denture sinks it will do so around a fulcrum axis that crosses the natural anterior teeth. A shift of the denture base stimulates both the periodontal and mucosal afferents in an integrated manner that requires a different response from that called forth by the separate periodontal feedback when crowns fitted to abutment teeth are contacted by opposing teeth. This separate contact of crowns may over-ride the feedback from the mucosa.

Fig. 14.4 illustrates an acrylic overdenture provided for a patient with severe attrition of her lower anterior teeth. The photograph was taken two years after the denture was fitted and it can be seen that the gingivae round the remaining teeth remained healthy. The fact that the denture was open-faced, and that the artificial teeth were adapted to fit the worn stumps of the natural teeth, ensured that the gingival health was better than if the natural teeth had been completely covered. Movement of dentures that completely cover the teeth tends to produce traumatic effects that encourage gingival hyperplasia, but these effects are reduced when the denture is left open-faced. Another advantage of this type of denture is that the denture space is not encroached upon by an additional labial flange in areas where there has been no alveolar resorption (*see Fig.* 14.5).

While the open-faced denture is indicated in the lower jaw, a choice must be made with regard to maxillary appliances. When the retention is dependent upon the physical forces that normally retain a complete upper denture, it is better to fit a labial flange, as leaving the denture open-faced reduces the retention. On the other hand, if it is possible to fit prefabricated retainers on the remaining teeth, the denture can be made open-faced and need not cover the whole of the patient's palate.

Choosing Abutments for Overdentures

Periodontics

Gingival inflammation and bony defects should be treated. Teeth selected as abutments should have adequate bone support and attached gingivae. The crown/root ratio in a natural tooth is approximately 1 : 2 and after crown modification or reduction, this ratio should be re-established or improved. Thus a tooth with little bony support and poor prognosis becomes a tooth with adequate support and good prognosis. It is best to select teeth with roots at least 3 mm apart for ease of cleaning, otherwise stagnation areas occur. At least a third of the root should be present to justify its retention in the mouth.

Endodontics

In some cases endodontic treatment may be unnecessary before crown reduction. Abrasion or attrition, for example, lead to pulpal recession and the crowns may be reduced to the required shape and size without endangering the pulp. The surface is then rounded and, in some cases, covered with either a base metal or gold alloy coping. It is usually sufficient to leave the prepared root surface uncovered unless thermal injury is foreseen. Fluoride gel protection is necessary.

When endodontic treatment is required, it

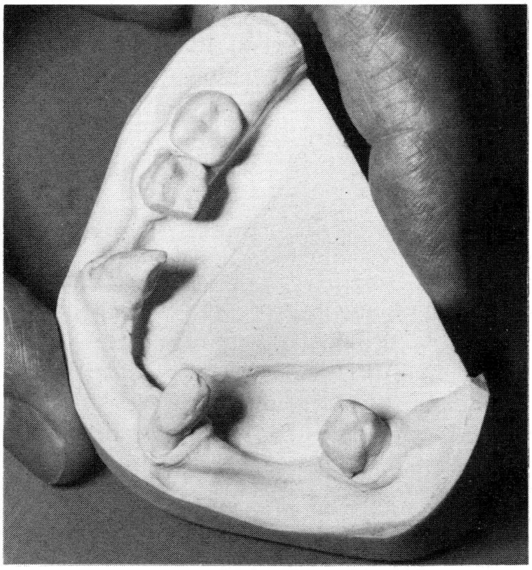

Fig. 14.6. Severe lingual inclination of canines and tilting of molars presents difficulties in designing a removable partial denture, which were resolved by removal of the crowns of the canines (*see Fig.* 14.7).

should be done very carefully to avoid future problems. Parkinson (1982) commented on the importance of good endodontic treatment. Endodontic treatment of selected abutment teeth makes it possible to reduce the crown length and improve the crown/root ratio. The interocclusal clearance is also increased and provides space for attachments and strengthens the denture.

Anatomy

Severe tilting may contraindicate the use of some teeth as abutments because of undercuts produced by the tilt. After blocking out these undercuts the flange of the denture no longer contacts the mucosa and spaces are left in which food accumulates. Appearance may also be adversely affected by this procedure, which increases the bulk at the denture periphery. However, these difficulties can sometimes be overcome by removing the crowns. *Figs.* 14.6 and 14.7 illustrate how reduction of the crowns of lingually-inclined canines and the placement of Dalbo studs on the shortened crowns make it possible to design a partial overdenture for a patient who had two badly tilted canine teeth.

Abutment Preparation

Several types of tooth preparation can be used for overdentures:

Crown Reduction with or without Coverage

This is the simplest approach to abutment preparation and is used mainly where the pulp has receded, the degree of which determines the reduction possible. The clinical crown is reduced without risking exposure or inflammatory damage of the pulp. The preparation may be rounded off and left. All undercuts must be eliminated and the tooth prepared either to a thimble shape or to a dome shape. Lateral load transfer is less with a dome-shaped preparation and for this reason it is preferred. If there is sufficient tooth substance the preparation may be covered by a coping, which may be made of either gold alloy or of composite resin (Renner and Foerth, 1978), but usually no restoration is placed as gingival health is better without a restoration.

Endodontic Treatment and Crown Reduction

Endodontic treatment is often required when space is needed for an overdenture. After crown reduction amalgam can be placed in a cavity cut in the preparation over the root filling. The surface is then rounded off and polished (*Fig.* 14.8). Alternatively, the canal is prepared and a gold post and diaphragm with a supragingival edge is cast to fit over the abutment.

Use of Attachments

Attachments for overdentures may be divided into two groups: intra-radicular anchors and supra-radicular anchors. An intra-radicular anchor is contained within the root of the tooth and so the tooth root must be large enough to accommodate it. The Zest is an example of this type of anchor (Preiskel, 1979). After endodontic treatment the root is prepared to accept the matrix, a hollow blind-end tube, which is cemented into place. The nylon patrix is contained within the partial denture and enters the tube in the root canal of

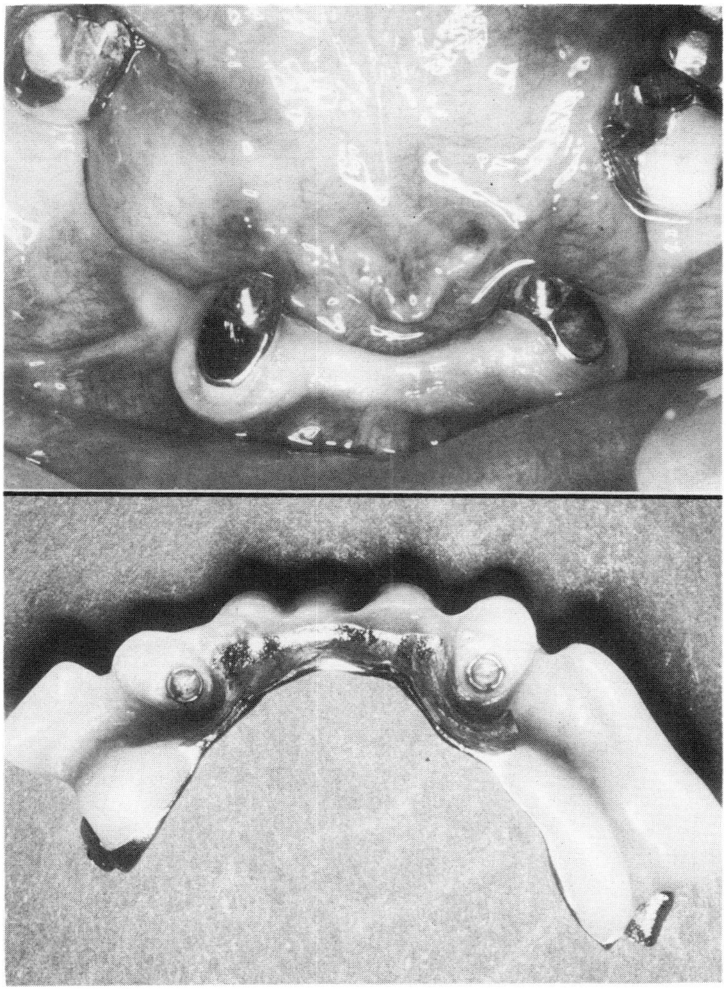

Fig. 14.7. The removal of the crowns of the canines shown in *Fig.* 14.6 and the fitting of Bona ball anchors 43.02.8 (Cendres et Metaux) provided a solution to a difficult problem.

the abutment tooth. The favourable crown/root ratio and low application of lateral forces make this a useful attachment. Detachment of the matrix and fracture of the nylon patrix can occur, but replacement is not difficult.

The Bona ball anchor is an example of a supra-radicular anchor (*see Fig.* 14.7). The patrix is a metal ball soldered to the root coping, which must incorporate a post in the root canal to provide sufficient retention. The matrix is a retentive socket incorporated into the denture. A similar attachment is the Gmür which is useful in partial overdentures because of its very small bulk as space is often limited (*Fig.* 14.9). The Gerber attachment is similar in principle to the Bona ball anchor, but the stud can be unscrewed from its base and replaced by a Schubiger ring and screw attachment to enable bar or other retainers to be used. Other examples of attachments for overdentures (Mensor, 1981) include the CEKA and the Rothermann eccentric anchor, the latter being especially useful when there is little vertical space. In some cases magnetic

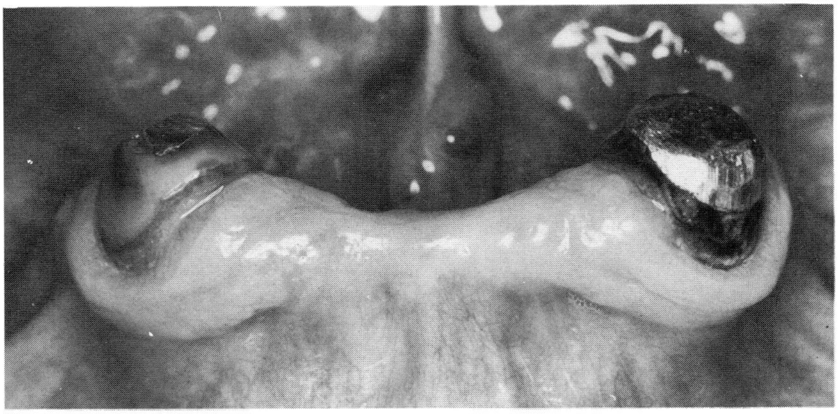

Fig. 14.8. Overdenture abutments. The canine crowns were reduced after endodontic treatment and the canals occluded with amalgam. Photograph taken nine years after treatment.

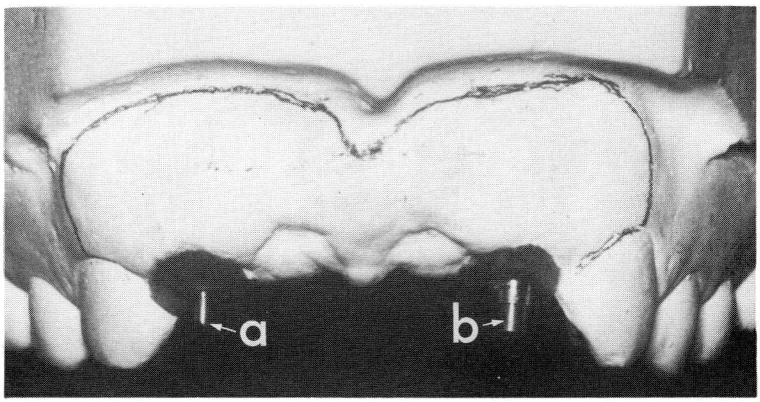

Fig. 14.9. The Gmür friction grip anchor (Cendres et Metaux) occupies little space and can be accommodated inside an artificial lateral incisor. (a), patrix. (b), matrix attached to patrix.

retainers may be incorporated in the root if sufficient space is available (Gillings, 1980).

Bar retainers connect two or more teeth or roots and provide retention by means of a clip set into the denture base. They give excellent support and bracing between abutments. Their bulk frequently makes it difficult to set the artificial teeth in their correct anatomical position. Types of bar retainers include the Andrews bar, the Gilmore bar, and the most popular Dolder bar (*see* Chapter 7).

Construction Principles

Overdentures are usually partly mucosa-supported and maximum tissue coverage is therefore required. If mechanical retention is not used, the techniques of complete denture construction should be meticulously carried out, including peripheral moulding and post-damming. The registration must be accurate, as any deflective or premature contacts cause movement of the base that produces an unsatisfactory result. It is also useful to take a check record to correct the occlusion of the dentures in the laboratory. During the processing stage a split cast technique should be used to correct processing changes.

Care of Partial Dentures

It is especially important that patients are instructed in the maintenance of a high standard of oral hygiene. After cleaning, to control caries one drop of fluoride gel should be applied once a week to each area in the overdenture contacting an abutment tooth. It has been shown by Fenton and Hahn (1978) that patients who did not apply fluoride to abutments had a higher incidence of caries than those who did.

Patients with overdentures should be seen frequently to assess their level of self-care and to make any adjustments to the dentures as wear and alveolar resorption occur. Toolson et al. (1982) have emphasized the importance of oral hygiene, adequate follow-up care and careful patient selection in treatment by overdentures. Failure in these respects can cause disastrous carious destruction of the abutment teeth and severe gingival damage.

Chapter 15

Appearance of partial dentures

When restoring the appearance of a patient with removable partial dentures, the aim is to replace all the lost tissues with a prosthesis that matches so exactly in form, colour and texture that it is undetectable. The morphological changes following tooth loss are discussed in Chapter 2, in which the design of partial dentures to replace the lost teeth and soft tissues is fully described. This chapter is devoted to further discussion of the selection and replacement of teeth. In Chapter 9 it was shown how the stated aim may conflict with other factors of denture design. For instance, it is clear that a patient's desire for complete restoration of appearance may conflict with the dentist's desire to make an appliance that does not cover the gingival margins and does not harm the remaining teeth and supporting structures. Thus, in all partial denture designing an element of compromise is necessary, and success depends on making the correct decisions for each patient.

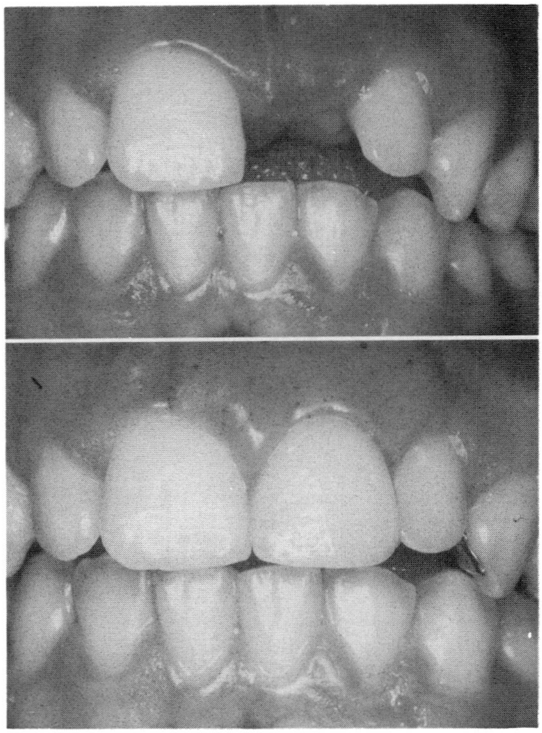

Fig. 15.1. Although the gap caused by the loss of the left central incisor has reduced in breadth, it is still possible to place a tooth of the correct size by fitting a flange and overlapping the left lateral incisor. Note that an attempt has been made to match the texture of the tooth with that of the right central incisor.

Tooth Size

The anterior teeth on a partial denture should always be of the same size as their natural counterparts. Even if the gap appears to be too small, in most cases it is possible to fit maxillary central incisors of the correct size by setting them further forward and overlapping them slightly (*Fig.* 15.1). An upper central incisor is usually about one-and-a-half times the breadth of the lower central incisor. This proportion should be kept in mind so that teeth of the correct size can be selected. A common error is to select artificial incisors that are smaller than the natural incisors. This is because the artificial teeth are positioned too close to the ridge and are set on too flat an arc (*Fig.* 15.2). The most labial portion of the central incisors is usually about 10 mm in front of a point at the middle of the incisive papilla and this measurement should be used to guide the positioning of the incisors and to ensure that they are set on an arch of the correct form. When this is done, incisors of the correct mesio-distal width can be set (*Fig.* 15.3). In cases of maxillary protrusion a large overjet may be present in the natural teeth, which should be duplicated in the artificial

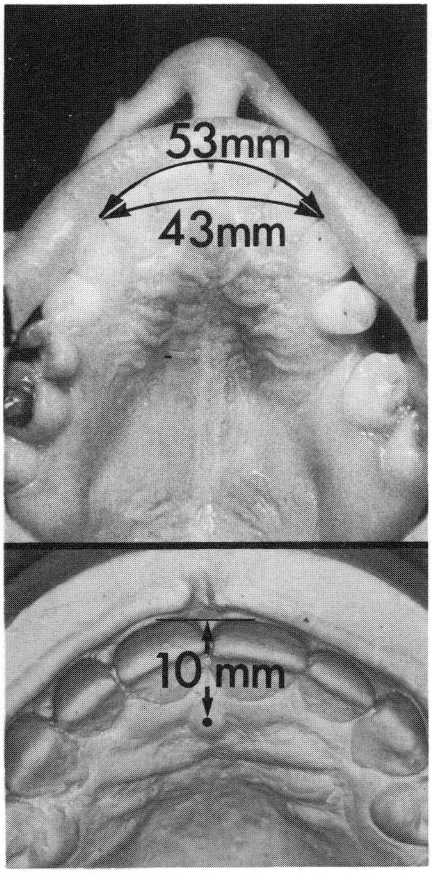

Fig. 15.2. *Upper,* The incisal edges of the incisors form an arc 10 mm longer than that traced along the residual ridge from canine to canine. Thus, incisors set 'on the ridge' are often much too narrow (*see Fig.* 15.3). *Lower,* The most anterior parts of the labial surfaces of the central incisors are usually about 10 mm anterior to the mid-point of the incisive papilla.

teeth in order to restore the appearance and produce a satisfactory lip form (*Fig.* 15.4).

Reduced Gaps

Bounded saddle areas that have been reduced through drifting of the adjacent teeth can sometimes be restored by orthodontic means before a prosthesis is fitted. If this is done, it is wise to fit fixed rather than removable prostheses, as these gaps are apt to become smaller during the night when a removable prosthesis is taken out of the mouth; the prosthesis therefore has to be wedged into

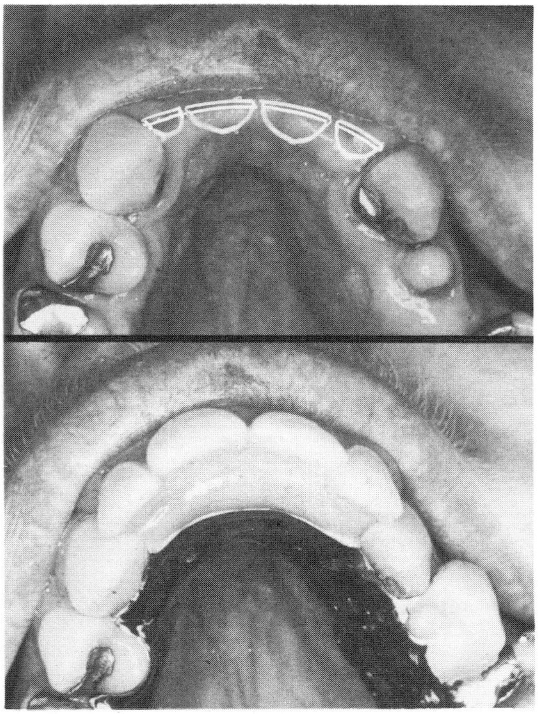

Fig. 15.3. Incisors set on the ridge occupy a much shorter arc than if they are set in their correct positions. The narrow teeth drawn on the photograph illustrate the disparity in size.

place the following morning, to the detriment of the periodontium of the abutment teeth. Sometimes, because of financial and other considerations, the patient is unwilling to have the gaps enlarged by orthodontic treatment and if the gap is unilateral some means must be sought to fill it with an artificial tooth that is the same size as its natural counterpart on the opposite side of the arch. A smaller tooth should seldom, if ever, be used as it looks artificial. It is sometimes possible to rotate an artificial tooth of the correct size in order to get it into the reduced gap or, alternatively, a tooth of the correct size can be placed slightly in front of the arch, overlapping one of the abutment teeth. Indeed, in most cases, if all the lost tissue is restored by an appropriately shaped flange, a tooth of the correct size and shape can usually be used (*see Fig.* 2.6). When the gaps are bilateral, it is permissible to use two smaller teeth as they do not spoil the symmetry of the arch.

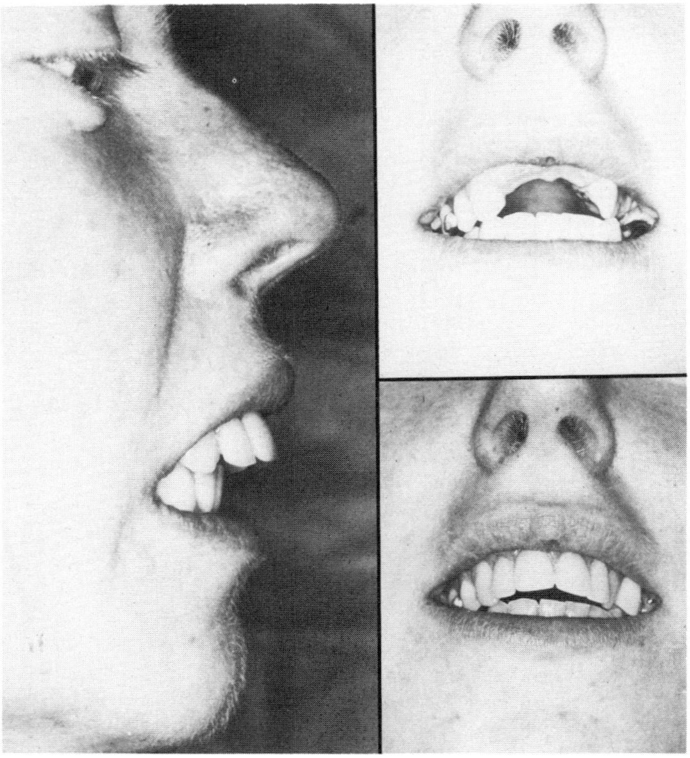

Fig. 15.4. The teeth on a partial denture for a patient who had a large overjet of the natural teeth are placed in the same position as the natural teeth in order to restore the appearance. Artificial teeth of the correct size were used. In the photographs on the right the camera angle was upwards to show the horizontal overjet.

Increased Gaps

Occasionally patients with large diastemas between their central incisors lose one central incisor and require its replacement. Provided the patient is happy to have a tooth replaced without closing the diastema, the problem can be solved as shown in *Fig.* 15.5, where the labial flange restores all the lost tissue. However, some wish to have the diastema closed and this can present quite severe problems. If the diastema is not very large, the remaining central incisor can be crowned with a slightly over-sized restoration and the lost central replaced by a pontic on a bridge. When a diastema is so large that this solution is not practicable (*Fig.* 15.6), it may be necessary to fill the gap with two central incisors and, by overlapping, the remaining natural central incisor can be made to look like a lateral incisor. A labial acrylic flange is necessary when this type of prosthesis is made.

Tooth Position

As already mentioned, when four maxillary incisors are missing, they are sometimes wrongly replaced by teeth that are narrower and smaller than the natural ones. These narrower teeth are selected because they fit between the two standing canines and are set close to the residual ridge. This produces a very flattened arch and spoils the patient's appearance, since the lip is not properly supported. Speech may also be affected by the incorrect position of the teeth.

The form of the lips is dependent on the position of the anterior teeth and knowledge of lip form can help one to decide where the anterior teeth should be placed. It has already been mentioned that the most labial part of the

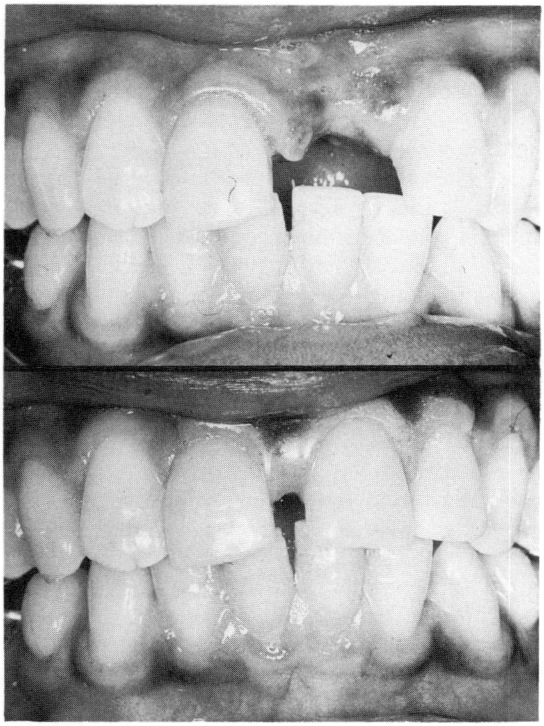

Fig. 15.5. *Upper,* A large gap caused by the loss of the left central incisor in a patient who had a median diastema. *Lower,* The tooth-borne removable partial denture to restore the gap has a labial flange which makes it difficult to detect in the mouth.

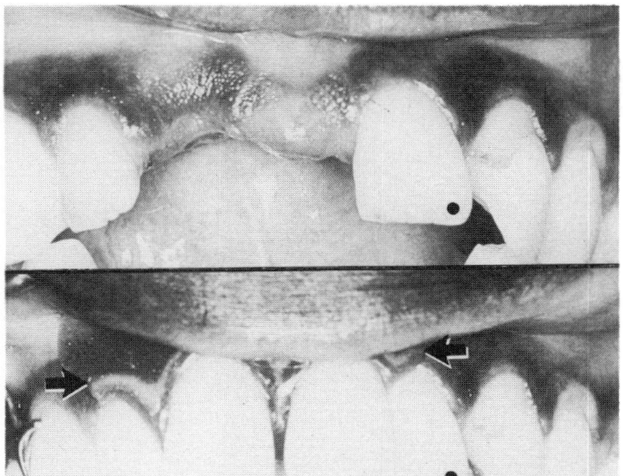

Fig. 15.6. A very large gap caused by the loss of the maxillary right central incisor in a patient with a very large median diastema. The gap was restored by a removable tooth-borne partial denture carrying two central incisors. The left central incisor overlapped the patient's own central incisor, so that it looked like a lateral incisor. In both photographs the dot is in the same position on the patient's central incisor. The arrows indicate the margins of the labial flange.

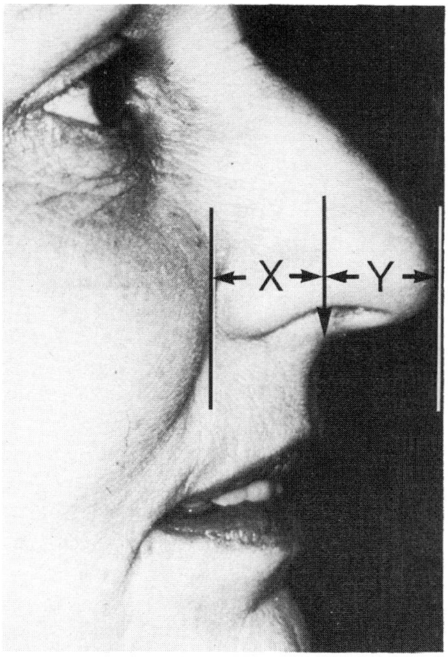

Fig. 15.7. When the lip is correctly restored by a denture, the middle of the curved junction between columella of the nose and philtrum of the lip lies half-way between the tip of the nose and the groove behind the ala. Measurement 'X' equals measurement 'Y'.

maxillary central incisors should be about 10 mm in front of the centre of the incisive papillae and this is perhaps the best guide to their positioning. If this measurement is less than 8 mm, the teeth have been set too far back in the mouth and the arch form should be modified to restore the contour of the arch and the support of the lip (*see Figs.* 15.2, 15.3, 15.4).

The following guides to lip form and tooth position are also helpful:

1. The middle of the curved junction between the columella of the nose and the philtrum of the lip should be half-way between the tip of the nose and the groove behind the ala (*Fig.* 15.7). If the nose is long the curved junction will be slightly nearer the ala, but the classic proportion is as stated.

2. In the classic Caucasian profile the angle between the columella of the nose and the philtrum of the lip is about a right angle and

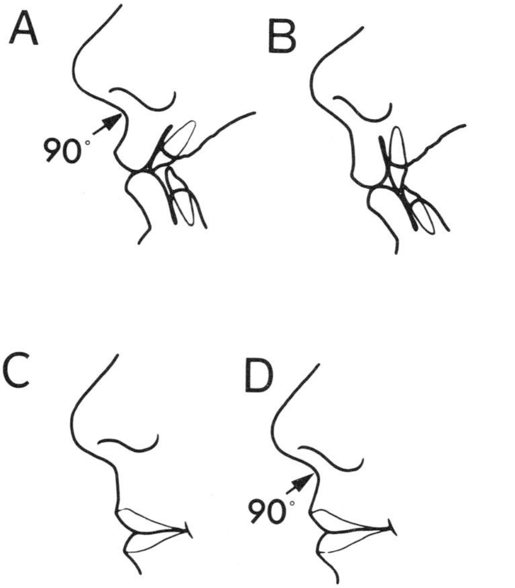

Fig. 15.8. The effect of tooth inclination and nose form on the nasolabial angle. **A**, When the teeth are proclined, the nasolabial angle is about 90° or less. **B**, When the teeth are retroclined, the nasolabial angle may be more than 90°. **C**, When the columella is prominent and the ala is high, the nasolabial angle is more than 90°. **D**, When the columella and ala are at the same level, the nasolabial angle is about 90°.

when ala and columella lie on the same level this is usually true. However, if the columella is prominent and the ala lies at a higher level, the nasolabial angle is usually greater than a right angle (*Fig.* 15.8C).

3. The angle of the teeth relative to the occlusal plane also affects the nasolabial angle. If the teeth are proclined the nasolabial angle is reduced, but if they are retroclined the nasolabial angle is increased (*Fig.* 15.8A, B).

4. When the upper incisors have been correctly positioned about 3 mm of the glossy oral mucosa, which contacts the lower lip to form the labial commissure, should be visible (*Fig.* 15.9). If the lip is incorrectly supported, only transitional epithelium will be seen as the lip folds inwards when unsupported.

5. The anterior teeth should be set on a curve that harmonizes with the curve of the natural arch and should so support the lip as to form a definite horizontal labial angle of between 90° and 120° (*Fig.* 15.9).

6. After setting the teeth, check the patient's speech and note that the incisal edges of the upper incisors hit the junction between the transitional epithelium and the glossy oral

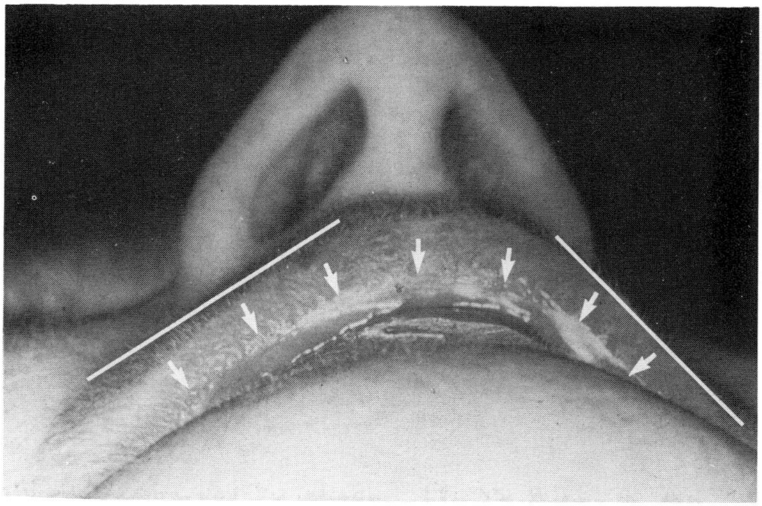

Fig. 15.9. When the lip is correctly supported (in this case by a record block), about 3 mm of glossy oral mucosa can be seen at the labial commissure. The arrows indicate the junction between the transitional epithelium of the red margin of the lip and the glossy oral mucosa. The horizontal labial angle between the sides of the lip (white lines) is between 90° and 120° in most people.

mucosa on the lower lip when the patient pronounces 'f' or 'v' very quickly.

7. In many patients the exact position of the anterior teeth is duplicated by immediate dentures, but some patients with prominent anterior teeth and deep anterior overbites want their incisors set further back so that they look less prominent than the natural teeth. This is usually a mistake as it causes thinning of the red margin of the upper lip. The best way to deal with this problem is to set the teeth at a higher level, but in the same forward position as the natural teeth occupied (*see Fig.* 15.20). The canine teeth might have to be shortened to accomplish this and this should be done carefully so that canine protection of the occlusion is not removed, but the appearance is improved.

8. The smile line. The upper anterior teeth should be set so that their incisal edges follow the curve of the smiling lower lip (*Fig.* 15.10). A pleasing effect is produced by this method of setting, because the line of the lower lip when the patient smiles is used as a visual reference line in the assessment of tooth position. Teeth that lie too near the lower lip are assessed as too long and those that lie too far away as too short. A common error in both fixed and removable partial dentures is that the incisors are set on a flat occlusal plane and this gives an artificial appearance to the appliance. Slight rotation of lateral incisors enhances the appearance by making each tooth separate from its neighbours. This gets rid of the 'all-of-a-piece' appearance that is so common, especially in fixed prostheses.

A more complete discussion of the setting of the anterior teeth and restoration of the lip is to be found in Watt and MacGregor (1976).

9. Dentists sometimes set teeth further back in the mouth to avoid the tilting forces caused by placing teeth in front of the ridge. This may be self-defeating, as putting the teeth closer to the residual alveolar ridge reduces the overjet. The lower incisors then contact the lingual surfaces of the upper incisors during speech and this dislodges the upper denture. In addition, the appearance of the patient is spoilt by the lack of upper lip support.

10. In patients with gum-fitted or open-faced dentures the lips are seldom supported correctly and it is usually wise to avoid these appliances unless tooth and bone loss are minimal.

11. When the lip is distorted by surgery or accident, the teeth should not be set regularly, but should follow the contour of the distorted upper lip. This is particularly important in cleft palate patients, as even if the lip is well repaired regular setting of the teeth looks artificial in these patients.

Tooth Form and Texture

The form and texture of the artificial teeth should match the remaining natural teeth (*Fig.* 15.11). Manufacturers' mould guides tend to concentrate our attention too much on the outline form of the teeth. It is just as important to select teeth that have the correct three-dimensional form. It is common to see artificial teeth that have a correct outline but incorrect body contour. Many moulds are too flat and it may be necessary to select a larger tooth with enough bulk to allow shaping to the correct contour without too much decrease in breadth. It is particularly important to select a tooth that has adequate breadth at its cervical margin. Artificial teeth of the correct breadth at the incisal edge are often much too narrow at the gingival margin, and a larger tooth should be selected and modified to match the breadth of the natural teeth at the gingival margin.

When selecting a tooth it is necessary to view the remaining natural teeth from all angles, especially from the side, so that the contour of the labial surface in the sagittal plane can be observed and matched (*Fig.* 15.12). When a tooth of the correct form has been selected, its texture should then be matched to that of the remaining natural teeth (*see Fig.* 15.1). A tooth of the right shade and the wrong texture may look more artificial than a tooth of the wrong shade but of the correct texture. The texture of tooth surfaces can be modified and individual characteristics can be added (Goldstein, 1976; Osborne et al., 1979; Eissmann et al., 1980; Martinelli and Spinella, 1981).

When examining the texture of the teeth, the light should be moved so that it strikes the teeth at different angles, and the highlights on

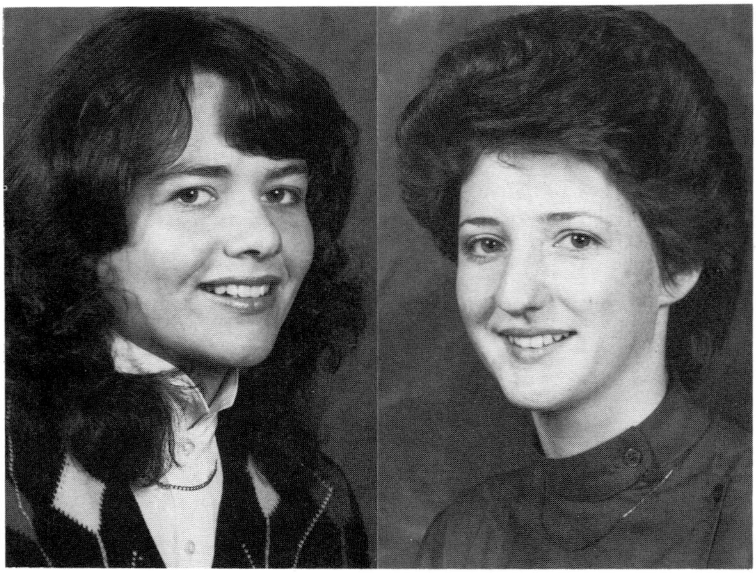

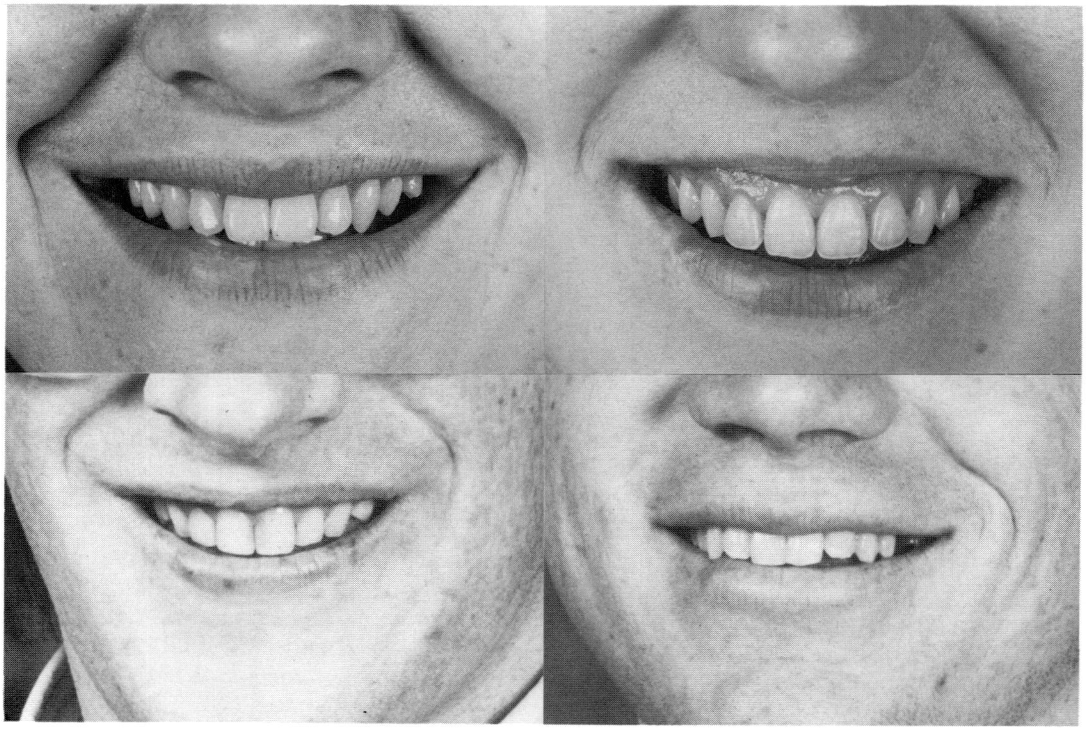

Fig. 15.10. In attractive smiles the incisal edges of natural teeth generally follow the curve of the smiling lower lip, which is used as a visual reference line in the assessment of tooth position. Note that in the bottom right photograph the right canine looks long and the left lateral looks short.

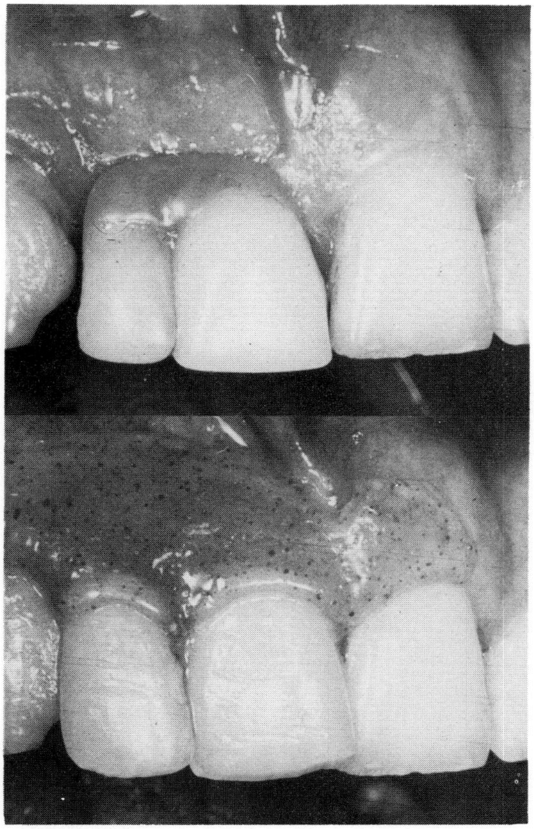

Fig. 15.11. *Upper,* How wrong can it be? Size, shape, shade, form, texture and position are all wrong in this inadequate denture. *Lower,* The replacement prosthesis is a marked improvement, but is spoilt by the mottled acrylic.

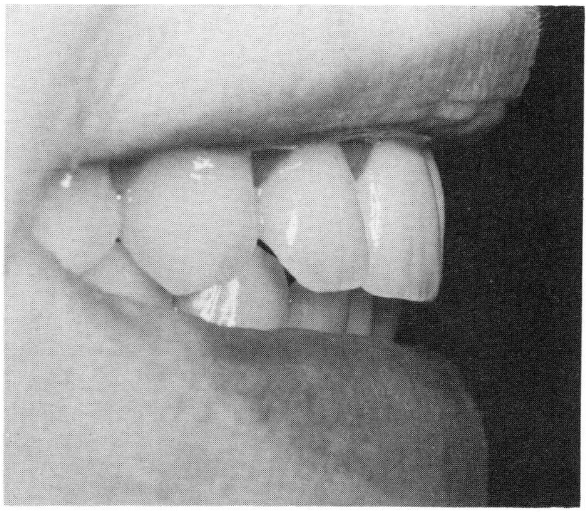

Fig. 15.12. When selecting an artificial tooth the remaining natural teeth should be viewed from all angles, especially from the side, so that the contour of the labial surface and the texture can be observed and matched.

the teeth should be examined closely to ensure that they are sufficiently broken up by the texture. Smooth highlights with unbroken edges usually look artificial. A very small round bur is used to put the appropriate texture on the tooth surface, which is then polished with tripoli on a cloth wheel.

Tooth Shade and Colour

The colour and shade of the tooth must match the adjacent natural teeth. Teeth are never pure white, but are cream-coloured, usually with a yellow, grey or bluish hue. There are three primary colours: blue, yellow and red. In varying proportions their mixture produces secondary colours. The 'hue' of a tooth is the distinctive quality of its colour. Each colour has a great many values. Tints are colour values that are lighter than normal and are made by adding white. Shades are colour values that are darker than normal and are made by adding black.

When matching the shade of artificial teeth, remember that the retina tires in about five seconds. After that time the ability to match subtle shades decreases. The teeth being matched should therefore be glanced at quickly; then the eyes should be averted to look at some neutral colour before again glancing at the teeth. The impression gained at the first glance is most likely to be accurate. The upper central incisors are usually lighter in shade than the laterals, which are usually greyer and more translucent. The canines are darker still and more opaque, and tend to be yellow rather than grey. The tendency is to select too light a colour and it is always wise to start at the dark end of the shade guide when selecting teeth. The teeth should be viewed from several angles before the final decision is made. Teeth that are darker than the natural teeth may make the natural teeth look artificial (*Fig.* 15.13). This is unsatisfactory and exact matching of shade and colour should be achieved. Illumination should be good when selecting shades.

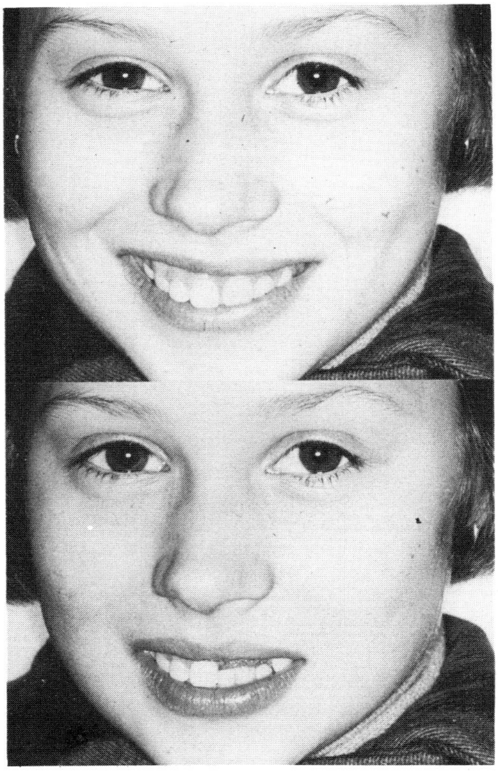

Fig. 15.13. The patient's right central incisor looks artificial because it is lighter than the left incisor on the prosthesis.

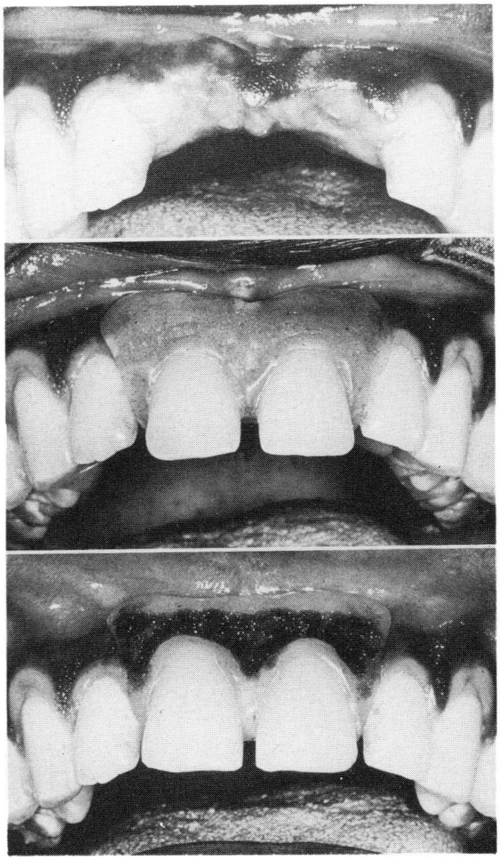

Fig. 15.14. The appearance of partial dentures is much improved by careful matching of gingival shade, colour and texture.

Daylight from a north-facing window is preferable, but a daylight type of artificial light is reasonably satisfactory. Avoid bright sunlight or ordinary artificial light, which is usually too yellow. Yellow light on a yellow tooth makes it look lighter. Hold the selected tooth against its natural counterpart. If the shade is correct, the one will merge with the other when your eyes are half-closed. Make a diagram of the tooth to be matched, indicate the basic colours from neck to incisal edge, and mark any cracks and stains that should be added to the artificial tooth.

The shade of the mucosa should be noted at the same time as the tooth shade. Various denture base materials can be mixed together in different proportions to produce almost any shade required. A shade guide for the denture bases should be made up in this way. Special colours can be produced by adding acrylic paints to the acrylic mix (*Fig.* 15.14).

Gingival Contour, Texture and Colour

Gingival margins of partial dentures should be contoured in the same way as gingival margins round natural teeth. The margin is furthest from the incisal edges at the most prominent part of the teeth and nearest the incisal edges at the least prominent parts of the teeth (*Fig.* 15.15), so that the buccal gingival margin of an upper incisor with a mesiobuccal rotation is highest towards its mesial margin and lowest towards its distal margin. The gingival margins of the central incisors are generally higher than those of the lateral incisors and the gingival margins of the canines are at a still higher level.

The texture of the gingivae is also important for patients who show their gingival margins

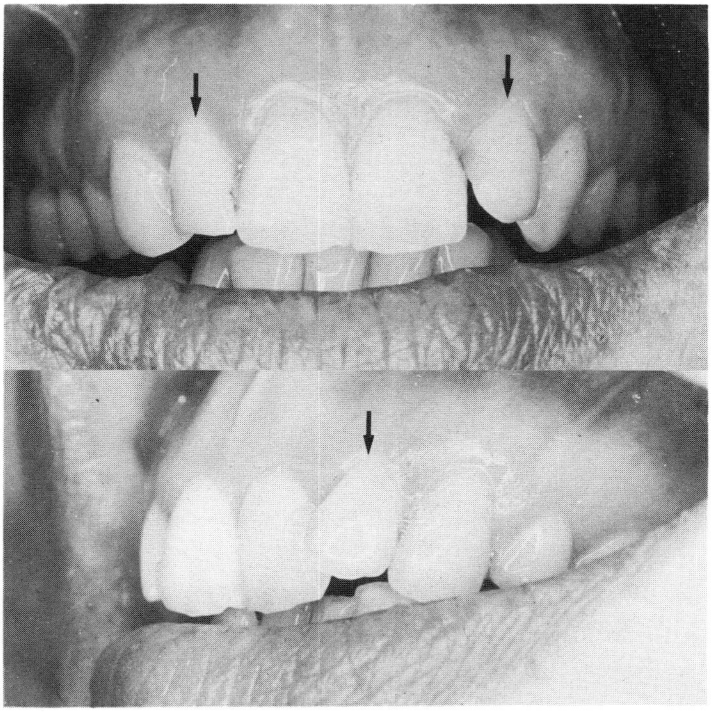

Fig. 15.15. Gingival margins are furthest from the incisal edges opposite the most prominent parts of the teeth and nearest the incisal edges at the least prominent parts of the teeth. The mesiobuccal rotation of both lateral incisors makes the gingival margins highest towards the mesial parts of these teeth (*arrows*) and lowest towards the distal parts.

when they smile (*Fig.* 15.16). The margin itself usually has little stippling on it, but about 2 mm from the margin stippling begins and is lightest opposite the most prominent part of the tooth and heaviest in the slight depressions between the teeth. In every case the gingival texture as well as the gingival shade and contour should be matched as closely as possible. Mismatches spoil the appearance of the denture. Few of the stock veined and mottled denture base acrylics are quite good enough, as they are apt to give a spotty or hairy effect (*Figs.* 15.11, 15.17) and some veined acrylics lose the included fibres and leave depressions on the surface of the denture.

How to avoid Clasps and other Alloy Components showing at the Front of the Mouth

A number of retentive systems other than clasps can be employed. Perhaps one of the simplest clasp retention systems for placing clasps out of sight at the back of the mouth is by using an oblique path of insertion for a labial flange that engages labial and mesiodistal undercuts in the incisor region. Molar clasps then provide retention posteriorly (*see Fig.* 8.2). The anterior flange lies firmly in the undercut in relation to the common path of displacement because of its oblique path of insertion. Thus, it retains the front of the

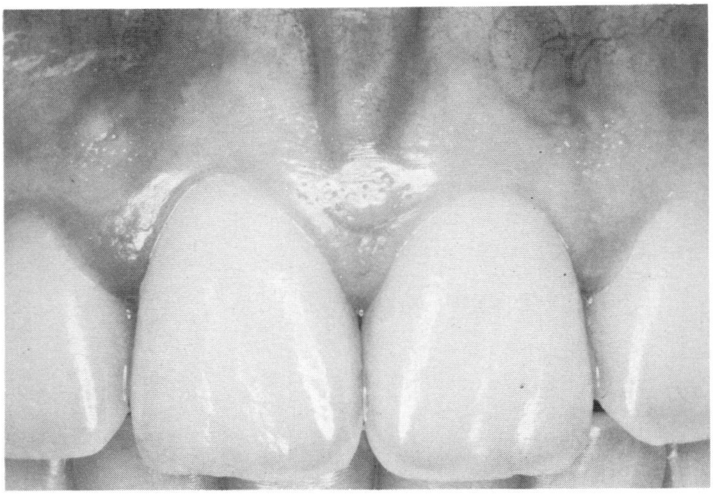

Fig. 15.16. The texture of the gingivae. The margin itself is fairly smooth, but stippling begins one or two millimetres beyond the margin and is most pronounced in the depressions between the teeth.

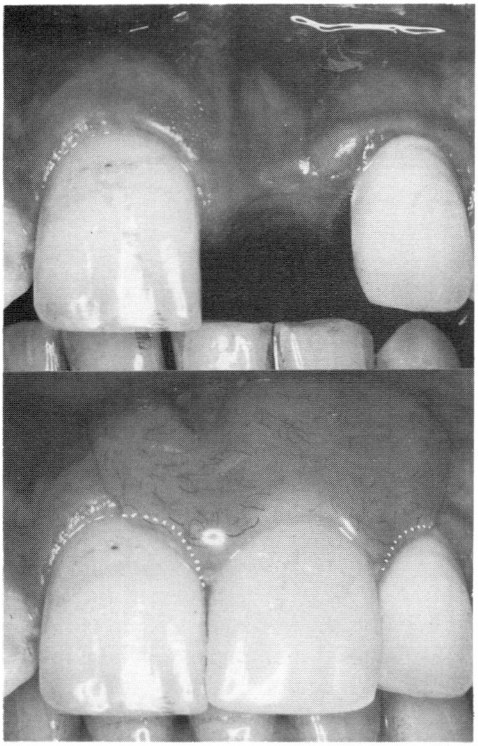

Fig. 15.17. The 'veins' in this acrylic flange are unsightly and the gingival texture and contour have not been duplicated. The dotted lines indicate the correct contour.

denture. Two-part and hinge-flange dentures provide an alternative method of retention that is virtually undetectable (*Fig.* 15.18). Internal precision attachments can also be used, but require the sacrifice of tooth substance and are sometimes difficult to hide in anterior teeth. It is usually better to use a system such as that illustrated in *Fig.* 7.23, when a channel shoulder pin preparation or a telescope crown is made in a posterior tooth to provide retention for a prosthesis replacing an anterior tooth. This has the advantage that a carious or heavily restored posterior tooth can be used without sacrificing sound tooth substance on teeth nearer the front of the mouth. When there are several gaps in the mouth and it is necessary to fit a removable partial denture, the remaining teeth that require endodontic treatment should not be crowned, but should have diaphragms and retentive studs or bars placed instead (*see Fig.* 7.17). The artificial teeth can then be placed on the partial denture (*see Fig.* 7.14) and the retainers can be hidden beneath them. This is better than making crowns (cf. *Figs.* 7.13, 7.14). Gerber attachments can be used on premolars, but are usually too bulky for upper canines, where Bona ball anchors, Rothermann or Zest attachments occupy less space.

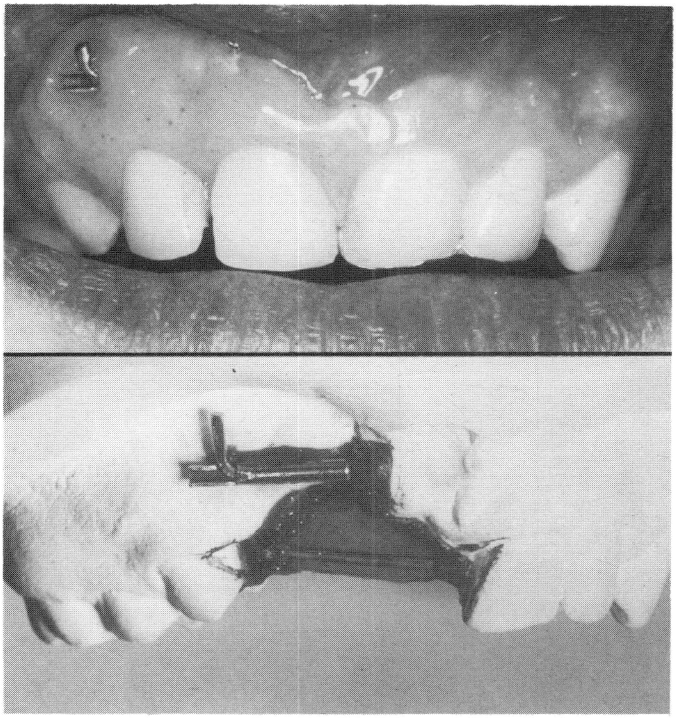

Fig. 15.18. A hinge flange denture for a cleft palate patient is virtually undetectable. The *lower* photograph shows the wax pattern with bolt and hinge mechanism prior to casting.

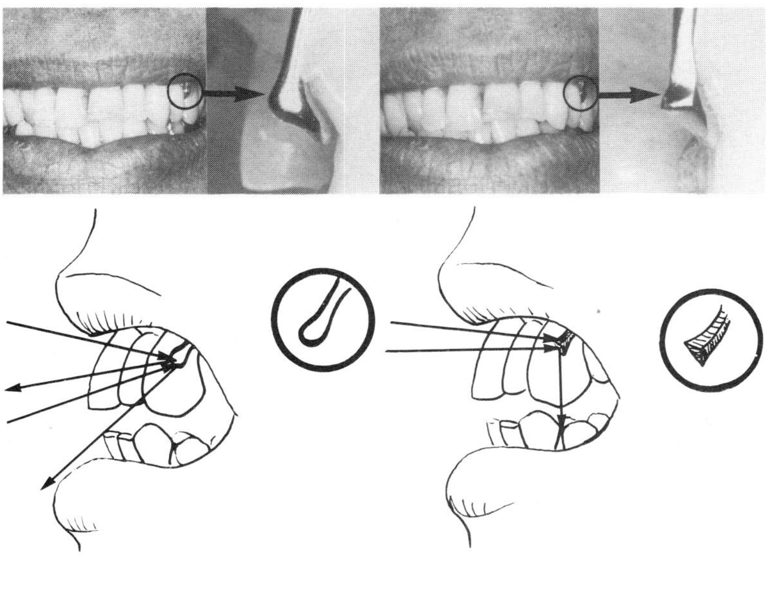

Fig. 15.19. *Left,* A clasp with rounded contour looks conspicuous because light striking it from almost any direction is reflected out of the mouth. *Right,* The clasp is made less conspicuous when facets that reflect the light into the mouth are cut.

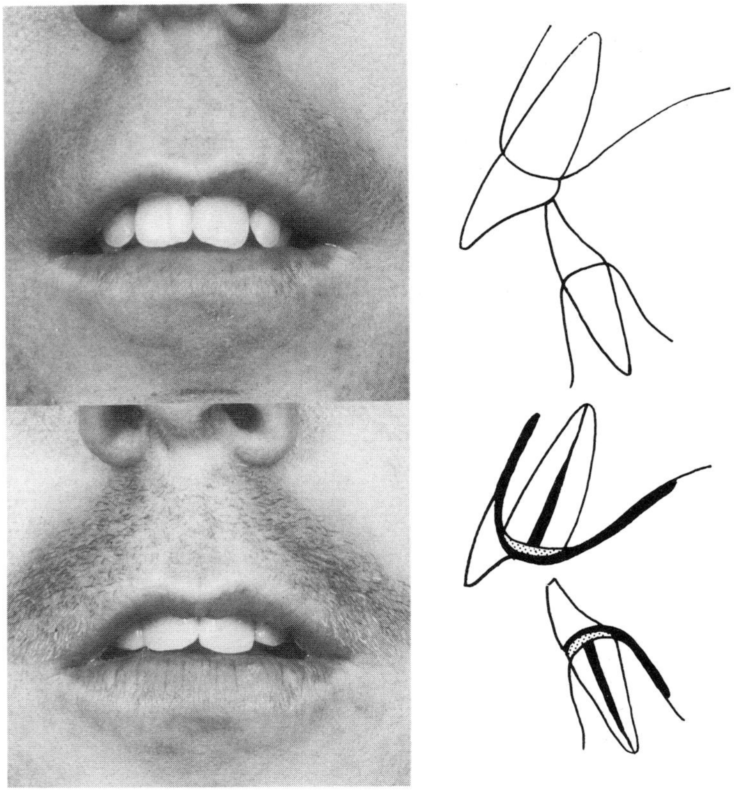

Fig. 15.20. Method of setting teeth for a patient with an Angle's Class II, division 1 malocclusion. The teeth are set in the same coronal plane, but at a higher level, and thus the lip form is preserved, although the teeth are less prominent. The procedure of root-filling and making overdentures is an alternative to orthodontic treatment or orthognathic surgery.

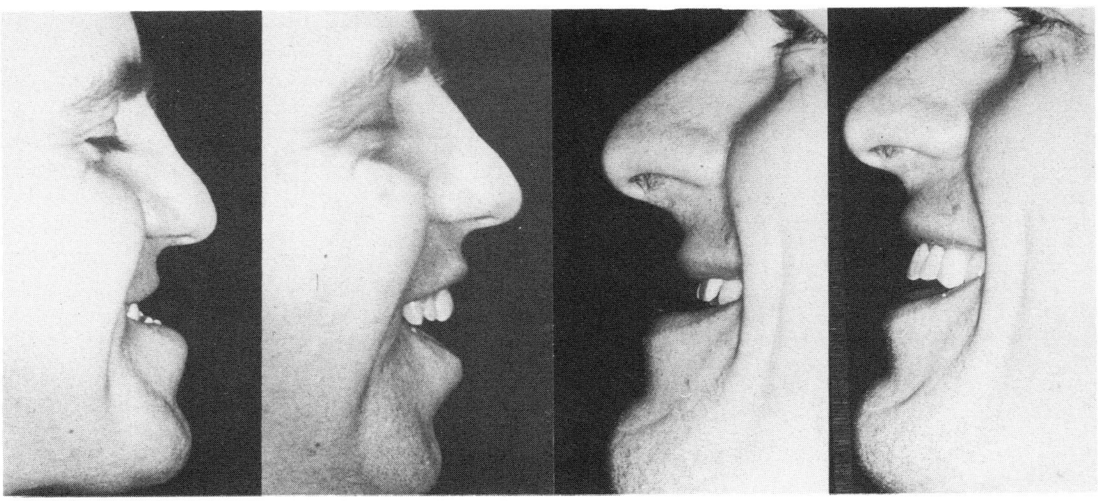

Fig. 15.21. The two photographs on the left show a patient before and after surgical reduction of mandibular prognathism. The two on the right show a patient without, and with, a removable overlay partial denture to correct a deficiency of the middle third of the face. The appliance is shown in *Fig.* 15.22.

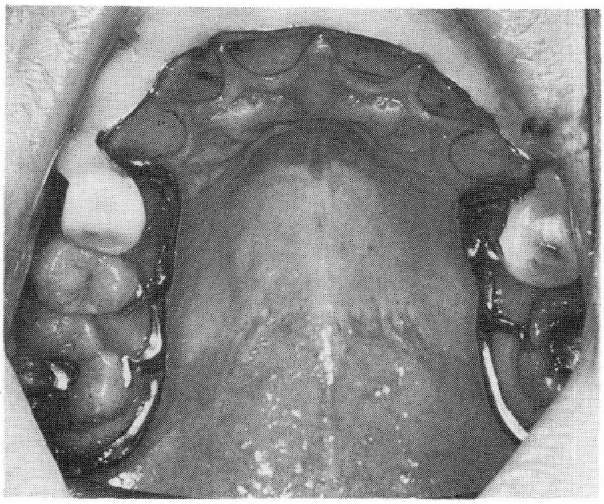

Fig. 15.22. Overlay removable partial denture to correct maxillary deficiency.

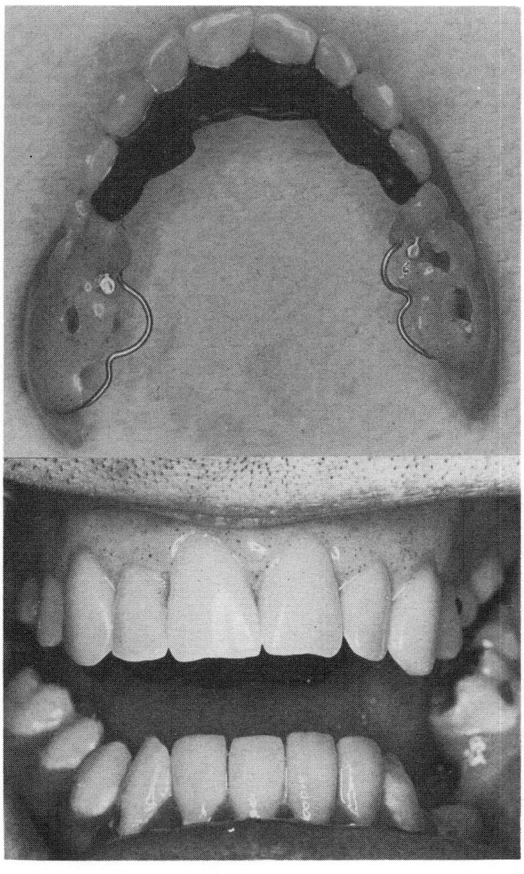

Fig. 15.23. A simple acrylic removable partial denture to correct deficiency in appearance caused by an underdeveloped maxilla. The natural incisors are masked with matt black acrylic.

Clasps can be made less conspicuous by forming them in such a way that light striking them is reflected into the mouth rather than back out again (*Fig.* 15.19). Avoid clasps of round or half-round cross-section at the front of the mouth, since light from almost any angle is reflected back out of the mouth. Clasp arms should be bevelled and faceted so that their surfaces face the dark interior of the mouth and thus any light striking them is reflected into the mouth and the clasp appears like a dark shadow.

Partial Dentures for Patients with Abnormal Jaw Relations

Maxillary Prognathism

Patients with superior prognathism occasionally ask dentists to remove anterior teeth and replace them with artificial teeth set further back in the mouth. Dentists usually resist such requests as they are aware of the long-term implications of loss of teeth, but occasionally the patient insists so strongly that the dentist extracts the teeth and makes a prosthesis with artificial teeth set further back. This has a disastrous effect on the appearance. The red margin of the upper lip becomes thinner and the lip loses its concave contour, and the nasolabial folds deepen, making the patient look much older (Watt and MacGregor, 1976).

An alternative treatment is to root-fill the upper teeth and remove the crowns and make an overdenture carrying artificial teeth at a higher level on the labial face of the gum (*Fig.* 15.20). This makes the teeth look less prominent, but does not spoil the youthfulness of the face. The patient is usually satisfied with the marked improvement in the appearance. The patient's appearance may not be the chief complaint. The main problem may be the lack of occlusion, when the lower posterior teeth do not meet the upper teeth, but pass lingual to them on closure of the jaws. Orthodontic treatment or orthognathic surgery can usually correct the defect, but, if financial or other considerations prevent this, removable partial dentures may be indicated. To provide occlusion for these patients, appliances either carry a lingual platform on the upper denture or a buccal platform on the lower denture. The latter solution is usually

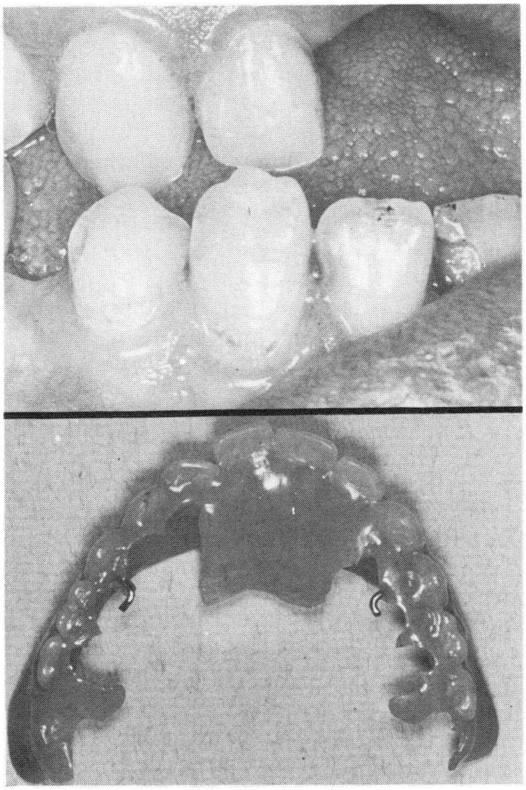

Fig. 15.24. *Upper,* Patient with marked inferior overjet and missing upper incisors. *Lower,* Simple acrylic partial denture to replace missing teeth and restore occlusion. (*See Fig.* 15.25.)

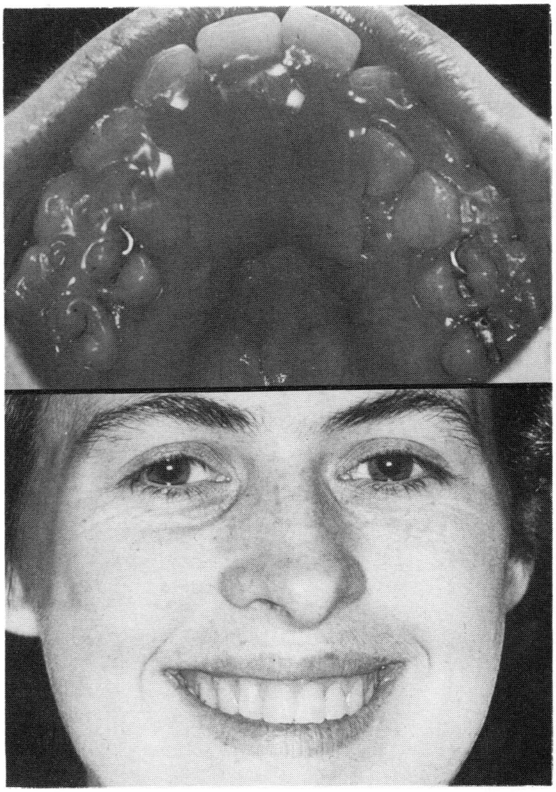

Fig. 15.25. The appliance in the mouth. The satisfied patient.

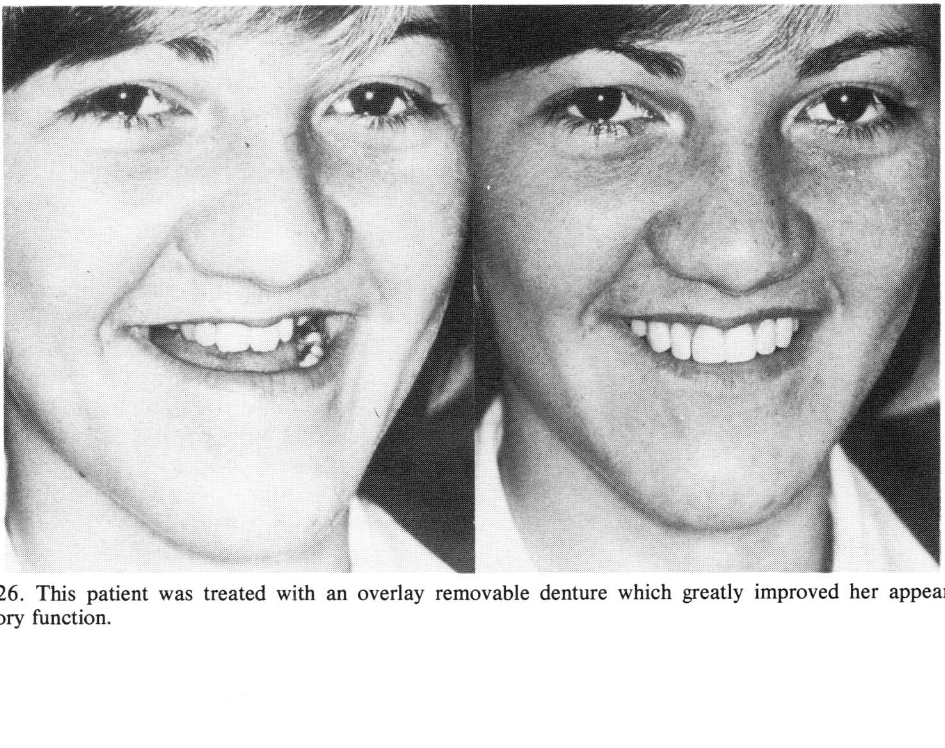

Fig. 15.26. This patient was treated with an overlay removable denture which greatly improved her appearance and masticatory function.

the more satisfactory, since the tongue space is not restricted as it would be with an upper lingual platform.

Techniques for the surgical correction of abnormal jaw relationships are now so well established that the wearing of permanent prostheses is unnecessary in most cases. Some patients refuse surgery and thus potentially damaging appliances have to be constructed. It is very important that the patient should have thorough instruction in oral hygiene and frequent topical applications of fluoride to avoid decalcification and caries of the teeth covered by the appliances.

Mandibular Prognathism

Surgical treatment of mandibular prognathism should not be undertaken lightly, as the fault in appearance is frequently caused by a small maxilla rather than by a large mandible. In these cases reduction of the mandibular prognathism produces a very radical change in the patient's appearance and the face may become weaker and more effeminate. While this might be acceptable in women, it is sometimes less acceptable in men. Thus, the patient often seeks advice as to how the appearance can be improved and it is usually wise to use a conservative approach to begin with, building out the maxillary arch to match the mandibular one (*Fig.* 15.21). The type of appliance usually depends on how much dentistry the patient is prepared to have done. A useful appliance is one that places a row of teeth in front of the patient's anterior teeth, supported on them by rests covering their incisal edges. The remainder of the appliance lies buccal to the arch with some lingual retainers. This design is usually quite easily tolerated by the patient (*Fig.* 15.22).

More extensive complex designs involving the preparation of telescopic crowns on the abutment teeth (*see Fig.* 7.20) or supporting bars (*see Fig.* 7.14) can be made if the patient is able and willing to have this done. A problem associated with the simpler appliance is that when the anterior teeth are placed in front of the natural teeth the lip tends to shorten and in order to preserve a reasonable appearance the artificial teeth must be set at a higher level than the natural teeth, which sometimes may show behind the artificial teeth and spoil the appearance. The obvious way to correct this defect is to reduce the crowns of the natural teeth and place retentive studs on them, but when the patient will only accept a simple appliance the teeth can sometimes be masked by covering with matt black acrylic (*Fig.* 15.23). Where the upper anterior teeth are missing this is not necessary (*Figs.* 15.24, 15.25).

In most of these patients a conservative approach with the prosthesis is tried before surgery is contemplated, and if the patient is not satisfied then surgery can be resorted to, but usually the restoration of the maxillary arch to match the mandibular one produces a satisfactory appearance (*Fig.* 15.26).

Appendix I

Oral hygiene

Dental Plaque

Dental plaque is the main aetiological factor in caries (Neff, 1967; Gibbons, 1968; Krasse et al., 1968) and gingivitis (Schei et al., 1959, Loe et al., 1965; Theilade et al., 1966; Jenkins, 1974). Dental plaque forms on tooth surfaces and restorative materials (Norman et al., 1972), usually adjacent to the gingivae and in the gingival sulcus (Cumming and Loe, 1973). Loe et al. (1965) have shown that plaque appears initially on the proximal surfaces of molars and premolars when oral hygiene is poor. Both clinical and experimental research have shown that inflammatory periodontal disease is more common in the interproximal aspects of posterior teeth (Lindhe et al., 1973). In fact, periodontal breakdown is usually found first in the mesial and distal aspects of posterior teeth, suggesting a relationship between plaque accumulation and disease. Research and clinical observation have shown that patients with low carbohydrate intake and plaque-free mouths demonstrate a very low incidence of new caries (Jenkins, 1974). Furthermore, the safe and predictable methods of water fluoridation and topical fluoride applications contribute significantly to caries prevention.

A high standard of oral hygiene prevents caries, gingivitis and destructive periodontal disease (Loe et al., 1965; Lindhe et al., 1973; Axelsson and Lindhe, 1974). The extensive literature on the prevention and control of caries and periodontal disease and the methods used to maintain good oral hygiene have been reviewed by Suomi (1971), but Theilade and Theilade (1976) emphasized that the impact of oral hygiene propaganda upon the prevalence of these diseases has been small.

If adults are given repeated instructions and prophylaxis, they will adopt the habit of good oral hygiene (Axelsson and Lindhe, 1978), while those patients who receive only symptomatic treatment will continue to have signs of gingivitis, lost periodontal tissue and recurrent caries. Results and comparisons like this indicate that routine dental treatment alone is ineffective as a means of curing caries and periodontal disease. The progressive breakdown of the periodontal support in marginal periodontitis is markedly retarded or inhibited by adequate periodontal treatment and plaque control, irrespective of the level to which the destruction has advanced (Suomi et al., 1971; Knowles et al., 1972; Nyman and Lundgren, 1973). A healthy periodontium without further destruction of marginal bone can be maintained with thorough plaque control. Bellini et al. (1981) reviewed the literature on the effect of oral hygiene on the prevention of caries and concluded that the quality of cleaning was probably more important than the frequency.

Damage Caused by Dentures

The few clinical longitudinal and follow-up studies that present material and methods of investigation correctly give evidence of tissue injury following the insertion of partial dentures. It is mostly the periodontal tissues that are traumatised, the changes being mainly seen as gingival inflammation and retraction of the gingiva. Caries and increased mobility of abutment teeth also occur. Inflammatory reactions of the mucosa covered by denture bases are often seen, as well as resorptive changes of alveolar ridges (Anderson and Lammie, 1952; Reichenbach and Kirchner, 1952; Wannenmacher, 1954; Anderson and Bates, 1959; Tomlin and Osborne, 1961; Carlsson et al., 1961, 1962, 1965; Derry and

Bertram, 1970). Koivumaa (1956) and Koivumaa et al. (1960) found that the incidence of inflamed gingival margins was 74 per cent in patients wearing dentures both day and night, but this figure dropped to 44 per cent in patients wearing them during the day only. In a group with no dentures the incidence of gingivitis did not rise above 3 per cent.

Brill et al. (1977) observed that, in an ecological sense, a profound change takes place in mouths with partial dentures. Addy and Bates (1979) provided further evidence of the potentially adverse effect partial dentures may have upon the supporting structures of the teeth when oral hygiene procedures carried out by the patient are inadequate. Common to many restorative procedures that encroach upon the periodontal tissues, partial dentures may have a harmful effect upon the very structures they are designed to preserve (Roberts, 1978, 1980; Ghamrawy, 1980). However, in a study of a selected sample of patients fitted with partial dentures, Bergman et al. (1977) did not support the general opinion that removable partial dentures cause periodontal and carious lesions. With careful planning of the prosthodontic treatment, and with adequate oral and denture hygiene, the remaining teeth will suffer little damage, if any. Fenner et al. (1956) and Dolder and Scharer (1961) discussed the differences in the traumatising effect of different designs of fixed and removable partial dentures, and Wetherell and Smales (1980) commented on the high rate of failure of partial dentures in a sample of patients and noted that few partial dentures survived for more than 5–6 years. More recently Lofberg et al. (1982) investigated changes in patients restored with partial dentures supported by bars fixed between canine abutments. They found that the clinical health of both hard and soft tissues was good after 3 years of wearing the appliances.

Removable partial dentures should be designed so that there is minimal accumulation of food debris and plaque on teeth and gingival margins. This is one of the benefits of streamlining, which has been emphasized in different parts of this book. As partial dentures are removable, cleaning the natural teeth and the denture should be a simple routine procedure, yet there are frequent occasions when dentures remain in the mouth for hours after a meal. Bearing this in mind, the design of partial dentures should avoid the intricate and complex in favour of the tidy and simple (Zarb et al., 1978).

Oral and Denture Hygiene

Proximal surfaces of abutment teeth accumulate the greatest amount of plaque and are the most difficult to keep clean. This can be shown by applying disclosing agents. Less plaque collects under minor connectors and clasp arms. Ghamrawy (1980) obtained plaque scores of the proximal surfaces of abutment teeth of patients wearing partial dentures. He concluded that, in spite of careful toothbrushing and appropriate oral hygiene instructions, deposition of plaque is a risk in any patient being treated with a partial denture.

Removable partial dentures should not be made for any mouth where the oral hygiene is poor. Patients should be given instruction in oral hygiene at the first consultation and then sent away to ensure maintenance of hygiene for a few weeks before impressions are taken. Hygiene of the mouth is particularly important if removable partial dentures are to be successful. The denture traps food against the remaining natural teeth and, even though it fits very closely, a solution of sugars and carbohydrates can be kept in constant contact with those parts of the teeth which the denture touches, encouraging plaque and acid decalcification of the enamel. It should be emphasised to patients that the usual method of toothbrushing (i.e. 30 seconds scrub round morning and evening) is quite insufficient to maintain the health of the teeth and the marginal periodontium, even when a partial denture is not worn, but when a partial denture is worn a particularly rigorous regimen of oral hygiene must be employed.

In addition to a normal toothbrush and pastes, special equipment must be used, such as interdental brushes, wood sticks, unwaxed dental floss and dental floss applicators. The latter should be inserted below bridge pontics in order to keep the undersurfaces clean and the gingivae around abutments healthy.

Regular visits for checking oral hygiene and for removal of plaque are part of an essential follow-up service for partial denture patients.

The Toothbrush

The use of the toothbrush has been described in various books and papers and in the plethora of literature produced by toothpaste manufacturers. Patients should be recommended to brush from the gingival margins towards the occlusal surfaces of the teeth with a rotating movement of the brush along the axis of its handle for the buccal and lingual segments of the posterior teeth. The same technique can be used for the lingual surfaces of the anterior teeth, but with the brush held vertically. There are many different techniques of toothbrushing in use, but no one method appears to be ideally suited to all patients; the roll technique is the most easily learned, but the attitude and manual dexterity of the patient must be taken into account. It seems that no one type of toothbrush can be recommended as superior to any other for general use by all persons.

Electric Toothbrush

There has been much interest in power versus manual brushing. Greene (1966) reviewed the literature on the subject and concluded that for well-motivated patients electric toothbrushes did not have any extra benefit, but for patients with less motivation tooth-cleaning was often more efficient with an electric toothbrush. Physically or mentally handicapped patients can often find great benefit from the use of electric toothbrushes and Ettinger and Pinkham (1977, 1978) have described various modifications of brushes for handicapped patients.

It is worth noting that there are no suitable powered denture brushes on the market. A rotary action with adequate torque would be an asset to some patients who find difficulty in cleaning their dentures properly.

Interdental Brush

Interdental or interspace brushes must be used with care to avoid damaging the gingival margins. These brushes must be carefully inserted between the teeth so that the wire does not prick or damage the gum. Brush heads are often interchangeable and should be changed frequently. Brushes with single tufts are useful in some situations where the 'bottle-type' brush cannot be inserted between the teeth, but they sometimes leave food debris untouched near the contact points.

Dental Floss

When properly employed, dental floss effectively cleans almost all proximal surfaces and contact areas (O'Leary, 1970). When interdental spaces are large, dental tape is even more effective. Unwaxed floss or tape is preferable as the wax, although acting as a pleasant lubricant, remains on the tooth surface and attracts further deposits of plaque. The floss or tape should be vigorously rubbed backwards and forwards and up and down on the proximal surfaces of the teeth; if there are particularly resistant areas of staining, a thin smear of toothpaste can be applied to the floss. Once established on the surface of a tooth, plaque cannot be removed by ordinary toothbrushing or flossing, but should be removed by the dentist or hygienist. Thereafter vigorous oral hygiene will prevent the re-establishment of plaque.

Wood Sticks and Rubber Points

The function of wooden sticks is partly to remove major food debris from between teeth where there has been considerable gingival recession, and partly to produce a stimulating massage of the gums to ensure keratinization of the interdental col. Where the interdental papillae are firm and fill the interdental spaces, use of wooden sticks is contraindicated as the gingivae are liable to be damaged. The fragile ends of the sticks tend to break off and become lodged in such spaces. Rubber points, often found at the handle end of some toothbrushes, should not be used as they may damage interdental papillae.

Water Spray Devices

A number of devices designed to clean the teeth and gums with water spray have appeared on the market (e.g. Water Pik, Teledyne Dental Products). The Council on Dental Materials and Devices of the American Dental Association has classified these irrigating devices as acceptable aids to good toothbrushing, but the general conclusion has been that these instruments are much less efficient than mechanical methods of cleaning the teeth.

Disclosing Agents

Disclosing tablets and solutions are important aids to oral hygiene as they indicate to the patient where the plaque is attached to the teeth. They can be used either before or after toothbrushing. If they are used before toothbrushing, the whole mouth is stained and the patient examines the mouth after toothbrushing to ensure that all the stains have been removed. If they are used after toothbrushing, thorough rinsing will wash away all the dye, except where plaque has been left on the teeth and it is on these areas that the patient should concentrate. The use of disclosing dyes is not widespread, however, and there is insufficient evidence in the literature to support the view that they have any significant effect on oral hygiene or periodontal health in partial denture patients.

Hygiene of Mucosa

All mucosal surfaces that are covered by the denture should be brushed each day with a soft natural bristle brush or, as the keratin layer builds up, an ordinary toothbrush can sometimes be used. The mucosa under dentures is protected from the massage normally provided by the tongue and food, and it is important that the patient should provide this massage each day by brushing in order to keep the mucosa healthy (Tautin, 1982).

Care of the Denture

Plaque collects on denture surfaces just as quickly and easily as it does on tooth surfaces, and patients should understand this. After cleaning the denture with brushes the patient should place disclosing solution on it, rinse it and note all the areas where plaque collects. The prevention of this plaque is of the utmost importance (Tarbet, 1982). It should be emphasized, however, that toothpastes should not be used for cleaning acrylic partial dentures, as they scratch the surface and make staining more likely to occur. However, toothpaste can be used to clean cobalt-chromium dentures without detriment, although a few drops of liquid detergent provide the best routine cleansing agent. Some parts of the fitting surfaces of partial dentures are difficult to clean with a normal denture brush, but can usually be reached with an interdental or interspace brush. The inner surfaces of clasp arms can be cleaned simply by attaching a loop of cotton string to a tap, coating the string with toothpaste and rubbing the clasp gently up and down along the string. Note that the wash-hand basin should be filled with water during this procedure so that if the denture is dropped it lands in the water and is not damaged. After a thorough cleaning of the denture, disclosing solution should be used again to check if any areas have been missed and particular attention should be paid to these. Patients should be asked to return to the dentist if they find some areas of plaque which they cannot remove by these means.

Denture Cleansers

Denture cleansers fall into four main groups:

1. *Denture cleansers containing chlorine.* These are chiefly based on sodium hypochlorite as used in household bleach. They are particularly useful for removing calculus from dentures, as the hypochlorite solution renders mucin soluble and the loss of this organic component from calculus makes it friable and easily dislodged. None of these cleaners should be used on stainless steel or cobalt-chromium alloy dentures, as they tend to corrode the surface and spoil the polish.

2. *Oxygenating agents.* Sodium perborate is one of the most popular of these agents, but if used too concentrated it can leave a deposit on the denture and, like the chlorine agents, can bleach the denture badly. Percarbonates can also be used. Hydrogen peroxide is occasionally used and also causes bleaching of the denture. None of these agents gets rid of calculus as efficiently as denture cleansers containing hydrochloric acid.

3. *Denture cleansers containing between 4 per cent and 6 per cent hydrochloric acid* are applied to the denture by brushing. This is a reasonably effective way of removing mild deposits of calculus, but these deposits

should not occur if the patient is cleaning regularly and correctly. Mild corrosion may result but, according to Combe (1981), a corrosion inhibitor may be present in some of these cleansers.

4. *Abrasive materials,* such as toothpaste and special denture powders, are popular means of cleaning dentures because they get rid of the stains very quickly, but they can cause severe abrasion and thinning of plastic denture bases and also spoil the appearance of acrylic teeth by removing the fine surface texture. They consist of chalk or fine pumice together with a flavouring. Some toothpastes contain essential oils that soften and damage the surface of the acrylic.

According to Combe (1981), work is being done on combinations of an enzyme, to render soluble the organic portion of deposits, and a chelating agent to affect the inorganic constituents. This is in the form of a solution in which the denture is left overnight. Augsburger and Elahi (1982) evaluated a number of proprietary denture cleansers which relied on soaking dentures, and Abelson (1981) found that an ultrasonic cleaner (Sonic Scrub, Clairol Inc.) produced good results.

Proprietary Denture Cleansers

1. *Oxygenating*
   Extradent (Corega)
   Steradent (Reckitt & Colman Ltd)
   Dental Cleansing Tablets (Boots Ltd)
   Superdent Tablets (E. R. Holloway Ltd)
2. *Hypochlorites*
   Milton (Richardson-Merrell Ltd)
   Dentural (Savory and Moore Ltd)
3. *Acid*
   Denclen (Richardson-Vick Ltd)
   Denture Cleansing Liquid (Boots Ltd)
   Steradent Brush-on (Reckitt & Colman Ltd)
4. *Pastes and Powders*
   Superdent Powder (E. R. Holloway Ltd)
   Denture Cleansing Powder (Boots Ltd)
   Dentu-Cream (Stafford Miller Ltd)
   Steradent Fresh (Reckitt & Colman Ltd)

Advice to Patients

The advice given to patients is not to use toothpaste on acrylic dentures, although it can be used sparingly on metal dentures. They should not use cleansers containing chlorine on metal dentures, although they are advantageous for occasional use by patients who find calculus collecting on acrylic dentures. In general the dentures should be cleaned with a little soap or liquid detergent with a bristle denture brush, which cleans better than nylon brushes as the ends of the nylon monofilaments are frequently rounded and have very little power to remove debris. The role of a detergent is that of wetting agent and emulsifier. Soap, the sodium salt of long-chain acids, was the principle detergent until superseded by synthetic detergents, which are usually sodium salts of alkyl sulphates or sulphonates.

Although a cloth can clean flat denture surfaces very thoroughly, it is dangerous to use a cloth on a partial denture carrying clasps as it can easily stick in the clasps and bend them. Patients should be particularly warned about distortion of the denture connectors and clasps during cleaning of their denture and the method of cleaning should be clearly demonstrated.

Appendix II

Preparation of the mouth for removable partial dentures

Oral Hygiene

Before partial dentures are made, your patients must show that they are capable of keeping their mouths and teeth very clean. This has been emphasized in Appendix I. In addition, patients should be told to massage the hard palate and the saddle areas with a toothbrush, so that the mucosa is firm and pink and capable of bearing the masticatory load on the saddles. If the patient is unable or unwilling to maintain this good oral care, then it is probably unwise to construct partial dentures.

Restorations

Caries and periodontal lesions must be eliminated before impressions are taken. Remove overhanging margins of restorations and replace faulty restorations. It is important that appropriate restorations should be made on abutment teeth. Porcelain jacket crowns should generally be avoided in partially edentulous mouths as they make very poor abutments. Teeth that have to be root-filled should not necessarily be crowned; instead, place Rothermann attachments, Dalla Bona or Gerber buttons on them to provide retention for the removable appliance. This arrangement is better than crowning, since it avoids clasps showing at the front of the mouth. Where the saddles are short-bounded, fixed prostheses are usually better than removable prostheses.

Guiding Surfaces

When surveying a cast before constructing a partial denture, use the analysing rod to identify as many parallel tooth surfaces as possible. Choose a path of insertion and removal that is also parallel to these guiding surfaces which guide removable partial dentures towards their final position in the mouth. Some believe that the advantages to be gained by using these parallel guiding surfaces or guide planes are such that the shape of teeth should be modified to increase the number of surfaces and ensure, as far as possible, a single path of insertion and removal for all the saddles of the denture. It is sometimes difficult to persuade patients to have teeth prepared to provide guiding surfaces for a removable partial denture. It is unwise to insist, as patients may feel that tooth preparation is unnecessary in the absence of caries and they may resent the treatment. Our usual advice is that if guiding surfaces are present, they should be used. If they are not present, it is usually unwise to prepare them, unless the teeth have already been restored or require restorations on which guiding surfaces can be built.

Rest Seats for Tooth-borne Partial Dentures

When planning the support of tooth-borne partial dentures, it is often necessary to grind teeth in order to provide space for occlusal rests and to ensure that the rests direct masticatory forces down the long axes of the abutment teeth. Rest seats should not be cut through the enamel. If deeper rest seats are required, restorations should be placed into which rest seats may be cut. Rest seats in enamel should always be self-cleansing. On the occlusal surfaces of posterior teeth they should be dish-shaped and on the marginal

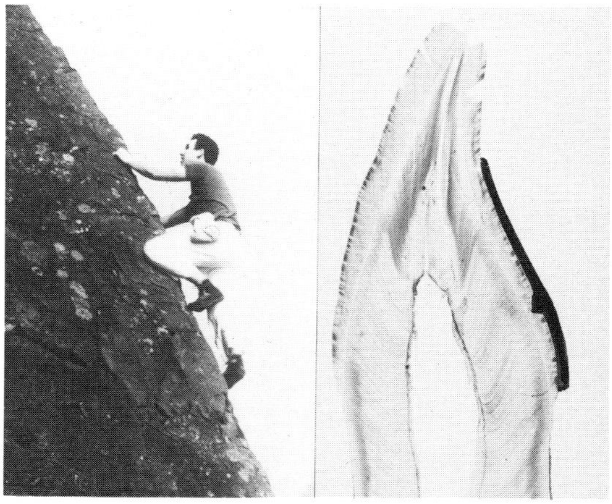

Fig. II.1. Just as tiny ledges prevent rock climbers slipping, so tiny rest seats prevent dentures slipping down the slippery slopes of the lingual surfaces of teeth. (*Photograph of climber by Allan Scott.*)

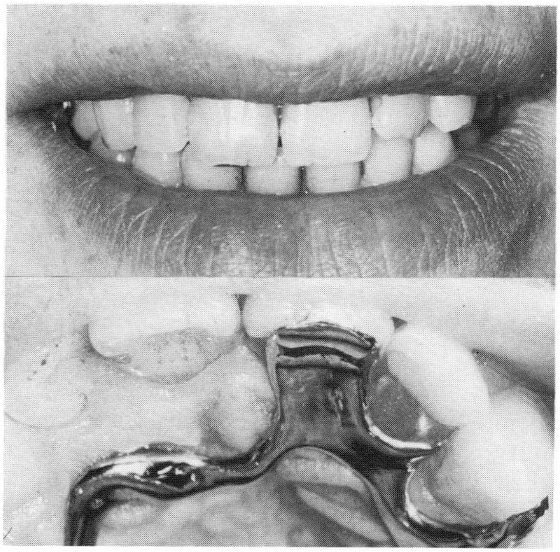

Fig. II.3. Incisal rest on right central incisor. Mirror image of denture in mouth.

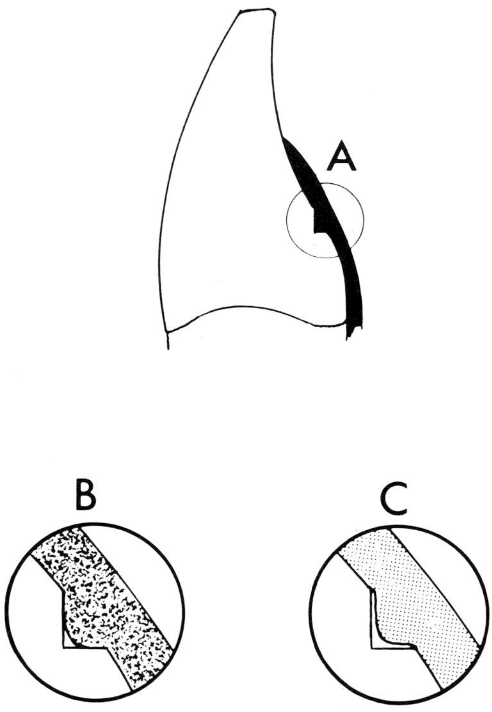

Fig. II.2. **A**, Dentures should enter the rest seats and fit them accurately. **B**, Casting shrinkage of cobalt-chromium alloys, or excessive polishing, can prevent a close fit. **C**, Careless use of separating medium when making acrylic dentures can also prevent a close fit of the denture to the rest seat.

ridges of anterior teeth narrow notches should be cut. The floors of these notches should be flat and at right angles to the long axis of the teeth. Just as tiny ledges provide adequate finger holds for a rock climber, so tiny notches prevent dentures slipping down the slippery slopes of the lingual surfaces of anterior teeth (*Fig.* II.1). It is essential that the occlusal rests on the denture base engage the rest seats. Contraction of alloy or acrylic denture bases on processing, excessive electropolishing, or using too much separating medium on the stone cast can easily prevent correct contact of the rests with the rest seats and hence defeat their purpose. This point should be carefully checked when the denture is fitted (*Fig.* II.2). Rest seats on anterior teeth can also be cut on the incisal edges. In this position they are usually made semilunar in shape and occupy only the lingual part of the incisal edge. The labial enamel remains intact and the incisal rest is hidden (*Fig.* II.3). Before cutting rest seats on maxillary anterior teeth, the parts of their lingual surfaces that are contacted by the lower incisors should be marked: place a piece of articulating paper between the anterior teeth and ask the patient to slide the jaws in occlusion from side to side and forwards and backwards (*Fig.* II.4), so that the whole contacting surface is shown. The articulating

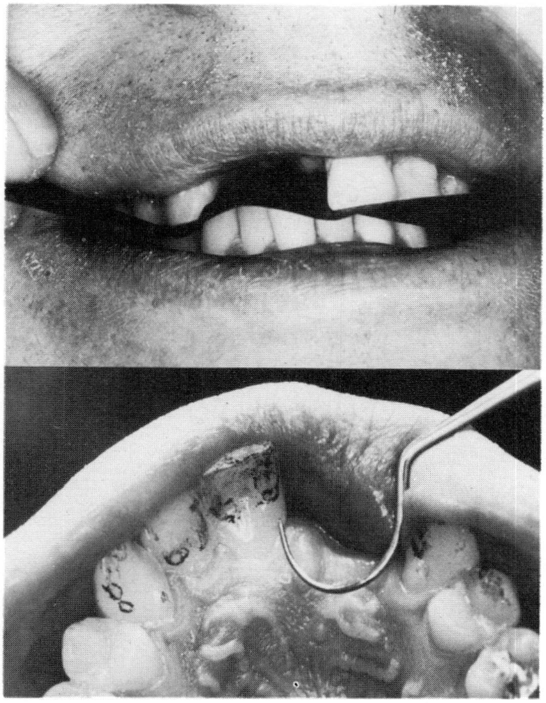

Fig. II.4. *Upper,* Marking the incisal contact area with thick articulating paper. *Lower,* (mirror image photograph). Probe indicates area available for rest seat.

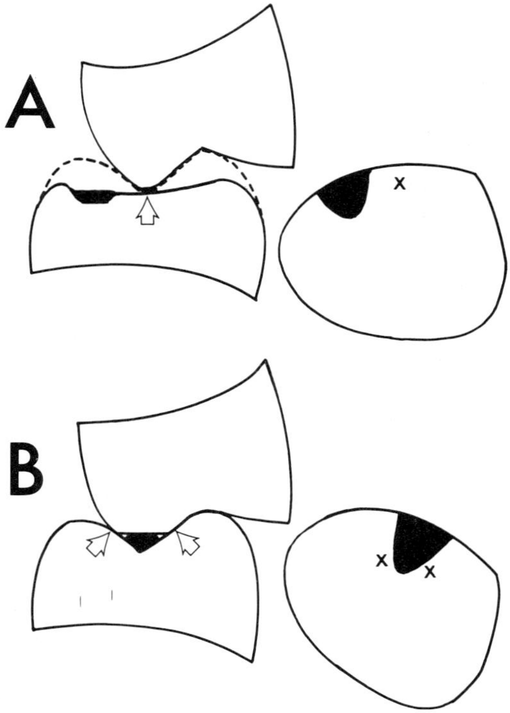

Fig. II.6. **A**, The rest seat should be cut on one side of the contact area of a supporting cusp so that the cusp does not enter the seat and cause tilting of the opposing tooth. **B**, It is sometimes possible to flatten the tip of a supporting cusp to allow room for a rest without endangering the occlusal contact of the cusp.

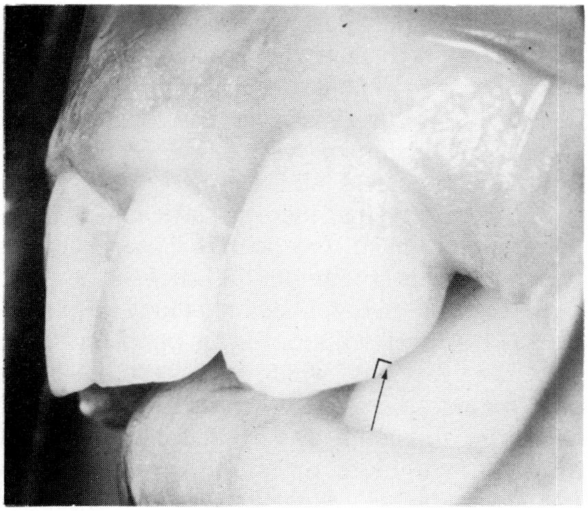

Fig. II.5. Where there is a deep overbite there is very little room to place occlusal rests on the incisors and the rest seats are cut at the disto-incisal angle of the canine.

paper should be held against the lower teeth when marking the upper teeth, as the paper moves with the lower teeth and rubs across the lingual surfaces of the upper teeth, producing better marks. Marking materials have been investigated by Kelleher and Setchell (1984). The rest seats should then be placed on unmarked parts of the teeth nearer the gingival margins. If incisal rests are used, their connectors must also lie on unmarked parts of the teeth. In cases where there is a deep overbite, there is sometimes very little room to place the rest seats on the incisors or canine teeth (*Fig.* II.5) and the first premolars may have to be used. If occlusal wax is used to determine the position of rest seats on upper incisor teeth, it should be pressed against their lingual surfaces before the teeth are rubbed together. The rest seats must then be cut on those parts of the incisors covered by intact wax.

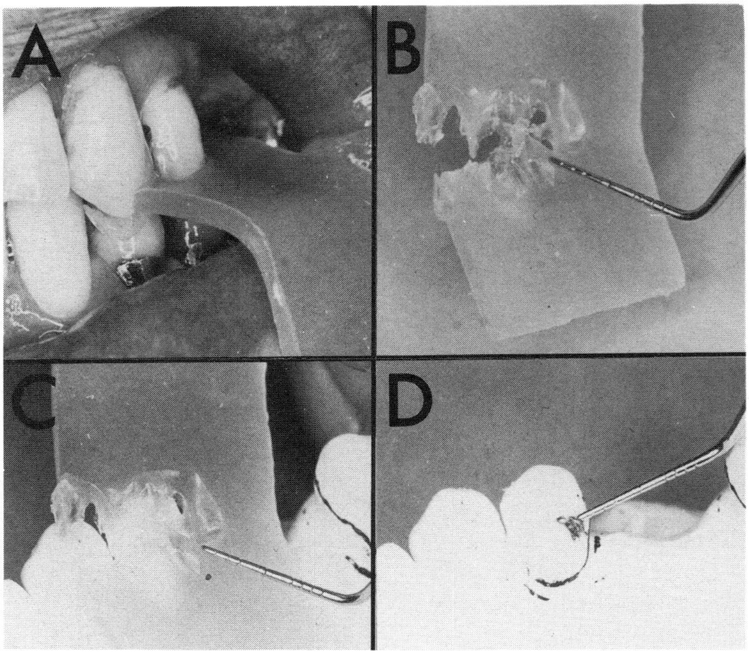

Fig. II.7. Base-plate wax is used to check that the rest seat is deep enough to provide room for an adequately strong rest. **A,** The patient chews on the wax. **B,** The probe indicates the part of the wax that lies in the rest seat. **C,** The wax positioned on the cast. **D,** The rest seat on the cast.

Rest Seats on Posterior Teeth

A similar technique can be used to outline non-contacting areas on posterior teeth, but it is sometimes found that there is insufficient room on the occlusal surfaces and room must be made by grinding the tooth. Several rules must be observed if the rest seats are to be effective:

1. Do not cut rest seats opposite supporting cusps, as the opposing teeth will change position and the space provided by the rest seats will be obliterated by the time the denture is fitted. If it is necessary to place rest seats near supporting cusps, place them a little to one side, so that at least parts of the cusps can contact the opposing teeth (*Fig.* II.6A). It is sometimes possible to flatten the tip of a supporting cusp (*Fig.* II.6B) to provide enough room for an occlusal rest, but yet allow the sides of the cusp to contact the opposing tooth at the edges of the rest seat.

2. Always check that the rest seat is deep enough to provide room for an adequately strong rest. This can be done by placing wax between the teeth and asking the patient to grind the teeth forwards and backwards and from side to side. At the end of this procedure remove the tattered piece of wax and identify the part that enters the rest seat. Examine it carefully and make sure that it would represent a strong enough rest when cast in metal (*Fig.* II.7). It is not enough to check that the rest does not interfere with centric occlusion; it should not interfere with any eccentric or protrusive occlusal slides.

3. Make sure that there is sufficient room to connect the rest to the denture base. There is often sufficient room on the occlusal surface for a rest, but the connector cannot be placed because of over-eruption of an opposing tooth into the gap for which the rest is being constructed (*Fig.* II.8). In these cases it is necessary to modify the contacting surface of the abutment tooth or of the opposing over-erupted tooth to provide enough space. Check with wax after modification has been completed.

4. Occlusal rests on isolated posterior teeth present a particular problem. Many of these

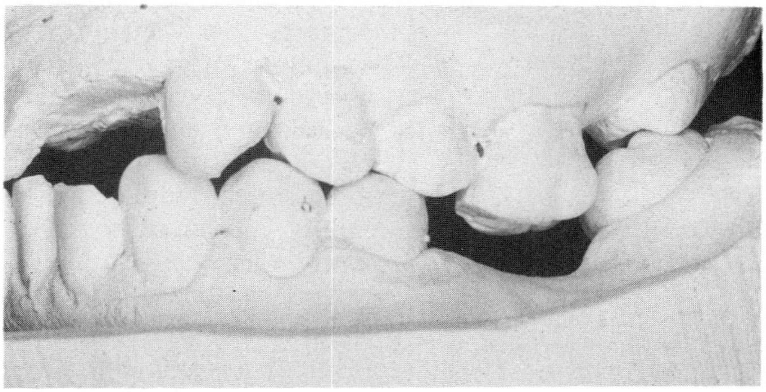

Fig. II.8. Preliminary casts showing over-erupted upper molar contacting the mesial surface of the lower molar. Although there is sufficient room for an occlusal rest on the lower molar, there is insufficient room for the connector. Preparation and crowning of the upper molar is necessary to improve the occlusion and make room for the connector.

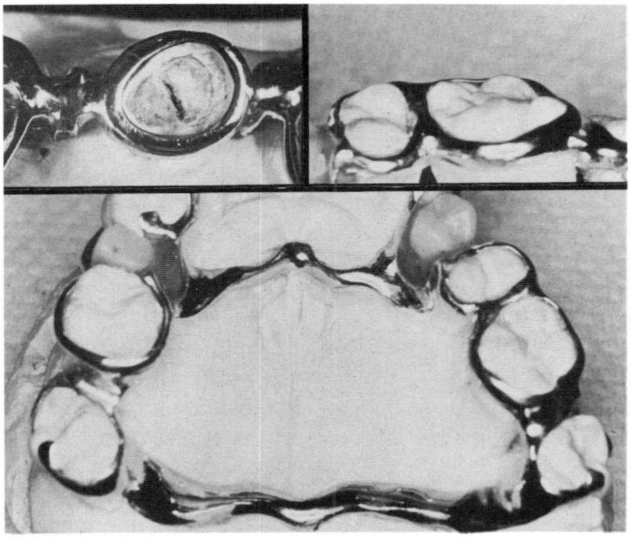

Fig. II.9. Examples of ring rests. These are particularly useful on isolated teeth as they distribute the load better than single occlusal rests and do not cover the occlusal surfaces of the teeth.

teeth are in firm occlusion with their opponents and any modification of their occlusal surfaces allows them to change position, either by tilting or by erupting further, and the space for the occlusal rest is lost, as already described. Ring rests are usually best for isolated teeth, provided there is sufficient area of tooth above the survey line to accommodate them (*Fig.* II.9). An additional advantage of ring rests is that they provide a better distribution of load to the abutment teeth (Geddes, 1958). In some cases it is necessary to prepare isolated teeth and fit telescope or full veneer crowns to improve the design of the appliance.

5. When molar abutment teeth are severely tilted, it is usually supposed that the occlusal rest should be placed on the part of the tooth furthest from the deepest undercut, in the belief that this will prevent further tilting of the tooth. Quite frequently an occlusal rest placed in this position requires quite a deep rest seat to accommodate it, since it lies on the part of the occlusal surface that is in contact with the

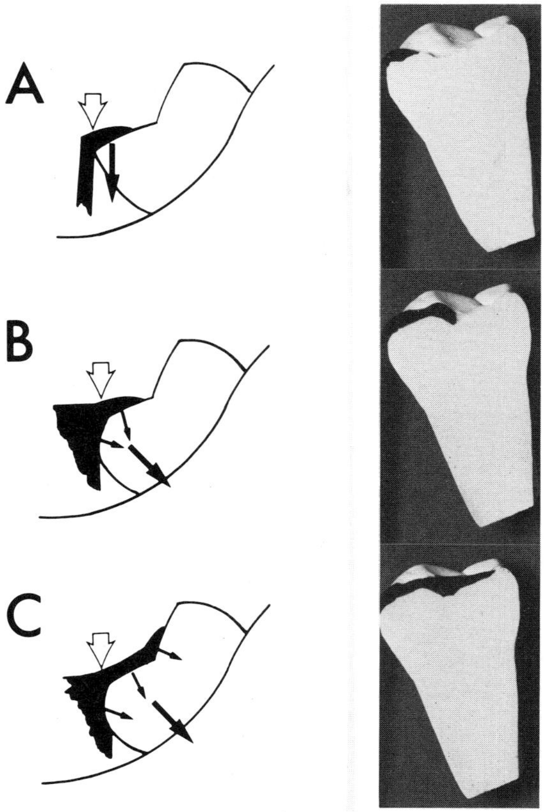

Fig. II.10. **A,** The occlusal rest tilts the molar mesially as there is insufficient contact of the connector with the mesial surface of the tooth. **B,** By adjusting the contour of the tooth, the resolved forces on rest and connector are directed in the long axis. **C,** Extension of the rest provides more resistance to mesial tilting of the tooth by shifting the resolved forces towards the centre of the tooth.

opposing teeth, whereas there is usually space on the side of the tooth to which it is tilted. Even the most cursory examination of the forces transmitted to the tooth by a rest on the side to which it is tilted will show that it is often possible to place a rest on that side without increasing the tilt of the tooth, provided the seat of the rest is at right angles to the long axis of the tilted tooth and provided that the saddle abuts on the tooth in such a way that it cannot tilt forward while the saddle is in place (*Fig.* II.10). It is not necessary to fuss about positioning rests on such teeth, since the hazard to the tooth is rather conjectural and in practice such teeth provide satisfactory abutments for fixed partial dentures over many years. An additional advantage of placing the rest on the mesial part of the occlusal surface is that its form can be adjusted to improve the occlusion, but before placing a mesial rest the contour of the tooth should be modified and the occlusal rest should be shaped so that it does not tilt the tooth.

The rest most likely to cause tilting is a simple rest that sits on the mesio-marginal ridge of a tooth that has a very high mesial survey line (*Fig.* II.10A) so that there is nothing to contact its mesial surface and prevent tilting. The most favourable form of tooth for a mesial rest is a tooth of rounded contour where the connector for the rest lies against a sloping mesial surface, preventing mesial rotation of the tooth.

6. It is difficult to cut adequate occlusal rest seats in teeth with severe attrition, as there is a danger of the enamel margins chipping off at the side of the rest seat. Increasing the vertical dimension by covering the occlusal surfaces of these teeth can be considered, but fixed bridges are better in these cases, since removable dentures that completely cover occlusal surfaces greatly increase the risk of dental caries.

7. Rest seats cut in premolars usually cross the central fissure of the tooth and may produce a food trap between the apex of the occlusal rest and the fissure. The occlusal rests should be carefully finished to minimize this risk. Rounding the end of the rest in the conventional manner leaves a pyramidal hollow between it and the fissure, whereas a slight pointed extension towards the fissure reduces this hollow and may decrease the risk of caries (*Fig.* II.11).

8. Occasionally it is necessary to cut rest seats on the buccal surfaces of lower second and third molars that are tilted mesiolingually. Rest seats in these positions are useful if they are kept clear of the buccal cusps of the upper molars. The clearance should be checked with articulating paper in much the same way as for rest seats on anterior teeth. Rest seats on lingual surfaces may present problems as they can irritate the tongue when the denture is out of the mouth. Therefore they should be kept small and if possible placed near the mesial or

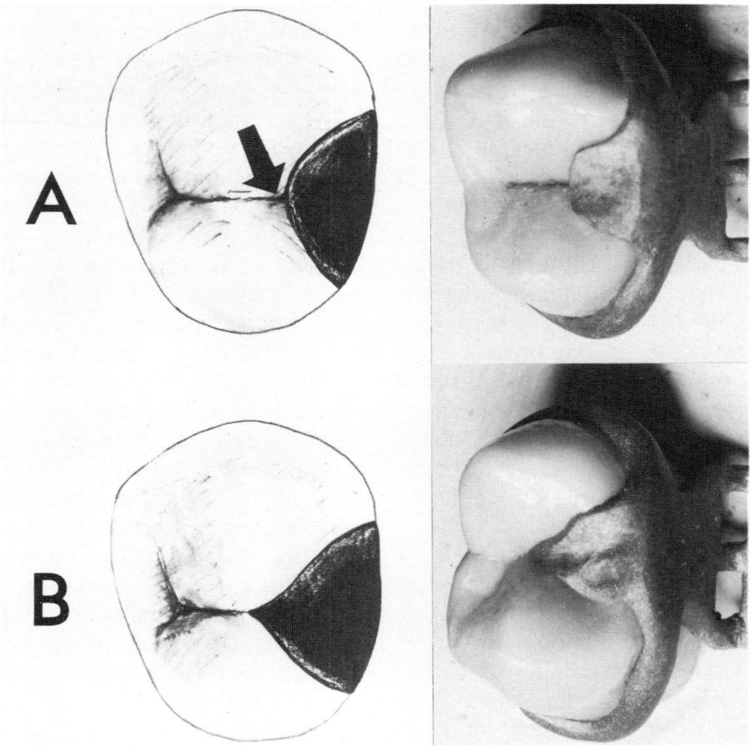

Fig. II.11. **A**, Rounded occlusal rest on premolar leaves food traps (*arrow*). **B**, Pointed extension on to the transverse ridge reduces the risk of food stagnation.

distal surfaces so that they are out of the way of the searching tongue.

9. Rest seats should be cut with a plain-cut tungsten carbide bur, rather than with a diamond instrument that leaves rough and scored surfaces on the rest seat. Tungsten carbide burs leave a smooth surface on the rest seat. After cutting, all rest seats should be thoroughly polished before impressions are taken.

Correction of Abnormal Tooth Contacts

The most retruded position of the mandible is not used in function. The findings of many workers in this field confirm that the intercuspal position is the most important functional position.

Investigations with ultra-high-speed cinematography and movement transducers show that during each chewing cycle the mandible pauses 0.24 sec in the intercuspal position. When the intercuspal position does not coincide with the muscle position (i.e. the position in which the mandible closes when the muscles are in optimum function), the patient has a malocclusion that is potentially pathological. The clinical problem is to establish a stable intercuspal position that coincides with a physiologically acceptable muscle position. By using the sounds of occlusion to monitor the occlusal correction, you can identify a patient's adaptive response to minor alterations of the occlusion and follow the progress towards occlusal stability. When the occlusion is unstable the teeth hit and slide into the intercuspal position and the sounds are muffled, but when the occlusion is stable the teeth make impact sounds of short duration as they close directly in the intercuspal position without any slide.

Once we have established, in the absence of muscle and joint pain, a stable occlusion (Class A) that is recognizable and reproducible by the patient, we have achieved our purpose. To define the position in anatomical terms is virtually impossible, as there may be a number of positions to which the patient can easily adapt and in which a satisfactory stable occlusion can be established. Nevertheless, in our present state of knowledge it would appear that retruded stable positions are generally more satisfactory than more anterior stable positions, although it is not uncommon to find patients who have used the latter satisfactorily for many years.

The clinical necessity of establishing a recognizable position for the mandible appears to oppose consideration of the self-regulating nature of physiological function. However, gnathosonic techniques, by enabling us to put occlusion on a time-base, can display the adaptive responses of our patients and lead, during the progress of treatment, to the recognition by both dentist and patient of a satisfactory stable intercuspal position.

With articulator techniques it is necessary to record, at a particular moment, a retruded mandibular position that is then taken as a reference position from which the occlusion is assessed and interceptive contacts diagnosed and corrected. However, each small alteration of the teeth is accompanied by an adaptive change in the position of the mandible, which the articulator cannot adequately reflect. As a result the dentist removes much more tooth surface in reducing contacts that intercept closure on the terminal hinge axis than would be necessary if the postural adaptation by the patient was taken into consideration.

What has been said so far may appear to be too vague to satisfy proponents of the hinge-axis techniques, but it is nearer physiological reality. Those who use gnathosonic techniques very soon find that they demand much greater precision than any articulator technique. The gnathosonic record is indeed a hard taskmaster.

The method the authors use to detect and remove abnormal contacts in order to establish a stable intercuspal position is as follows:

1. Relieve the patient's symptoms of muscle and joint pain with a temporary occlusal splint on the maxillary arch. This is purely a diagnostic appliance; by removing the cuspal guidance it allows the mandible to occupy the muscle position and hence produces relaxation of the muscles. The splint should present a smooth surface to the mandibular teeth. If possible ensure that the cusp tips of all these teeth contact but do not indent the appliance, so that tooth movement is minimal.

Other methods of relaxing the muscles can be used (heat, ethyl chloride spray, injection of local analgesic, biofeedback, physiological pulsing techniques).

2. After completing the diagnosis when the muscles are relaxed, start the treatment phase, locating and removing intercuspal contacts.

3. Place the patient in the supine position with the teeth apart, or with the occlusal splint in the mouth, so that no tooth-to-tooth contact takes place. (Tooth contact would cause the patient to adapt to the malocclusion and this is undesirable at this stage of treatment.)

4. Ask the patient to open and close the jaws several times without tooth contact and then, after the splint has been removed, request that the teeth are brought gently together into light contact. Before this, warn the patient to note which tooth contacts first.

5. As the patient closes into contact, listen with the stereostethoscope so that you can confirm on which side the contact occurs.

6. Ask the patient to open the mouth again and place thin articulating paper or occlusal indicating wax on the maxillary teeth.

7. Ask the patient to close gently until the same contact is again felt. Observe this contact and modify the tooth accordingly.

8. Continue with this procedure until you have achieved all round stable contact of teeth in this position. Almost invariably the patient notices an improvement when stability is reached. This stability can be checked quite easily with a stereostethoscope.

9. Raise the chair until the patient is in an upright position and correct the occlusion in the same way as previously and stabilize it in this position also.

Do not make any attempt to force the jaw into a retruded position, but simply use the posture of the patient to place the mandible in its physiologically retruded position. Only grind one or two contacts at each session as adaptations to the new occlusion take place between sessions. In this way a stable position can be achieved with minimal grinding.

This concept of occlusion is closer to physiological reality than concepts based on the terminal-hinge-axis of the mandible as a reference position. It is helpful to think of the intercuspal position in terms of the 'brain end' of occlusion rather than in terms of the 'dental end'. By this is meant that when a stable reproducible position has been achieved the afferent impulses from periodontium, joints and muscles will produce a reproducible and recognizable engram within the brain which represents the base line from which masticatory activity takes place. We believe that food between the teeth distorts this engram and calls forth the appropriate muscular responses to deal with the food during mastication. However, if a recognizable and reproducible pattern of intercuspal occlusion is not present, the deflective tooth contact also distort the engram and incoordinated occlusal activity results as shown by large variations in occlusal sound duration (*see Fig.* 3.8). When you have removed abnormal contacts interfering with the path of closure of the mandible into the intercuspal position, repeat the procedure to remove abnormal contacts interfering with the eccentric occlusal positions. It is particularly important to remove premature contacts on the non-working side (overbalancing contacts) as they cause symptoms more often than cuspal interferences on the working side.

Appendix III

Surveying dental casts

Surveying is an essential step in the design and construction of partial dentures. By means of a surveying instrument, lines can be drawn on a cast so that the dentist can be sure that no rigid portion of a partial denture will lie in an undercut in relation to its path of insertion and removal. The lines on the cast are also a guide to the positioning of clasp arms, and the surveyor can be used to eliminate unwanted undercuts. The surveyor in this Appendix is a simple one, but more complex instruments are available that have attachments for milling and drilling metal (*see Fig.* 5.2).

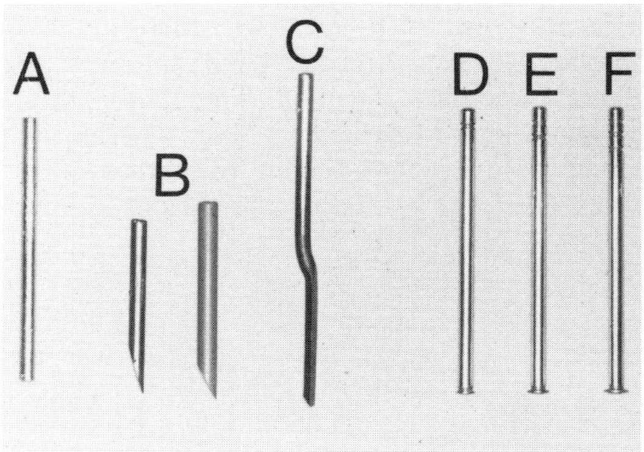

Fig. III.2. Various pieces can be put into the screw chuck of the cast surveyor:
A, Analysing rod
B, Marking rods (black and red)
C, Trimming knife
D, 0·25 mm undercut gauge
E, 0·50 mm undercut gauge
F, 0·75 mm undercut gauge

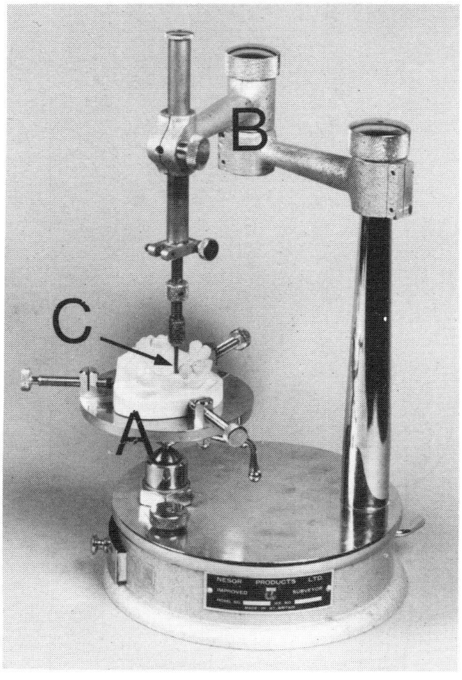

Fig. III.1. This instrument is a simple surveyor.
A, A table that can be tilted at different angles.
B, A movable arm with specially constructed parallel joints.
C, A marking rod held vertically in a screw chuck attached to the movable arm. The vertical marking rod is used to indicate the greatest horizontal width of the object being surveyed.

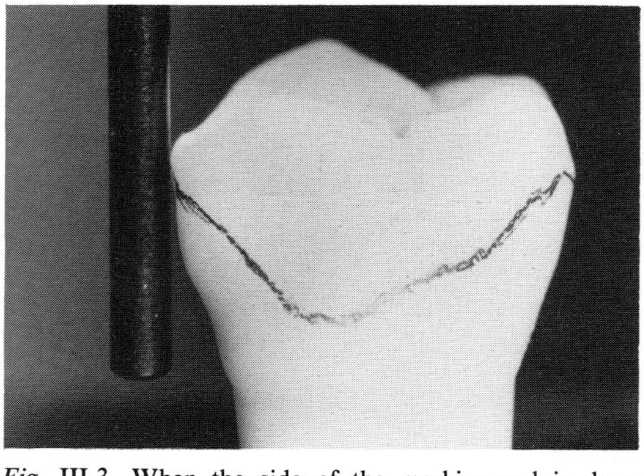

Fig. III.3. When the side of the marking rod is drawn round a model of a tooth placed on the table of the surveyor, it marks the greatest diameter of the tooth. The line produced by the marking rod is called the *survey line* and the area below the survey line is the *undercut area*.

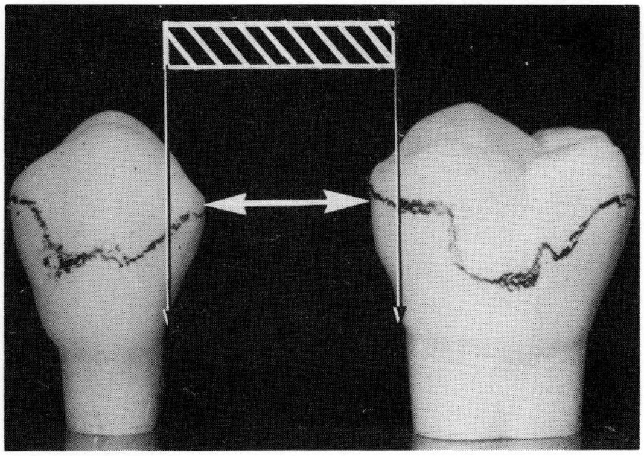

Fig. III.4. A block of greater width than the minimum distance between two teeth cannot be passed into the undercut area by moving the block vertically downwards from above. The minimum distance between the teeth is opposite the survey line on each tooth.

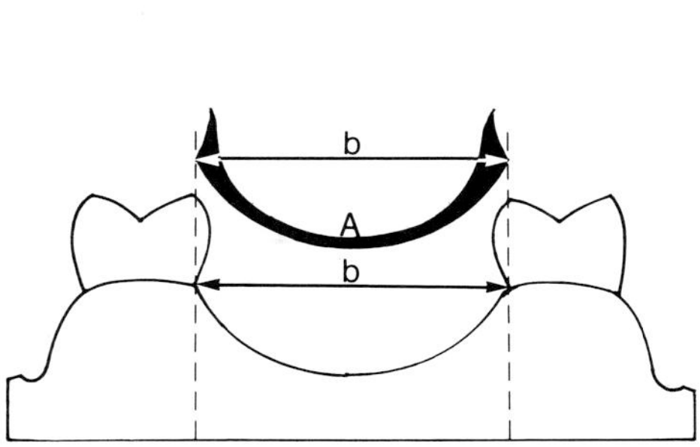

Fig. III.5. Similarly, a denture base (A) made on this cast could not be fitted in the mouth, as the width (b) between the gingival portions is greater than that between the maximum convexities of the teeth.

Elimination of Undercuts (blocking out)

A cast is mounted on the table of the surveyor so that the path of insertion of the denture is parallel to the marking rod.

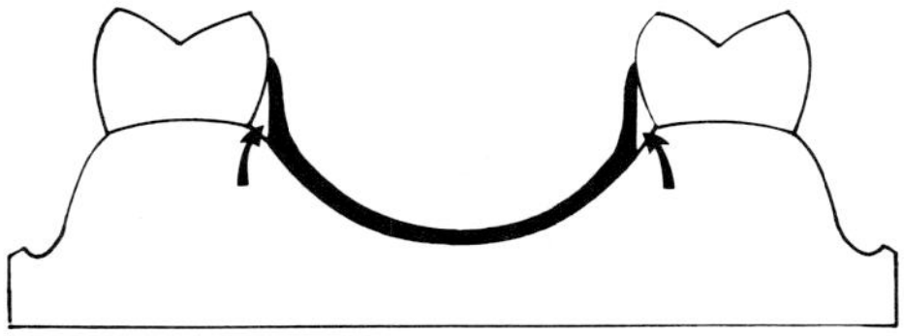

Fig. III.6. However, if the undercut areas (*arrows*) on the cast are filled up (blocked out) with plaster before making the base, then it can be fitted without difficulty.

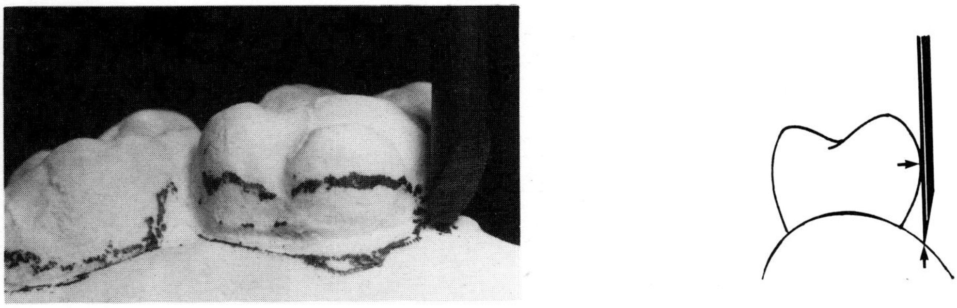

Fig. III.7. This cast is being surveyed to show the undercut areas of the teeth in relation to the path of insertion. The marking rod is bevelled on one side to form a chisel point, so that it traces a second line vertically below the survey line made by the side of the marking rod on the tooth. Arrows in the diagram indicate the borders of the undercut area.

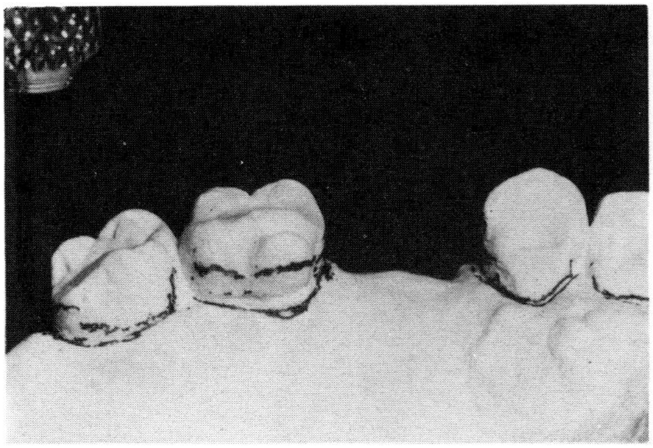

Fig. III.8. The complete undercut area is therefore outlined.

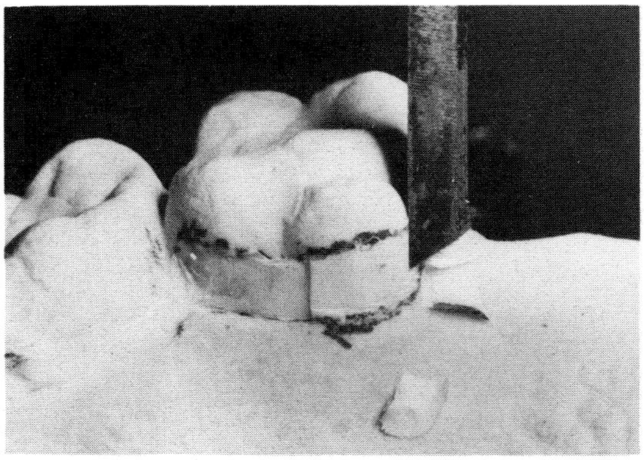

Fig. III.9. The undercut areas are then blocked out with wax or plaster that is trimmed with a knife attached to the arm of the surveyor. Plaster is used when the denture is processed on the master cast, but wax may be used (as illustrated) when the cast is prepared for duplication.

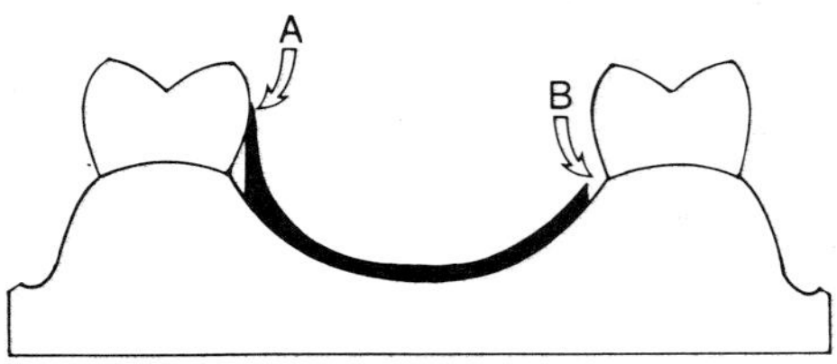

Fig. III.10. It is essential to bring the denture base up to or slightly above the survey line (as shown as 'A'). Otherwise a space is produced (as at 'B') that causes the base to be ill-fitting and food debris can easily pack into the space and damage the gingivae.

Use of Undercuts (Retention)

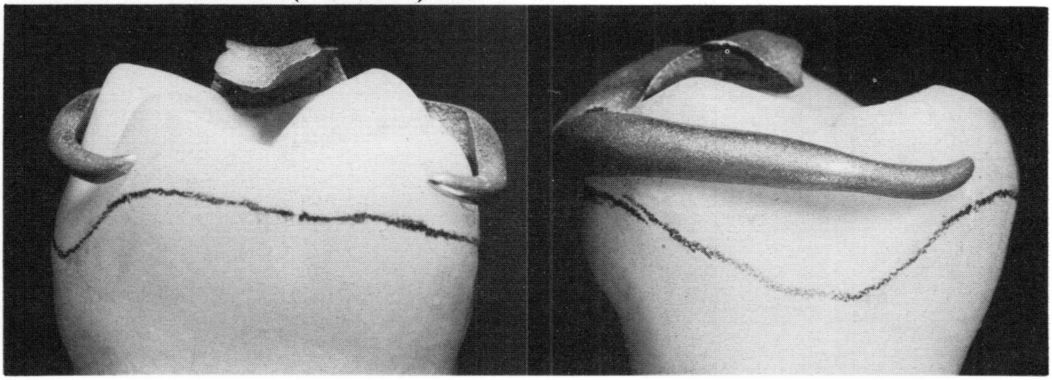

A

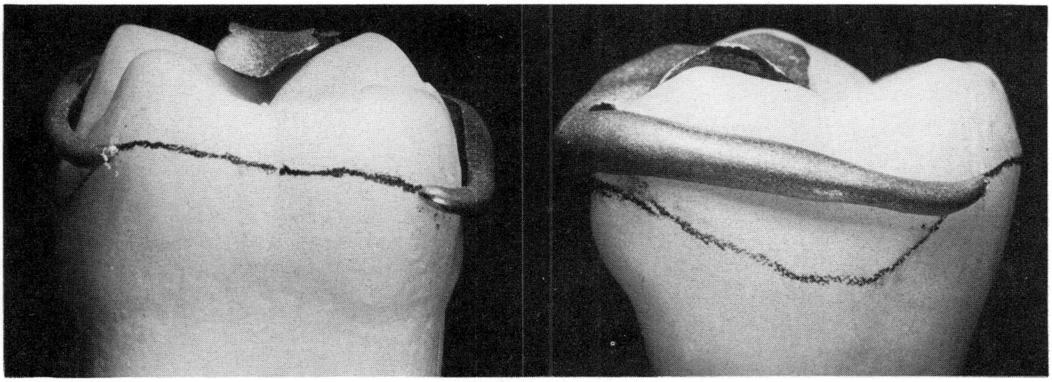

B

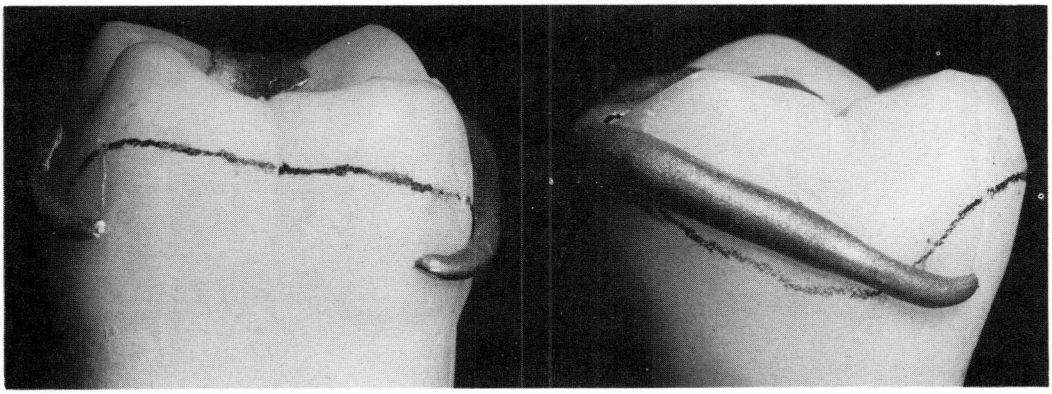

C

Fig. III.11. Partial dentures are retained by clasps placed in undercut areas of teeth.

A, This clasp has been placed on a tooth, but has not yet been pressed past the 'equator' of the tooth into the undercut and the tips of the clasp arms lie passive.

B, The clasp is now opposite the survey line. The distance between the tips of the clasp arms is greater than in 'A'.

C, The clasp has now passed beyond the survey line into the undercut. Once again the distance between the tips of the clasp arms indicates that the arms are passive against the tooth when the clasp is in its final position. Any attempt to remove the clasp from this position would require sufficient force to spread the arms to pass over the survey line.

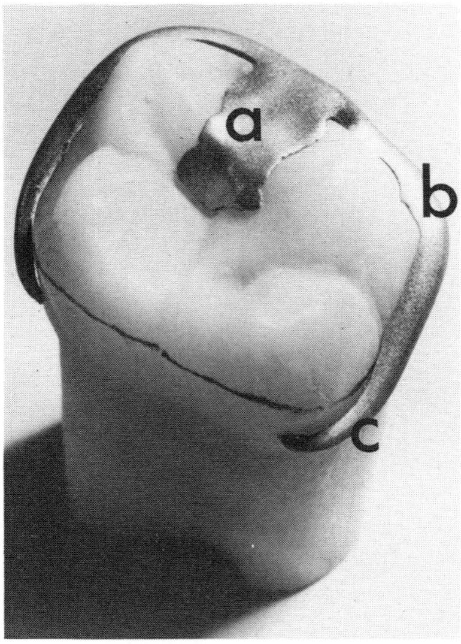

Fig. III.12. This is an occlusally-approaching clasp. There is an arm on each side of the tooth and an occlusal rest on the occlusal surface. The occlusal rest (a) provides support for the appliance. The stiff parts (b) of the clasp arms provide bracing against lateral thrusts, and the slender distal thirds (c) of the arms provide retention.

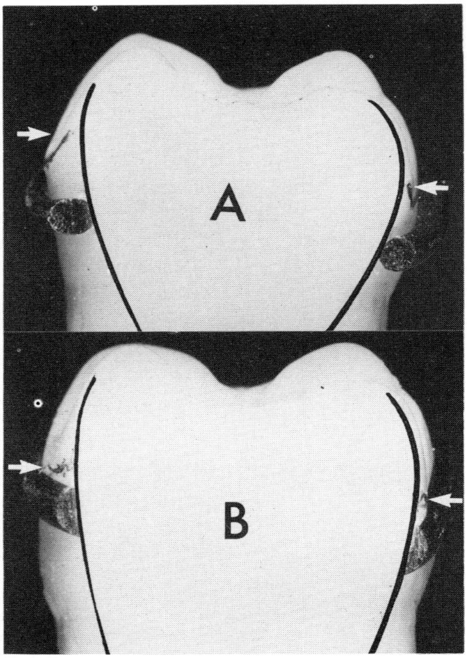

Fig. III.14. Buccolingual sections through premolars. The horizontal undercuts at given distances below survey lines (*white arrows*) vary according to the shape of the tooth. The amount of horizontal undercut to be engaged by a clasp arm depends on the type of metal used to make the clasp. For example, as wrought wire is more flexible than cast cobalt-chromium alloy, it can spring into (and out of) bigger horizontal undercuts (**A**). The undercut engaged by a cobalt-chromium clasp is smaller (**B**).

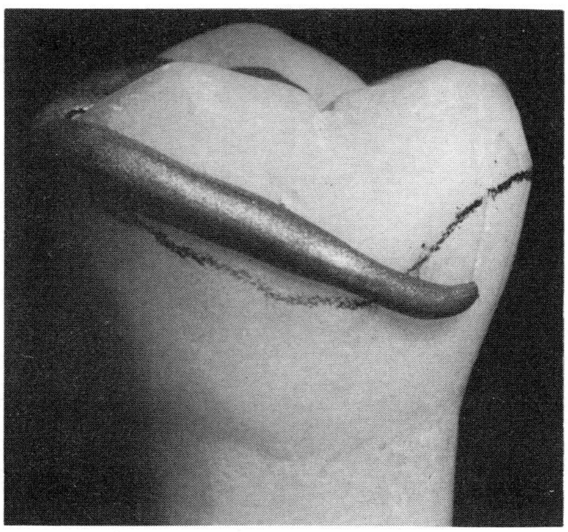

Fig. III.13. The clasp arms taper away from the supporting area, pass over the maximum convexity of the tooth (shown by the survey line) and the tips engage in the undercut area. The taper of the arm must be regular to allow smooth distribution of stress when flexion takes place. The tip of the arm should be thin to allow most flexion. This is the portion of the clasp that has to pass over the greatest diameter of the tooth to engage the undercut where it lies passively, but resists upward displacement.

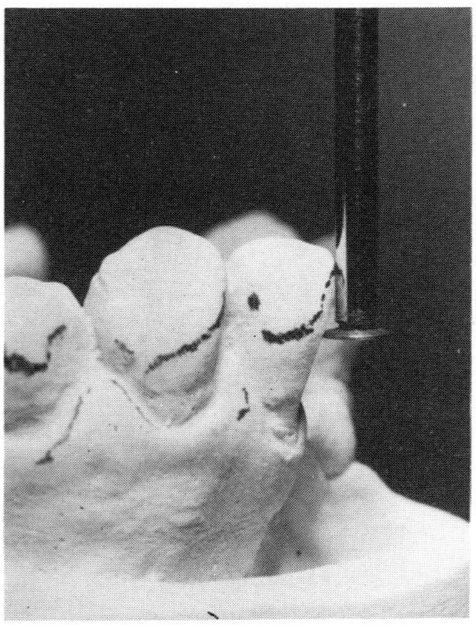

Fig. III.15. Undercut gauges are used to measure the amount of horizontal undercut required. The gauges are fitted to the arm of the surveyor to ensure that both the side of the rod and the edge of the disc touch the tooth. The edge of the disc then indicates the horizontal undercut.

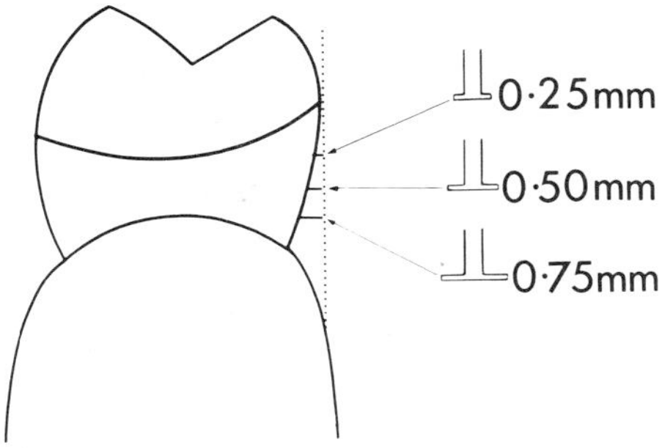

Fig. III.16. The gauges are graded in three sizes (0·25 mm, 0·50 mm, 0·75 mm) and are selected according to the flexibility of the metal. For instance, a 0·25 mm gauge for cobalt-chromium, 0·50 mm for cast gold, and 0·75 mm for stainless steel wire.

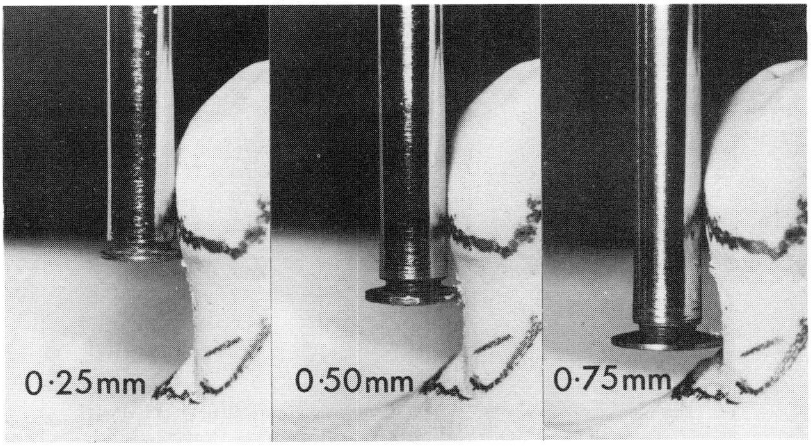

Fig. III.17. Undercut gauges of different sizes on the same tooth. The largest gauge (0·75 mm) contacts the tooth at a point furthest from the survey line when the rod is in contact with the line.

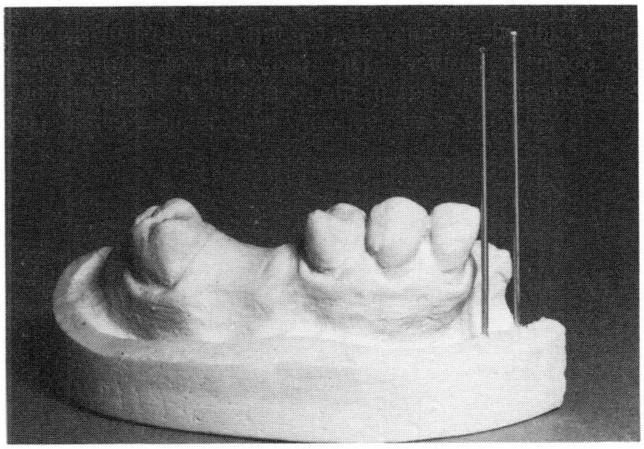

Fig. III.18. If the denture is inserted along a vertical path it is necessary to block out the mesial undercut on the lateral incisor and to block out the mucosal undercut in the labial sulcus.

Insertion and Removal of the Denture Base using an Inclined Path

The choice of a path of insertion and removal of the denture is discussed in Chapter 5. Circumstances may make it necessary to insert and remove the denture on an inclined path. It is sometimes better if the path of insertion/removal and the common path of displacement are not the same.

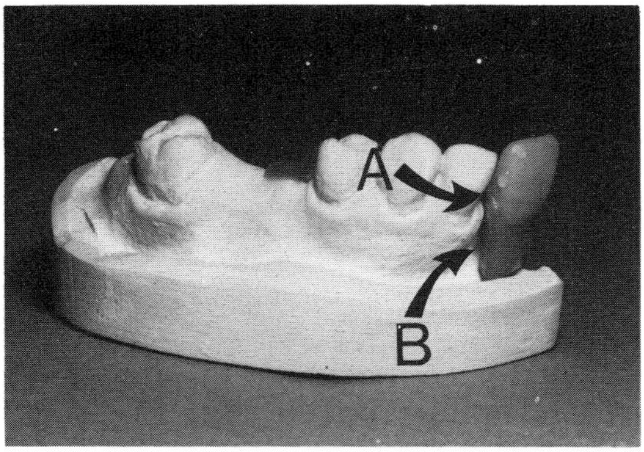

Fig. III.19. This produces an unsightly gap (A) between the central and the lateral incisor, and another (B) between the flange and the mucosa.

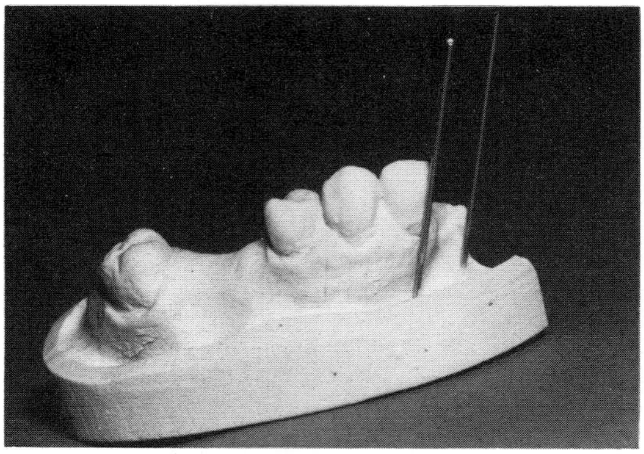

Fig. III.20. These spaces can be eliminated by tilting the cast before surveying, thus using an angled path of insertion for the denture.

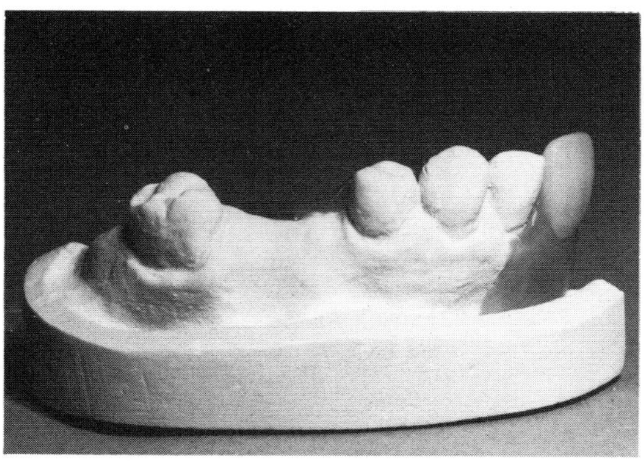

Fig. III.21. As a result, the labial flange fits snugly against the lateral incisor and into the sulcus. The denture looks better and does not drop down anteriorly as it engages the soft tissue undercut.

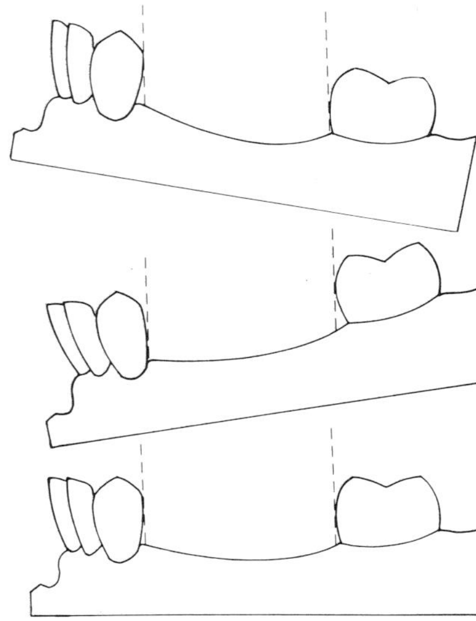

Fig. III.22. The apparent size of undercuts can be altered by tilting the cast (e.g. the front of the cast is raised to produce greater distal undercuts and smaller mesial undercuts). However, these undercuts are not necessarily useful for retention. Only the undercuts in relation to the common path of displacement should be used to provide retention of the denture.

The common path of displacement of a denture is at right angles to the occlusal surface, as this is the direction of the displacing forces exerted on the denture by sticky food. Clasp arms must therefore engage undercuts relative to the common path of displacement to provide retention of the denture. If there are no undercuts relative to this path, the denture will not be retained.

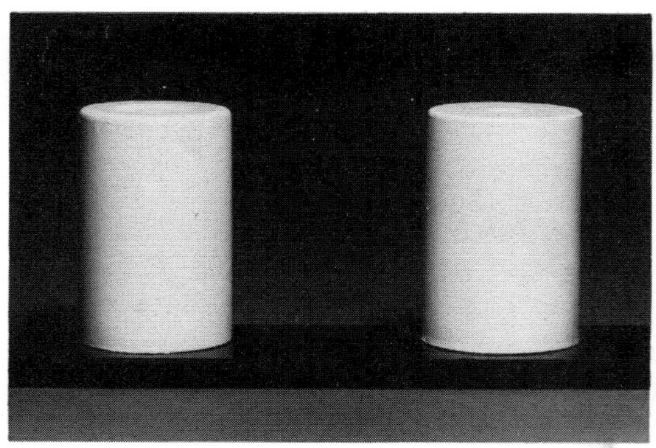

Fig. III.23. These cylinders represent teeth with parallel-sided crowns that have no undercuts in relation to the common path of displacement.

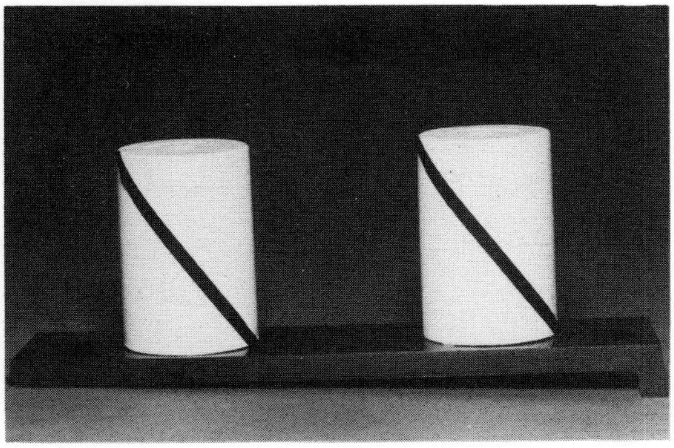

Fig. III.24. If the cylinders are tilted, undercuts appear beneath the survey lines, but these undercuts provide no resistance to displacement of an appliance along the common path of displacement, and are therefore useless for retention. Tilting of the cast produces 'false' undercuts.

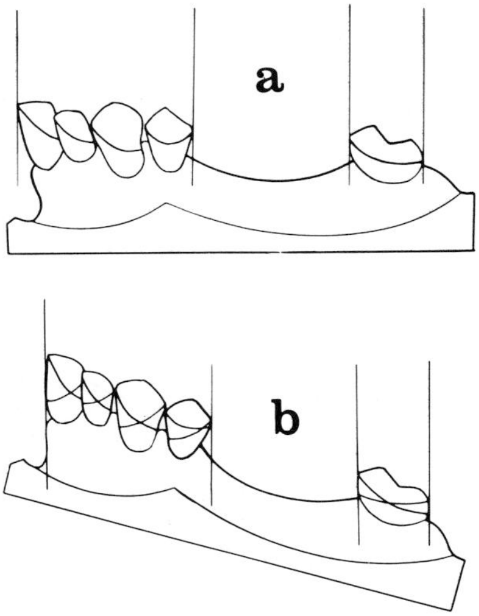

Fig. III.25. The cast must therefore first be surveyed vertically (**a**) to find out the undercut areas that would provide resistance to vertical displacement. The cast should then be tilted to the desired angle (**b**) and surveyed again, using a different coloured marker to show the areas of resistance to removal of the appliance in the path chosen.

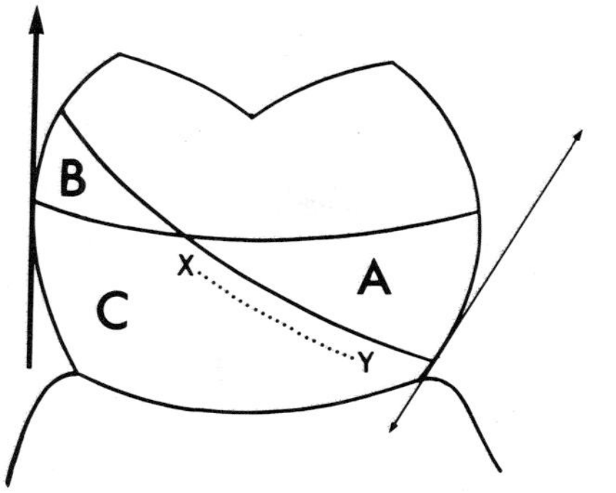

Fig. III.26. The two survey lines should then be examined more closely to ascertain the significance of the dual survey. Area 'A' resists vertical but not angled displacement (*thin arrow*). Area 'B' resists angled but not vertical displacement (*thick arrow*). Area 'C' resists both vertical and angled displacement (*thick* and *thin arrows*). How far the tip of a clasp can be placed into an undercut depends on its flexibility, so if the clasp is cobalt-chromium alloy the tip must be placed somewhere along the line between 'X' and 'Y' as this line represents the depth (0·25 mm) selected below the survey line related to the path of insertion and removal (*thin arrow*). However, the deeper the arm lies in an undercut in relation to the vertical path of displacement (*thick arrow*), the greater is the resistance to removal in a vertical direction. At point 'X' resistance to vertical displacement is equal to that along the tilted path of insertion and removal, but the nearer the tip of the clasp is placed to point 'Y', the greater is the resistance to vertical displacement. Ideally, the tip of the clasp should be placed at point 'Y' to give maximum resistance to vertical displacement. (For example, when the jaws are opened after biting into a sticky substance, the vertical forces trying to displace the denture will be strongly resisted.)

Further Considerations

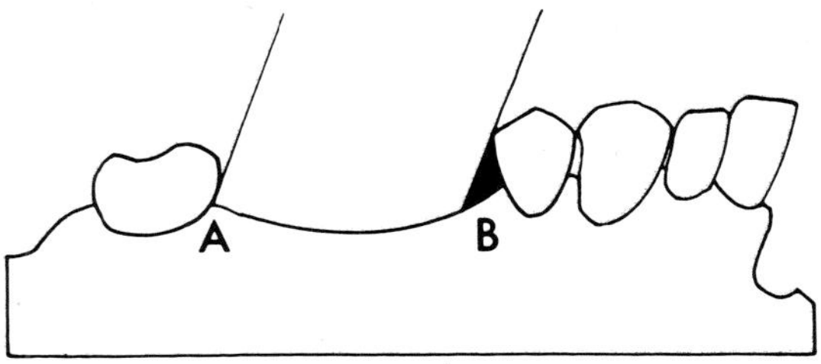

Fig. III.27. By inserting the denture at an angle, part of it can be placed in an undercut in relation to the vertical common path of displacement and can be used for retention. To do this, the cast should be tilted until the analysing rod enters 'A'; it should be surveyed in this path and the undercut at 'B' should be blocked out. However, this has the disadvantage of creating a zone of displacement (*see Fig.* III.29).

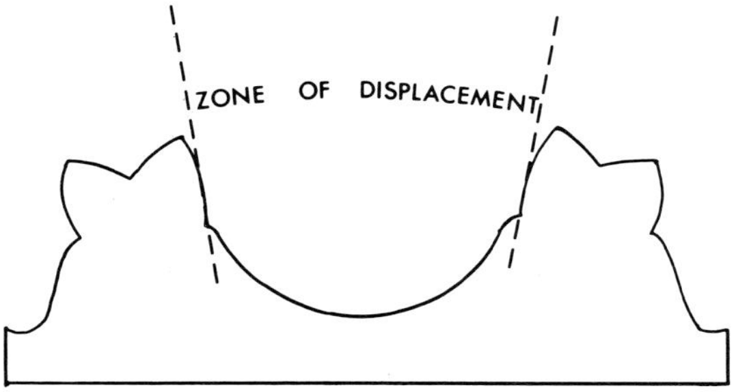

Fig. III.28. If the abutment teeth are divergent, this also creates a zone of displacement from which the denture can be displaced at any angle between the diverging lines.

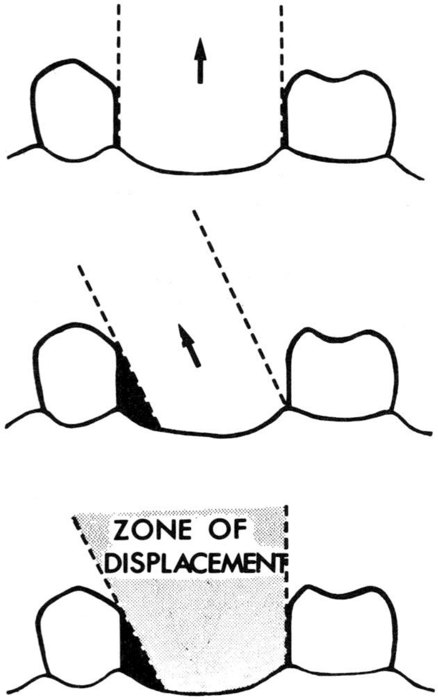

Fig. III.29. A zone of displacement can be created inadvertently in the following way:
Upper, There are no vertical undercuts against the abutment teeth and if a vertical path of insertion is chosen the saddle can be displaced only in one direction.
Middle, However, where there is an anterior saddle, for the sake of appearance it may be necessary to angle the cast and thus block out the distal undercut produced on the premolar.
Lower, The denture can then be displaced at any angle between the vertical path and the chosen path, giving rise to an undesirable zone of displacement.

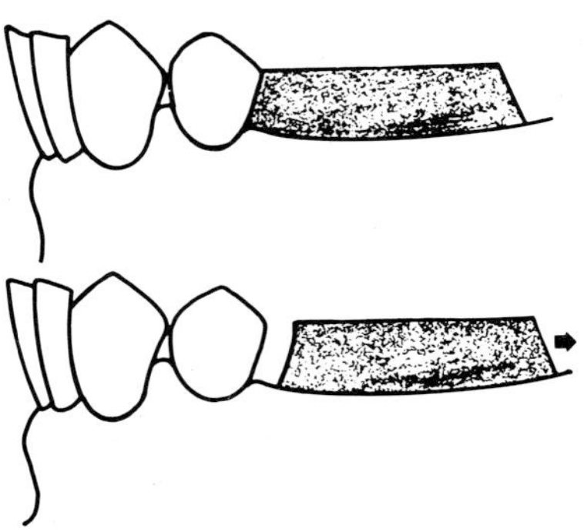

Fig. III.30. Distal displacement of free-end saddles can occur unless there is adequate retention (*see Fig.* III.31).

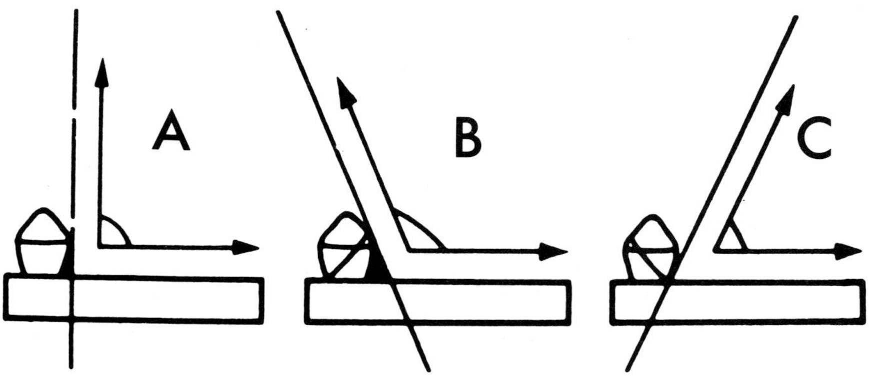

Fig. III.31. **A**, The angle within which displacement can occur when the cast is surveyed vertically. **B**, The angle when the anterior part of the cast is raised and the undercut on the distal side of the premolar is blocked out. **C**, The angle when the posterior part of the cast is raised. This is the most satisfactory path of insertion as it produces the smallest possible zone of displacement.

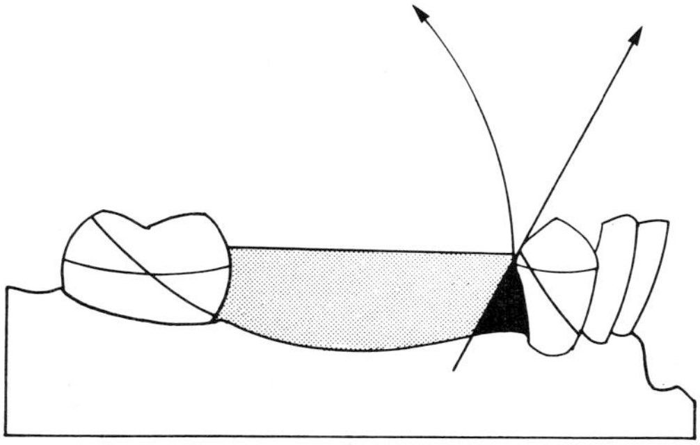

Fig. III.32. It must not be forgotten that certain rotational paths of displacement may develop. In *Fig.* III.27 it can be seen that the anterior part of the saddle could be rotated out, the posterior part hingeing against the molar. The greater the tilt employed, the greater the zone of displacement anteriorly and the clasping must be designed accordingly.

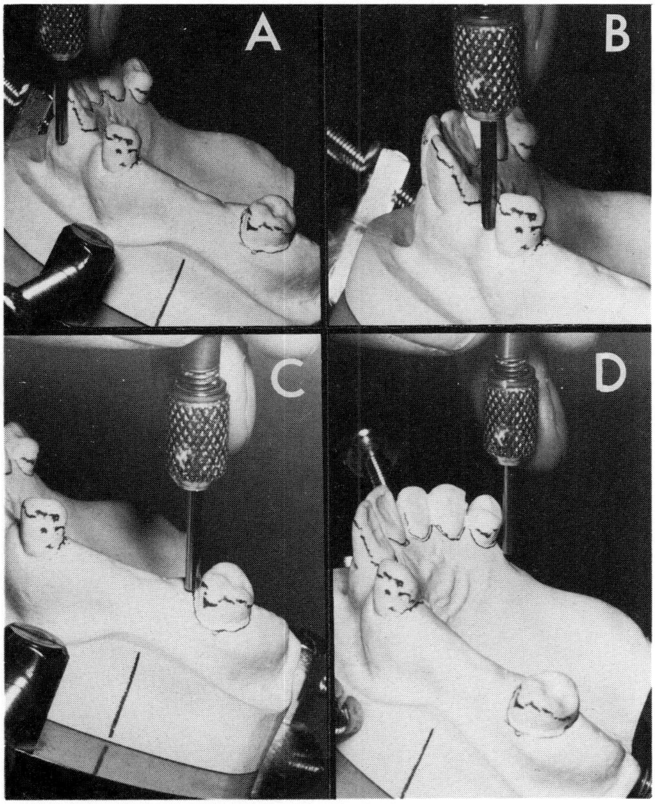

Fig. III.33. After surveying in relation to the common path of displacement, the marking rod on the surveyor should be replaced by a metal analysing rod before a path of insertion and removal is selected. The cast should then be examined at various tilts and the best path of insertion chosen without making marks on the cast that might be confusing later. **A** and **B**, The cast is tilted to eliminate the distal undercut on the right central incisor and the mesial undercut on the right canine. Thus the buccal flange of the denture can replace the missing interdental papillae and engage the undercut in relation to the common path of displacement. **C**, This tilt of the cast also enables the denture base to engage the mesial undercut on the right molar. **D**, The disadvantage of this path of insertion is that it creates a large undercut on the distal side of the left premolar. This undercut would have to be blocked out and might produce a food trap. Once the path of insertion and removal has been chosen, the marking rod can be put back on the surveyor (instead of the analysing rod) and the final lines can be drawn on the cast.

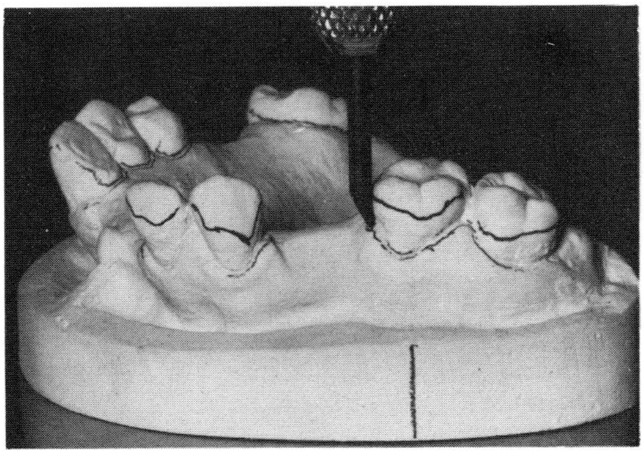

Fig. III.34. Surveying the cast with the black marking rod in relation to the vertical common path of displacement.

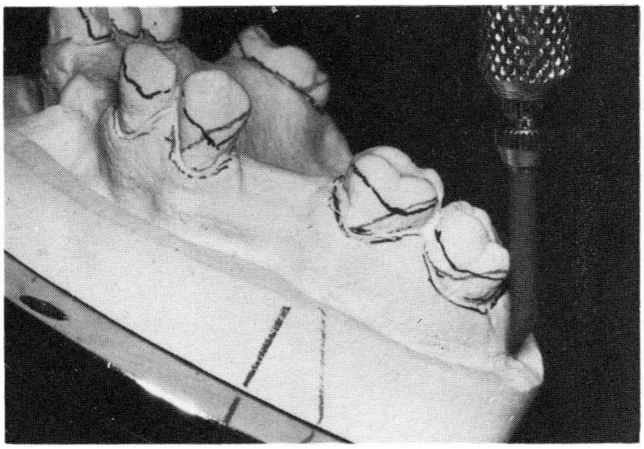

Fig. III.35. Using the red marking rod to survey the cast in relation to the chosen path of insertion and removal. The undercut area below both lines is used for retention.

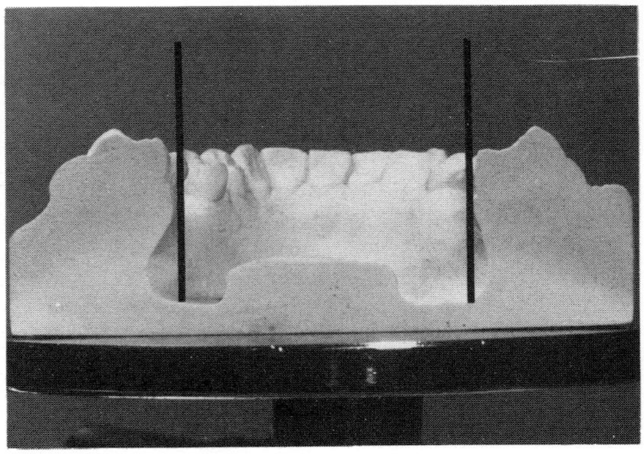

Fig. III.36. Sectioned cast illustrating large soft tissue undercuts on the lingual side in the lower molar region.

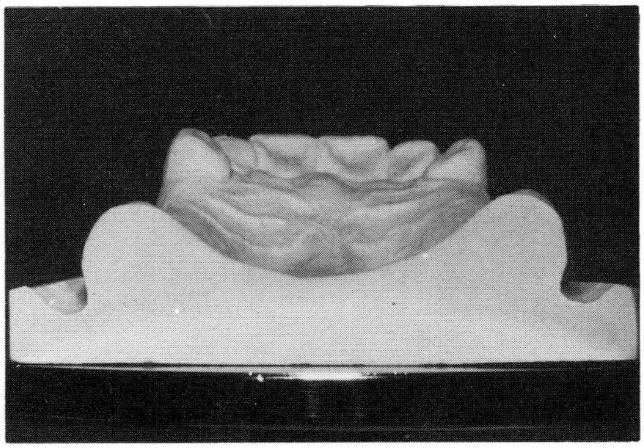

Fig. III.37. It may be necessary to block out these bilateral undercuts to enable the denture to be inserted, although the resilience of the soft tissue may allow small undercuts to be engaged.

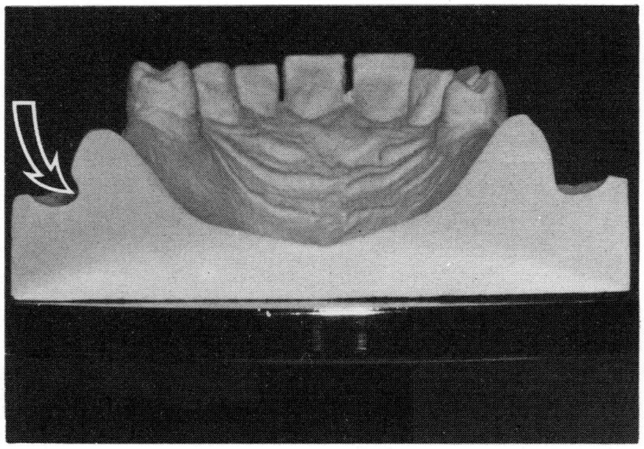

Fig. III.38. Sectioned cast illustrating unilateral undercut in the right upper molar region (*arrow*). In this case it is not necessary to block out the undercut as the denture can be inserted at an angle to engage the undercut before being finally seated.

Soft tissue undercuts should also be surveyed and may have to be blocked out to permit the insertion and removal of the denture.

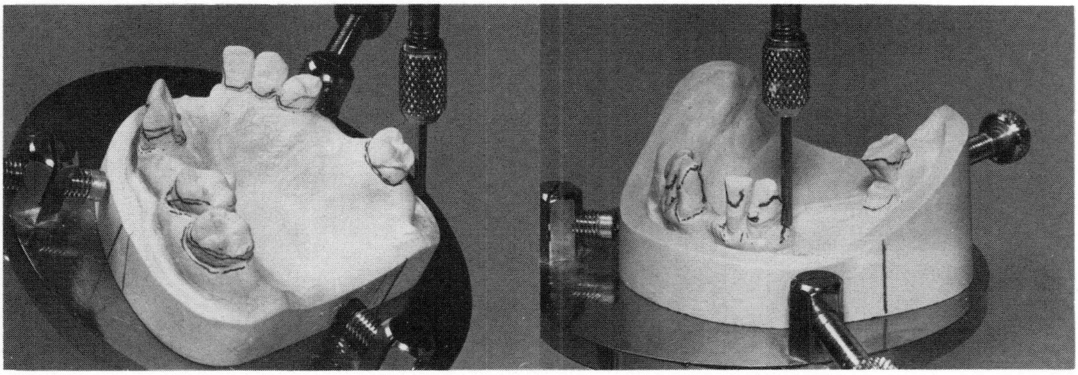

Fig. III.39. To sum up, the surveyor should be used to indicate the presence of undercuts, both those required for retention and those that must be blocked out to enable the denture base to be inserted and removed. If an angled path is used, it is essential that the cast should first be surveyed vertically to ensure that there are undercuts to resist displacement in that direction.

Use of the Surveyor for Fixed and Complex Partial Dentures

When constructing fixed partial dentures or fixed abutment pieces for complex partial dentures, the cast should be surveyed in order to discover the best method of preparing the remaining abutment teeth. Here the surveying method differs from that described for removable partial dentures, inasmuch as the long axes of teeth are being considered rather than the guiding planes of the tooth surfaces since the preparations are largely made symmetrically round the long axes of teeth.

After mounting the duplicate cast on the surveying table, the analysing rod is used to identify groups or pairs of abutment teeth. whose long axes are parallel. Then with a long tapered milling cutter each pair or group of teeth is milled in a semblance of the preparation that will be finally carried out in the mouth (*Fig.* III.40).

It is important to do minimum

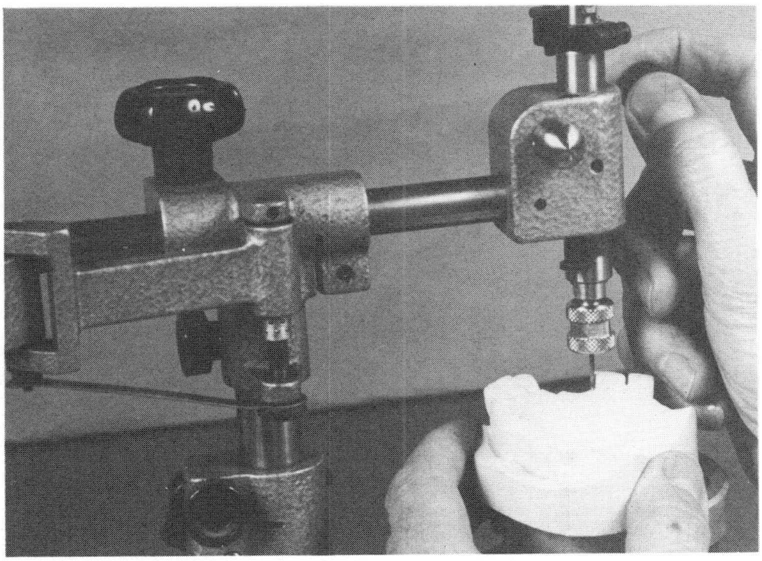

Fig. III.40. Milling cutter being used to make parallel minimum preparations on stone cast.

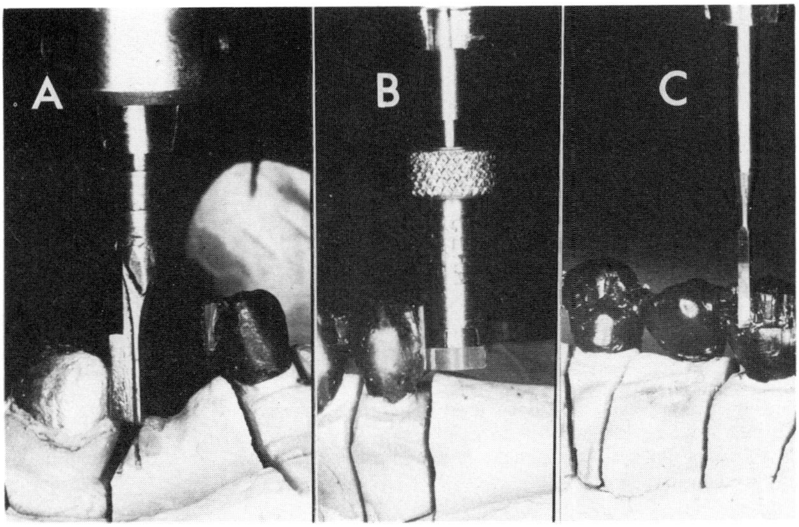

Fig. III.41. Three uses of the surveyor in the construction of complex partial dentures. **A**, Mandrel for positioning a precision lock. **B**, Positioning a Ceka attachment with a special mandrel. **C**, Carving a recess in a wax full veneer crown.

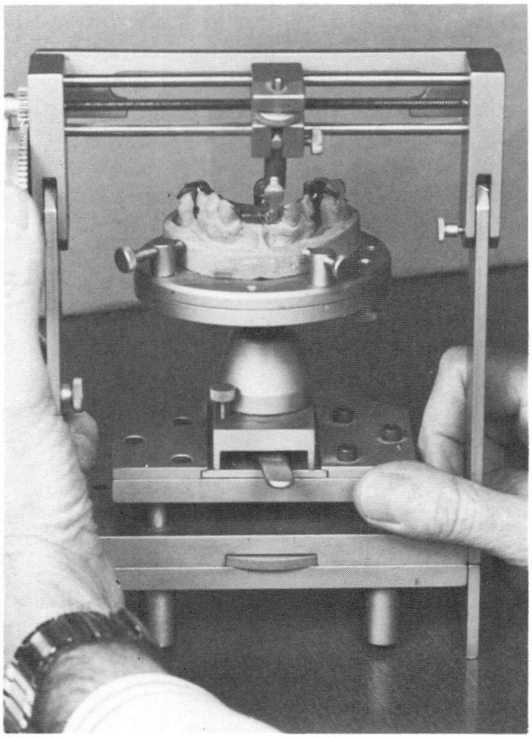

Fig. III.42. P–W rotary surveyor marketed by Metrodent Ltd. At the top the hinged 'goalpost' allows a fixed horizontal rotational axis. By means of a hinge axis locator and an adjustable analyser, the trimming blade attached to the cross-bar enables curved surfaces of variable radii to be carved (Pullen-Warner and L'Estrange, 1978, pp. 85–88).

preparations on the plaster teeth so that the appropriate teeth are left larger than the actual preparations will be in the mouth. Castings can then be designed that have common paths of insertion in the pairs of teeth, although there might be wide disparities of the path of insertion between one pair of teeth and the other pair. This does not affect the final result since by using a mandrel on the surveyor it is quite a simple matter to position a precision lock on one casting that is precisely in the path of insertion of another casting (*Fig.* III.41). The first casting with the lock in it is cemented and the second casting is inserted in a different path and the lock engages the first casting.

In this way much tooth substance can be saved, since the preparations do not have to be parallel. Quite commonly a single tooth may be out of alignment with others to be included in the fixed partial denture and this will be taken into consideration in making the preparation, but it will carry a lock on its abutment piece which will be parallel to the remaining castings in the mouth (*Fig.* III.41**A**).

Any teeth whose value as abutments may be in doubt, but yet are being included in the overall treatment plan, may be isolated from the rest of the bridgework by placing screw locks so that should they fail as abutments at a later date the locks can be undone, the tooth extracted and replaced by a pontic that is locked in place by the remaining attachments on the bridge. Even where all abutments are considered to be healthy, it is usually wise to divide full cover bridgework into segments which are locked together. These locks would normally occur as required by the different paths of insertion of the various parts of the bridge.

Another approach to full cover bridgework, where the teeth subtend different angles to each other, is to prepare each tooth individually on the duplicate cast in the most appropriate manner, preserving the maximum amount of tooth structure. Then build up full veneer crowns on the teeth and use the surveyor to carve the wax (*Fig.* III.41**C**). In this way a recess is prepared for an overall locking piece that is screwed in place later and provides the necessary continuity for the full cover bridgework.

The surveyor is also used to position external and internal precision attachments for complex partial dentures (*Fig.* III.41**A** and B). Special mandrels to hold the attachments are supplied by their makers (e.g. Ceka). The surveyor ensures that the attachments are placed parallel to each other.

A special surveying method for use for sectional and two-part dentures has been described by Pullen-Warner and L'Estrange (1978), who have devised a rotary surveyor for this purpose (*Fig.* III.42).

Appendix IV

Classifications of partial dentures

In 1968 Osborne and Lammie stated that

> 'An examination of the literature reveals that several criteria have formed the basis of partial denture classification. Classification in itself facilitates case history recording and the exchange of views between practitioners, always provided there is general acceptance of the particular system. It is felt, however, that a classification should do more, and also give an immediate clue to the main problem of treatment involved in the particular case.'

Over the years many attempts have been made to classify partial dentures or partially edentulous mouths. Cummer (1920) classified partial dentures into four types, depending upon the position of the direct retainers:

1. Diagonal—two retainers diagonally opposite one another.
2. Diametric—two retainers diametrically opposite one another.
3. Unilateral—two or more direct retainers on the same side.
4. Multilateral—three (or rarely four) direct retainers in a triangular (or rarely a quadrilateral) relationship.

Cummer subtitled his paper 'A little excursion in partial denture mathematics' and cited the vast array of possible saddle positions.

Unlike Cummer, Kennedy (1928) did not classify dentures, but classified 'partially edentulous arches'. His classification related the edentulous spaces to the remaining teeth:

Class 1: Bilateral free-end saddles with various modifications, e.g. Mod. 1: one additional bounded saddle; Mod. 2: two additional bounded saddles; Mod. 3: three additional bounded saddles.

Class 2: Unilateral free-end saddle with modifications as necessary.

Class 3: Unilateral bounded saddle with modifications.

Class 4: Single bounded saddle anterior to abutment teeth (no modifications).

The following points were noted:

1. The most posterior edentulous area determined the class.
2. Additional edentulous areas were called 'modifications'.
3. The size of the modification was not important.
4. If a third molar was missing, and not to be replaced, it was not considered in the classification.

The Kennedy classification is positional or anatomical and conveys a picture of certain tooth/saddle relationships, but gives little more information than do the teeth present on a cast and their relative positions.

Bailyn (1928) produced a classification based on the available support. He used the descriptive letters 'A' and 'P':

A Anterior restorations, where there were saddle areas anterior to the first bicuspid (premolar).

P Posterior restorations, where there were saddle areas posterior to the canines.

and in addition:

Class I Bounded saddle (not more than 3 teeth missing).

Class II Free-end saddle (no distal abutment).

Class III Bounded saddle (more than 3 teeth missing).

Thus, for example, if all the posterior teeth between the canines and third molars were missing, together with the lateral incisors, the classification would be 'AI PIII'.

Class I should be tooth-supported.

Classes II and III should be supported by mucosa.

Bailyn's classification was the first to emphasize the importance of support of partial dentures by the remaining tissues.

Neurohr (1939) also classified according to the type of support available, but the system was unnecessarily complex. Many of his denture designs did not match his principles of classification.

He wrote as follows:

'Class I Tooth-bearing.

Unilateral or Bilateral.

A case falls under the above classification when there are teeth posterior to all spans, and when there are no more than four teeth missing in any space.

Variation I—Missing posteriors predominate.

a. Posteriors missing, anteriors in place.

b. Posteriors missing, some anteriors missing.

Variation 2—Missing anteriors predominate.

a. Anteriors missing, posteriors in place.

b. Anteriors missing, some posteriors missing.

Class II Tooth-and-tissue-bearing.

A Unilateral or Bilateral case falls under the above classification when there are no teeth posterior to one or more spans, or when there are more than four teeth (which include a canine) in one or more spans.

Division I—When there are no teeth posterior to one or more spans.

Variation 1—Missing posteriors predominate.

a. Posteriors missing, anteriors in place.

b. Posteriors missing, some anteriors missing.

Variation 2—Missing anteriors predominate.

a. None.

b. Anteriors missing, some posteriors missing.

Division II—When there are teeth posterior in all spans, but when there are more than four teeth (including a canine) in any one or more spans.

Variation 1—Missing posteriors predominate.

a. None.

b. Posteriors missing, some anteriors missing.

Variation 2—Missing anteriors predominate.

a. Anteriors missing, posteriors in place (bilaterals only).

b. Anteriors missing, some posteriors missing.

Class III Tissue-bearing (complete dentures).'

The complexity of Neurohr's classification is obvious and it is seldom used.

Mauk (1942) proposed a classification based on the number, length and position of the spaces, and the number and position of the remaining teeth.

Wild (1949) proposed a simple but self-explanatory classification, little known in the English dental literature;

Class 1 Interruption of the dental arch (i.e. bounded)

Class 2 Shortening of the dental arch (i.e. free-end)

Class 3 Combination of 1 and 2.

Godfrey (1951) used a system based on the location and size of the edentulous spaces.

Friedman (1953) introduced his A B C classification: 'A' for anterior, 'B' for bounded posterior, and 'C' for cantilever (free-end).

Beckett (1953) and Wilson (1957) based their ideas on Bailyn's classification (1928) and felt that the following must be considered when deciding the proportionate amount of support provided by teeth and tissue (the word 'tissue' meant mucosa and underlying bone):

a. The quality of abutment support.

b. The magnitude of the occlusal support.

c. The harmony of the occlusion.

d. The quality of the mucosa and residual ridge.

They believed that every effort should be made to avoid tissue support alone.

Class I Bounded saddle: abutment teeth qualified to support the denture. Mucosa not used for support.

Class II Free-end (a) tooth-and-tissue-borne.
(b) tissue-borne.

Class III Bounded saddle: abutment teeth not so well qualified to support the denture as in Class I.

Wilson (1957) elaborated further:
Mandibular Class III should be treated as Class I.
Maxillary Class III should be treated as Class I or II.

Craddock (1954) classified partial dentures as follows:

Class 1 Saddles supported at both ends by substantial abutment teeth.

Class 2 Vertical biting forces applied to denture resisted entirely by soft tissue.

Class 3 Tooth-suported at only one end of the saddle.

Skinner (1959) was obviously influenced by Cummer and formed a classification with five classes, characterized in most cases by the anatomical or positional relationship of the remaining teeth. Some of the five classes were curiously similar.

Austin and Lidge (1957) pointed out that there were over 65000 possible combinations of teeth and edentulous spaces and suggested a classification that described the position of missing teeth:

'1. Class A—Missing Anteriors
   a. A1 Missing anteriors one side (unilateral construction)
   b. A2 Missing anteriors both sides *c.*
   c. ABi Missing anteriors with bilateral posterior construction.
2. Class P—Missing Posteriors
   a. P1 Posteriors missing one side (unilateral construction)
   b. P2 Posteriors missing both sides
   c. PBi Posteriors missing one side with bilateral construction.
3. Class AP—Missing Anteriors and Posteriors
   a. AP1 Missing anteriors and posteriors one side (unilateral construction)
   b. AP2 Missing anteriors and posteriors both sides
   c. APBi Missing anteriors and posteriors one side with bilateral construction.

Any combination of the above may be possible, such as A2P1 or A1P2.'

Watt et al. (1958) stated that there were three possible methods of supporting partial dentures:

1. Entirely tooth-borne.
2. Entirely tissue-borne.
3. Partly tooth-borne and partly tissue-borne.

A partial denture should fall into one of these three classes.

Applegate (1960) proposed modifications to the Kennedy classification and enumerated six classes:

Class I All remaining teeth anterior to the bilateral edentulous areas.

Class II Remaining teeth of either right or left side anterior to the unilateral edentulous area (unilateral free-end).

Class III The edentulous space bounded by teeth both anteriorly and posteriorly.

Class IV The edentulous space anterior to the remaining teeth, which bound it both to the right and left of the median line.

Class V A space bounded by remaining teeth at its posterior and anterior terminals. (There was an essential difference between Class V and III, viz. in Class V the space was long and the anterior tooth 'very weak'.)

Class VI Same as Classes III and V, but in Class VI conditions were such that the restoration could be made entirely tooth-borne.

Confusion in this classification is highlighted by three of the six classes having the same anatomical landmarks. There is little advantage over Kennedy's classification, except that the class is determined after deciding which abutment teeth can be used.

Fiset (1973) suggested the addition of four extra classes to make a total of ten classes in the Applegate classification.

Another altered Kennedy classification was described by Terkla and Laney (1963) who used the original Swenson classification (Swenson and Terkla, 1955). They named the Kennedy Class II a Swenson Class I (unilateral free-end) and the Kennedy Class I a Swenson Class II (bilateral free-end). In addition, the modifications in all four Kennedy classes were completely changed. The end result was another descriptive classification without much contribution to the problem.

Avant (1966) proposed a classification based on the anterior and posterior segments of the dental arch; this was also reminiscent of Kennedy's classification, without any obvious improvement.

Costa (1974) proposed yet another descriptive classification of partially edentulous arches based on anterior, lateral and terminal spaces.

Osborne and Lammie (1974) quoted a classification based on support of a denture as a whole:

Class I Mucosa-borne.
Class II Tooth-borne.
Class III Combination of mucosa-borne and tooth-borne.

Summary

Many classifications of partial dentures and their designs have been proposed by different clinicians. The confusion is not yet resolved and there is no universally accepted classification. A classification is either one that describes the various tooth and saddle positions, like those of Kennedy and others, or one that looks more closely at the available support, like those of Bailyn and others. A classification like Kennedy's is useful when describing the basic outlines of any particular case. However, while it helps to form a common 'partial denture' language among colleagues, it does not take into account the available support upon which the success or failure of any partial denture or bridge ultimately depends. For this reason a support classification is preferable.

Glossary

We have defined the following terms, as our use of them in the text differs from the definitions that are to be found in the *Glossary of Prosthodontic Terms* prepared by the Academy of Denture Prosthetics (1977) and also from the definitions in the *British Standard Glossary of Dental Terms* prepared by the British Standards Institution (1983). We do not imply that our definitions are better, but include them only to avoid misunderstanding.

ABNORMAL TOOTH CONTACT
A contact to which the patient is unable to adapt without symptoms or pathological change.

ABUTMENT PIECE
That part of a fixed or complex partial denture which is cemented to the abutment tooth. The abutment pieces for fixed partial dentures (bridges) are sometimes called retainers, but the use of this term can be misleading because, although the crowns and inlays on the abutment teeth provide retention, they also provide support for the appliance. For this reason we prefer to use the term 'abutment piece' for the 'retainers' of fixed partial dentures.

ABUTMENT TEETH
The teeth that provide support and/or retention for fixed or removable partial dentures.

ARTICULATION
The dynamic sliding contact of cusps of upper and lower teeth that takes place during closed grinding movements of the mandible. Articulation is a continuous change from one occlusal position to the next.

BALANCED MUSCLE ACTIVITY
Symmetrical masticatory muscle activity that closes the jaw in a centric position.

BRACING
The resistance to horizontal forces on a partial denture. We must distinguish between the means whereby the forces are transmitted to the teeth (e.g. the bracing elements of clasps, connectors and saddle flanges) and the resistance provided by the teeth and periodontium which can be thought of as 'horizontal support' as opposed to 'vertical support'.

BRACING ELEMENT
That part of a denture which transmits horizontal forces to the supporting structures.

CENTRIC JAW RELATION
The jaw relation when the condyles are in the most posterior position in the glenoid fossae at the occluding vertical dimension.

COMMON PATH OF DISPLACEMENT
The path along which a denture is most likely to be displaced during function. This path is at right angles to the occlusal surfaces of the teeth, since sticky food tends to dislodge the denture along this path when the jaws are opened.

COMPLEX PARTIAL DENTURE
Partial denture with some fixed parts (abutment pieces or bridges) and some removable parts.

COMPRESSION OF MUCOSA
A uniform reduction in volume of mucosa without distortion.

CONNECTOR
A part of a partial denture which joins its components. *Major Connector:* A saddle connector. *Minor Connector:* A clasp or rest connector.

CONTINUOUS CLASP
A bar that contacts the lingual surfaces of the teeth and provides bracing and indirect retention for partial dentures. It is normally used in conjunction with a lingual bar, but if made strong enough can be used as a major connector. It is sometimes called a 'continuous bar retainer'.

DENTURE SPACE
The space in the mouth formerly occupied by the teeth and the supporting tissues that have since been lost.

DE VAN CLASP
A gingivally-approaching clasp that hugs the denture margin. Designed by De Van (1935) who called it 'an embrasure saddle clasp'.

DIMPLE HINGE
Laboratory-made hinge attachment for tooth-and-mucosa-borne partial dentures in which a pair of dimples provides the axis for the hinge. This allows a change in position of the fulcrum axis of the denture in order to distribute the occlusal load more favourably to the supporting tissues.

DISJUNCT DENTURE
A denture in which there is complete separation (disjunction) between the tooth-borne part and the mucosa-borne part. The tooth-borne part splints the remaining teeth and provides only retention for the mucosa-borne part.

DISPLACEMENT OF MUCOSA
Distortion of mucosa with or without uneven reduction in volume.

EXTRA-ANATOMICAL PART OF A DENTURE
Part of a prosthesis that goes beyond the boundary of the natural part replaced by the prosthesis. The extra-anatomical part lies beyond the denture space and is an addition to the normal anatomical contour.

FIXED PARTIAL DENTURE (BRIDGE)
A dental prosthesis fixed to abutment teeth in such a way that it cannot be removed by the patient.

FLANGE
Part of a partial denture that replaces lost buccal or lingual mucosal contour.

FULCRUM AXIS
The axis round which a tooth-and-mucosa-borne denture tends to rock when the mucosa-borne saddles are loaded. It normally passes through the occlusal rests nearest the mucosa-borne saddles. When the force is in the opposite direction, so that the saddles are lifted from the mucosa, the axis passes through the tips of the clasp arms nearest the saddles.

FUNCTIONALLY-GENERATED OCCLUSAL SURFACE
The surface of an occlusal rim which has been contoured by the natural chewing movements of the opposing teeth.

GINGIVALLY-APPROACHING CLASP
A clasp that approaches an undercut on a tooth from the gingival side of the survey line.

GNATHIC DYSFUNCTION
Impaired functioning of the jaws that may arise from malocclusion of the teeth, diseases of the joints or abnormal muscle activity. This general term is preferred to such terms as 'temporomandibular joint syndrome' or 'temporomandibular joint dysfunction', as many of the dysfunctions arise from adaptive responses to malocclusion rather than from joint disease. *Myofascial pain dysfunction syndrome* also comes within the general heading of 'gnathic dysfunctions', but has a more restricted meaning.

GNATHOSONIC RECORD
A record of the sounds made by the masticatory mechanism.

GNATHOSONICS
The study of sounds made by the masticatory mechanism.

GUIDING SURFACES
Surfaces of teeth that guide removable partial dentures towards their final position in the mouth. It is advantageous if the guiding surfaces are parallel to each other, but this is seldom possible as the surfaces of the teeth are curved. For this reason we prefer the term 'guiding surfaces' to the term 'guiding planes'.

HABITUATION
Adaptation to a repeated stimulus.

HYBRID DENTURE
A type of overdenture that looks like a complete denture, but is retained and supported by natural teeth for which prefabricated or precision attachments have been made.

INDIRECT RETAINER
A supporting element of a denture that lies on one side of a line drawn between the direct retainers and provides (indirect) retention for the part of the denture on the opposite side of the line.

INDIRECT SUPPORTER
A direct retainer that lies on one side of the fulcrum axis through the occlusal rests nearest a mucosa-borne saddle and provides indirect (cantilever) support for that saddle.

INTERCUSPAL POSITION
The most elevated position of the mandible when there is maximum engagement of the cusps of the upper and lower teeth.

MALOCCLUSION (FUNCTIONAL)
When 'muscle position' and 'tooth position' do not coincide and the teeth slide into the intercuspal position from their first contact in the path of closure.

MALOCCLUSION (MORPHOLOGICAL)
A malrelationship of the teeth caused by an anatomical abnormality of the arch form or jaw relationship. In spite of the abnormal arrangement, the functional occlusion of the teeth may be stable.

MILLED ATTACHMENTS
Laboratory-made attachments produced by milling cast abutment pieces on a parallelometer. They usually depend on friction between the accurately milled pieces to provide retention.

MUCOCOMPRESSIVE IMPRESSION
An impression made under load such that the mucosa is uniformly reduced in volume and is evenly condensed.

MUCOGINGIVAL LINE
The line of junction between the attached and reflected mucosa of the mouth.

MUCOSAL SUPPORT
Support from the mucosa and underlying bone.

MUSCLE BALANCE
The relationship between the denture and the investing musculature, such that the forces exerted by tongue, lips and cheeks do not dislodge the denture during functional movements of the mouth with the teeth out of contact.

MUSCLE POSITION
The position to which the mandible closes when the muscles are acting in an optimum symmetrical manner.

OCCLUSAL REST
A rigid extension of a partial denture which rests on the occlusal surface of a tooth.

OCCLUSALLY-APPROACHING CLASP
A clasp that approaches an undercut on a tooth from the occlusal side of the survey line.

OCCLUSION
The static closed relationship of cusps or masticating surfaces of upper and lower teeth. *Occlusion (Ideal):* A morphologically normal occlusion in which muscle position and tooth position coincide. *Occlusion (Normal):* the maximum intercuspation of the teeth achieved

without muscle pain, periodontal or joint trauma.

OVERLAY DENTURE
A removable partial denture that has a metal casting or an acrylic extension on or over the occlusal or incisal surfaces of natural teeth.

PATH OF INSERTION AND REMOVAL
The path along which a partial denture is inserted and removed from the mouth.

PATHS OF DISPLACEMENT
All possible paths along which all or part of the denture may be displaced during function.

POSTURAL ADAPTATION
A change in the path of closure of the mandible to avoid a premature tooth contact or a change in mandibular posture to enable the teeth to meet evenly all round the dental arch.

PREFABRICATED ATTACHMENT
Attachment manufactured separately and fixed to a denture to provide retention and/or support.

PREMATURE TOOTH CONTACT
A tooth contact that occurs before the occlusal surfaces of the other teeth meet.

PROSTHESIS
An artificial replacement of a natural part. *Dental Prosthesis:* A prosthesis that supplies artificial substitutes for lost natural teeth and their related structures.

RECORD BLOCKS
Appliances used to record the jaw relationship and the dimensions of the denture space.

REMOVABLE PARTIAL OVERDENTURE
The design is similar to a partial denture, except that some parts cover natural teeth that have been prepared or modified for that purpose. It derives its support and retention from a combination of abutment teeth, retained roots, alveolar bone and mucosa.

RESTLESS OCCLUSION
Where there is no stable occlusal position, each unstable occlusion calls forth a postural adaptive response that produces a different unstable occlusion that in its turn causes a further adaptive response and another unstable occlusion. This restless occlusion causes jiggling forces on the teeth.

RETAINER
Any type of clasp, attachment or device used for the anchorage of a prosthesis. In the text we use the term ‘abutment pieces’ for retainers for fixed bridges.

RETENTION
The resistance of a denture to removal from the mouth in a direction at right angles to the occlusal surface.

RETRUDED CONTACT POSITION
The position of the mandible when its condyles are in their retruded position in the glenoid fossae and there is occlusal contact of the teeth or occlusion rims. This is the most retruded position that is right for the patient.

RETRUDED FUNCTIONAL POSITION
The relation of the mandible to the maxilla when a relaxed supine patient with neck extended closes the mandible in an unstrained manner. This is the most retruded position that the mandible is likely to adopt in function.

RING REST
A complete ring of metal that surrounds a tooth on the occlusal side of the survey line and acts as an occlusal rest.

R/L RATIO
The ratio of the *R*emaining tooth support to the *L*ost tooth support. It is calculated by dividing the sum of the periodontal areas of the abutment teeth by the periodontal areas of the teeth that have been lost from the gap.

RPI SYSTEM
Rest, plate, I-bar system of retention described by Kratochvil (1963).

SADDLE AREA
The area of mucosa in a gap in the dental arch caused by the loss of teeth.

SECTIONAL DENTURE
A denture made in two or more sections which are then fixed together with bolts or other devices. As the sections have different paths of insertion, rigid portions of these appliances engage undercuts and ensure the retention of the appliance.

SMILE LINE
The curve of the smiling lower lip that provides a visual reference line against which maxillary anterior tooth position is judged. The upper anterior teeth should be set so that their incisal edges follow this line.

STABLE OCCLUSION
An occlusion of the teeth when muscle position and tooth position coincide. All the occlusal sounds are impact sounds of short duration.

STABLE TOOTH CONTACT
A non-sliding first contact of teeth in the position of maximum elevation of the mandible.

STEREOSTETHOSCOPE
A stethoscope with two chest-pieces, one connected to each ear-piece, that enable the user to hear sound stereophonically.

STREAMLINED PARTIAL DENTURE
A partial denture that is shaped so that it produces minimal distortion of the denture space and has as few extra-anatomical parts as possible.

STRESS-BREAKER
A special connector intended to distribute the stress between a tooth-borne part and a mucosa-borne part of a partial denture. The term 'stress-distributor' is preferred by some.

SUPPORT
The foundation on which the denture rests. It comprises the hard and soft tissues that bear the loads of mastication and clenching applied to the denture.

SUPPORT DEFICIT
The difference between the periodontal area of an extracted tooth and the area of healed mucosa remaining in the gap.

SUPPORTER
An occlusal rest or other element of a partial denture that transmits the occlusal loads to the supporting teeth and tissues.

SURVEY LINE
A line drawn round the greatest girth of a tooth in relation to the common path of displacement or to the path of insertion and removal of the denture.

SWINGLOCK PARTIAL DENTURE
A type of partial denture devised by Simmons (1963). A labial bar is hinged at one side of the mouth and locks at the other side to provide retention.

TERMINAL HINGE AXIS
A line between the mandibular condyles around which the mandible rotates when it is in the most retruded position possible.

TOOTH POSITION
The position of maximum intercuspation of the teeth.

TOOTH SUPPORT
Support from the teeth and periodontium. It is sometimes helpful to think of the support in relation to vertical and horizontal forces, although the forces on the teeth are multi-directional.

TWO-PART DENTURE
A term sometimes used for a *Sectional Denture* or for a *Disjunct Denture.* It literally means a denture made in two parts, but we prefer the terms 'sectional denture' and

'disjunct denture' as they are more closely defined.

UNBALANCED MUSCLE ACTIVITY
Asymmetrical muscle activity that closes the jaws in an eccentric position.

UNDERCUT
Dental: The part of a tooth which lies between the survey line and the gingivae.
Soft tissue: The part of the mucosal surface of a cast that lies between the survey line on the mucosa and the line marked by the tip of the surveying rod.

UNSTABLE OCCLUSION
All the occlusal sounds are prolonged, sliding or muffled sounds, indicating that all the occlusal contacts are unstable.

ZONE OF DISPLACEMENT
The zone that encompasses all the possible paths of displacement of a partial denture.

Envoy

We hope that you have enjoyed this book and that it has provided you with some food for thought and discussion. Compromise is inevitable when designing partial dentures, and skill in designing them depends on an ability to select the most important factors for each individual patient, so that the partial denture you produce will not only please the patient with its appearance and comfort, but will also please you because it does not harm the mouth. Our intention has been to provide a guide to the selection of what is important for good design of partial dentures and we hope that you have found it useful and practical.

References

Abelson D. C. (1981) Denture plaque and denture cleansers. *J. Prosthet. Dent.* **45,** 376–379.

Academy of Denture Prosthetics (1977) *Glossary of prosthodontic terms.* 4th ed. *J. Prosthet. Dent.* **38,** 66–109.

Addy M. and Bates J. F. (1979) Plaque accumulation following the wearing of different types of removable partial dentures. *J. Oral Rehabil.* **6,** 111–117.

Agerberg G. and Carlsson G. E. (1973) Functional disorders of the masticatory system. II. Symptoms in relation to impaired mobility of the mandible as judged from investigation by questionnaire. *Acta Odontol. Scand.* **31,** 335–347.

Agerberg G. and Carlsson G. E. (1981) Chewing ability in relation to dental and general health. *Acta Odontol. Scand.* **39,** 147–153.

Anderson D. J. (1956a) Measurement of stress in mastication I. *J. Dent. Res.* **35,** 664–670.

Anderson D. J. (1956b) Measurement of stress in mastication II. *J. Dent. Res.* **35,** 671–673.

Anderson J. N. (1958) Dimensions of cast palatal and lingual bars. *Dent. Practit.* **8,** 270–274.

Anderson J. N. and Bates J. F. (1959) The cobalt-chromium partial denture: a clinical survey. *Br. Dent. J.* **107,** 57–62.

Anderson J. N. and Lammie G. A. (1952) A clinical survey of partial dentures. *Br. Dent. J.* **92,** 59–67.

Ante I. H. (1926) The fundamental principles of abutments. *Mich. State Dent. Soc. Bull.* **8,** 14–23 (quoted in Tylman S. D. (1954) *Theory and Practice of Crown and Bridge Prostheses.* 3rd ed. London, Kimpton, p. 183).

Antos E. W., Renner R. P. and Foerth D. (1978) The swing-lock partial denture: an alternative approach to conventional removable partial denture service. *J. Prosthet. Dent.* **40,**3, 257–262.

Applegate O. C. (1960) The rationale of partial denture choice. *J. Prosthet. Dent.* **10,** 891–907.

Appleton I. E. (1980) Restoration of root-resected teeth. *J. Prosthet. Dent.* **44,** 150–153.

Ash M. M. and Ramfjord S. P. (1982) *An Introduction to Functional Occlusion.* Philadelphia, Saunders.

Atkinson W. H. (1861) Plates over fangs. *Dent. Register* **15,** 213–216.

Atkinson H. F. and Ralph W. J. (1973) Tooth loss and biting force in man. *J. Dent. Res.* **52,** 225–228.

Augsburger R. H. and Elahi J. M. (1982) Evaluation of seven proprietary denture cleansers. *J. Prosthet. Dent.* **47,** 356–359.

Austin K. P. and Lidge E. F. (1957) *Partial Dentures.* St. Louis, Mosby, pp. 17–21.

Avant W. E. (1966) A universal classification for RPD situations. *J. Prosthet. Dent.* **16,** 533–539.

Avant W. E. (1973a) A study of some factors associated with denture retention. *J. Prosthet. Dent.* **29,**4, 383–389.

Avant W. E. (1973b) A comparison of the retention of complete denture bases having different types of posterior palatal seal. *J. Prosthet. Dent.* **29,**5, 484–493.

Axelsson P. and Lindhe J. (1974) The effect of a preventive programme on dental plaque, gingivitis and caries in school children. Results after one and two years. *J. Clin. Periodontol.* **1,** 126–138.

Axelsson P. and Lindhe J. (1978) Effect of controlled oral hygiene procedures on caries and periodontal disease in adults. *J. Clin. Periodontol.* **5,** 133–151.

Bailyn C. M. (1928) Tissue support in partial denture construction. *Dent. Cosmos.* **70,** 988–997.

Basker R. M. and Tryde G. (1977) Connectors for mandibular partial dentures: use of the sublingual bar. *J. Oral Rehabil.* **4,** 389–394.

Bates J. F. (1980) Retention of partial dentures. *Br. Dent. J.* **149,** 171–174.

Beam E. M. (1973) Effect of different occlusal profiles on the masticatory forces transmitted by complete dentures: An evaluation. *Br. Dent. J.* **134,** 7–10.

Becker C. M. and Bolender C. L. (1981) Designing swinglock partial dentures. *J. Prosthet. Dent.* **46,**2, 126–132.

Beckett L. S. (1953) The influence of saddle classification on the design of partial removable restorations. *J. Prosthet. Dent.* **3,** 506–516.

Bellini H. T., Arneberg P. and Fehr F. R. von der (1981) Oral hygiene and caries: a review. *Acta Odontol. Scand.* **39,** 257–265.

Bergman B., Hugoson A. and Olsson C. O. (1977) Caries and periodontal status in patients fitted with removable partial dentures. *J. Clin. Periodontol.* **4,** 134–146.

Bhaskar S. N. and Orban B. (1955) Experimental occlusal trauma. *J. Periodontol.* **26,** 270–284.

Bien S. M. (1966) Hydrodynamic damping of tooth movement. *J. Dent. Res.* **45,**3, 907–914.

Black G. V. (1895) In: *G. V. Black's Operative Dentistry* (revised by Robert E. Blackwell), Vol. 1, 8th ed., 1948. London, Kimpton.

Bolender C. L. and Becker C. M. (1981) Swinglock removable partial dentures: where and when. *J. Prosthet. Dent.* **45,** 4–10.

Brewer A. A. and Morrow R. M. (1980) *Overdentures.* 2nd ed., Ch. 13. St Louis, Mosby.

Brill N. (1955) Adaptation and the hybrid-prosthesis. *J. Prosthet. Dent.* **5,** 811–824.

Brill N. (1967) Factors in the mechanism of full denture retention—a discussion of selected papers. *Dent. Pract. Dent. Rec.* **18,**1, 9–19.

Brill N., Tryde G., Stoltze K. and Ghamrawy E. A. (1977) Ecologic changes in the oral cavity caused by removable partial dentures. *J. Prosthet. Dent.* **38,** 138–148.

British Society for the Study of Prosthetic Dentistry (1981) Guides to standards in prosthetic dentistry. *Br. Dent. J.* **150,**6, 167–169.

British Standards Institution (1983) *British Standard Glossary of Dental Terms.* BS 4492.

Burras T. H. (1861) Ueber das Kauen und die Artikulation kunstlicher Gebissstüke. *Der Zahnarzt.* **16,**11, 343–348.

Carlsson G. E., Hedegård B., Koivumaa K. (1961) Studies in partial dental prosthesis. II. An investigation of mandibular partial dentures with double extension saddles. *Acta Odontol. Scand.* **19,** 215–237.

Carlsson G. E., Hedegård B., Koivumaa K. K. (1962) Studies in partial dental prosthesis. III. A longitudinal study of mandibular partial dentures with double extension saddles. *Acta Odontol. Scand.* **20,** 95–119.

Carlsson G. E., Hedegård B., Koivumaa K. K. (1965) Studies in partial dental prosthesis. IV. Final results of a four year longitudinal investigation of dentogingivally supported partial dentures. *Acta Odontol. Scand.* **23,** 443–472.

Catena D. L. (1972) Radiologic changes associated with tooth movement. *Dent. Clin. North Am.* **16,**3, 549–557.

Cerny R. (1978) Magnetodontics. The use of magnetic forces in dentistry. *Aust. Dent. J.* **23,**5, 392–394.

Chick A. O. (1953) The correct location of clasps and rests on dentures without stress breakers. *Br. Dent. J.* **95,** 303–309.

Clayton J. A. (1966) A Measurement of Clasp Forces on Teeth. M.S. Thesis, School of Dentistry, University of Michigan.

Combe E. C. (1981) *Notes on Dental Materials.* 4th ed. Edinburgh, Livingstone, pp. 296–299.

Costa E. (1974) A simplified system for identifying partially edentulous dental arches. *J. Prosthet. Dent.* **32,** 639–645.

Crabb J. J. and Wilson H. J. (1974) A method of measuring root areas of extracted teeth. *J. Dent.* **2,** 171–174.

Craddock F. W. (1954) Trends and needs in prosthetic dentistry. *Int. Dent. J.* **4,** 507–526.

Cummer W. E. (1920) Possible combinations of teeth present and missing in partial restorations. *Oral Health* **10,** 421–430.

Cumming B. R. and Loe H. (1973) Consistency of plaque distribution in individuals without special home care instruction. *J. Periodont. Res.* **8,** 94–100.

De Boever J., McCall W. D., Holden S. and Ash M. M. (1978) Functional occlusal forces: An investigation by telemetry. *J. Prosthet. Dent.* **40,** 326–333.

De Franco R. (1977) Overdentures. *Dent. Clin. North Am.* **21,** 379–394.

De Van M. M. (1935) The embrasure saddle clasp—its principle and design. *J. Am. Dent. Assoc.* **22,** 1352–1362.

Dennis G. J. (1893) A study of the masticating force of the jaws. Trans. World's Columbian Dent. Cong., Chicago, 786–790.

Derry A. and Bertram U. (1970) A clinical survey of removable partial dentures after two years' usage. *Acta Odontol. Scand.* **28,** 581–598.

Dietz K. (1920) Die Funktion einer nicht operierten Pseudarthrose des Unterkiefers. Dissertation, Tubingen.

Dolder E. and Scharer P. (1961) Die Steg-Gelenk-Prothese. *Dtsch. Zahnarztl. Z* **16,** 358–363.

Driessens F. C. M. (1977) Chemical adhesion in dentistry. *Int. Dent. J.* **27,**4, 317–323.

Eckermann R. (1911) Physiologische Bedeutung der Kieferbelastung und ihre Ermessung. *Dtsch. Mschr. Zahnheilk.* **29,**9, 681–691.

Eissmann H. F., Rudd K. D. and Morrow R. M. (1980) *Dental Laboratory Procedures.* Vol. 2. St Louis, Mosby.

Ettinger R. L. and Pinkham J. R. (1977) Dental care for the homebound—assessment and hygiene. *Aust. Dent. J.* **22,**2, 77–82.

Ettinger R. L. and Pinkham J. R. (1978) Oral hygiene and the handicapped child. *J. Int. Assoc. Dent. Child.* **9,** 3–11.

Farrell J. H. (1956) The effect of mastication on the digestion of food. *Br. Dent. J.* **100,** 149–155.

Farrell J. H. (1969) Partial denture tolerance. *Dent. Pract.* **19,** 162–164.

Farrell J. H. (1971) *Partial Denture Designing.* 2nd ed. London, Kimpton, pp. 17–20.

Fenner W., Gerber A. and Muhlemann H. R. (1956) Tooth mobility changes during treatment with partial denture prosthesis. *J. Prosthet. Dent.* **6,** 520–525.

Fenton A. H. and Hahn N. (1978) Tissue response to overdenture therapy. *J. Prosthet. Dent.* **40,** 492–498.

Fiset J. (1973) A classification utilised in the treatment of exceptional or terminal dentitions. *J. Prosthet. Dent.* **30,** 526–532.

Fish S. F. (1970) Partial dentures. 6. Free end saddle dentures. *Br. Dent. J.* **128,** 495–502 (6th paper in a series).

Frantz W. R. (1975) Variations in a removable maxillary partial denture design by dentists. *J. Prosthet. Dent.* **34,** 625–633.

Friedman J. (1953) The A B C classification of partial denture segments. *J. Prosthet. Dent.* **3,** 517–524.

Galler C., Selipsky H., Phillips C. and Ammons W. F. (1979) The effect of splinting on tooth mobility. *J. Clin. Periodontol.* **6,** 317–333.

Garner L. D. and Kotwal N. S. (1973) Correlation study of incisive biting forces with age, sex and anterior occlusion. *J. Dent. Res.* **52,** 698–702.

Gates G. M. and Nicholls J. I. (1981) Evaluation of mandibular arch width change. *J. Prosthet. Dent.* **46,**4, 385–392.

Geddes M. (1958) Investigations of the biological and mechanical factors in the design of tooth-borne dentures. *Int. Dent. J.* **8,** 32–34.

Geissler P. R. (1968) Disjunct dentures. *Dent. News* **5**,2, 1–5 and **5**,3, 6–8.

Geissler P. R. (1973) The disjunct partial denture. *Edin. Dent. Hosp. Gazette* **12**,3, 15–20.

Geissler P. R. and Watt D. M. (1965) Disjunct dentures for patients with teeth of poor prognosis. *Dent. Practit.* **15**,11, 421–423.

Ghamrawy E. (1980) Plaque recordings as a guide to the prognosis for partial denture treatment. *J. Oral Rehabil.* **7**, 117–121.

Gibbons R. J. (1968) Formation and significance of bacterial polysaccharides in caries etiology. *Caries Res.* **2**, 164–171.

Gibbs C. H., Mahan P. E., Lundeen H. C., Brehnan K., Walsh E. K. and Holbrook W. B. (1981) Occlusal forces during chewing and swallowing as measured by sound transmission. *J. Prosthet. Dent.* **46**,4, 443–449.

Gibson T., Kenedi R. M. and Daly C. H. (1965) Bioengineering studies of the human skin. Part 2. In: Kenedi R. M. (ed.) *Biomechanics and Related Bioengineering Topics.* Oxford, Pergamon, pp. 147–158.

Gillings B. R. D. (1977) Intraradicular anchorage of overlay dentures using cobalt rare earth magnets. *Aust. Soc. Prosthodont. Bull.* **7**,2, 27–32.

Gillings B. R. D. (1980) Magnetic retention for the overdenture. In: Brewer A. A. and Morrow R. M. (ed.) *Overdentures.* 2nd ed. St Louis, Mosby, pp. 376–397.

Glantz P. and Nyman S. (1982) Technical and biophysical aspects of fixed partial dentures for patients with reduced periodontal support. *J. Prosthet. Dent.* **47**, 47–51.

Glickman I. (1963) Inflammation and trauma from occlusion, co-destructive factors in chronic periodontal disease. *J. Periodontol.* **34**, 5–10.

Glickman I. and Smulow J. B. (1962) Alterations in the pathway of gingival inflammation into the underlying tissues induced by excessive occlusal forces. *J. Periodontol.* **33**, 7–13.

Godfrey R. J. (1951) A classification of removable partial dentures. *J. Am. Coll. Dent.* **18**, 5–13.

Goldman H. M. and Gianelly A. A. (1972) Histology of tooth movement. *Dent. Clin. North Am.* **16**,3, 439–448.

Goldstein R. E. (1976) *Esthetics in Dentistry.* Philadelphia, Lippincott.

Gomes B. C., Renner R. P., Antos E. W., Baer P. N. and Carlson M. (1981) A clinical study of the periodontal status of abutment teeth supporting swinglock removable partial dentures—a pilot study. *J. Prosthet. Dent.* **46**,1, 7–13.

Gottlieb B. and Orban B. (1931) Tissue changes in experimental traumatic occlusion with special reference to age and constitution. *J. Dent. Res.* **11**, 505–510.

Greene J. C. (1966) *Workshop in Periodontics.* Univ. Michigan, Ann Arbor, USA, p. 422.

Haber G. (1926) *Die Aufgaben der Kaudruck-messung und der Zahndruckprüfung.* Berlin, Haber.

Hallett G. E. M. and Farrell J. H. (1956) Nylon denture base. *Dent. Practit.* **6**, 239.

Hargreaves A. S. (1971) Nylon as a denture base material. *Dent. Practit.* **22**, 122–128.

Hay G. E. (1939) The equilibrium of a thin compressible membrane with application to the periodontal membrane. *Can. J. Res.* **17**, Sec.A:7, 123–140.

Heartwell C. M. and Rahn A. O. (1974) *Syllabus of Complete Dentures.* 2nd ed. London, Lea & Febiger.

Hekneby M. (1969) Distribution of load with the lower free-end partial denture. *Acta Odontol. Scand.* **27**, suppl. 52.

Helkimo E., Carlsson G. E. and Helkimo M. (1977) Bite force and state of dentition. *Acta Odontol. Scand.* **35**, 297–303.

Henderson D. and Steffel V. L. (1981) *McCracken's Removable Partial Prosthodontics.* 6th ed. St Louis, Mosby.

Henking J. P. A. (1982) Overdentures. *J. Dent.* **10**, 217–225.

Hibberd J. L. (1981) A quantitative study of the relationship between severity of dental diseases and the decisions to extract teeth with special reference to the role of chronic periodontal disease. PhD Thesis, University of London.

Hobkirk J. A. and Strahan J. D. (1979) The influence on the gingival tissues of prostheses incorporating gingival relief areas. *J. Dent.* **7**,1, 15–21.

Holt J. E. (1981) Guiding planes: When and where. *J. Prosthet. Dent.* **46**,1, 4–6.

Hopkins C. (1981) An immediate cantilever Rochette bridge. *Br. Dent. J.* **151**,9, 292–295.

Howell A. M. and Manly R. S. (1948) An electronic strain gauge for measuring oral forces. *J. Dent. Res.* **27**, 705–712.

Izikowitz L. (1976) A long-term prognosis for the fixed saddle-bridge. *J. Oral Rehabil.* **3**, 25–40.

Jacobson T. E. and Krol A. J. (1982) Rotational path removable partial denture design. *J. Prosthet. Dent.* **48**,4, 370–376.

Jenkins G. N. (1974) The biochemistry of plaque and caries with special reference to fluoride. In: *Forum Medici, Metabolism and Cariogenicity of Dental Plaque.* Nyon, Zyma, Switzerland.

Jepsen A. (1963) Root surface measurement and a method for X-ray determination of root surface area. *Acta Odontol. Scand.* **21**, 35–46.

Johnson D. L. and Stratton R. J. (1980) *Fundamentals of Removable Prosthodontics.* Chicago, Quintessence, pp. 271–273.

Johnston J. F., Phillips R. W. and Dykema R. W. (1971) *Modern Practice in Crown and Bridge Prosthodontics.* 3rd ed. Philadelphia, Saunders.

Jumber J. F. (1981) *An Atlas of Overdentures and Precision Attachments.* Chicago, Quintessence.

Kantorowicz G. F. (1979) *Inlays, Crowns and Bridges: A Clinical Handbook.* 3rd ed. Bristol, Wright.

Kelleher M. G. D. and Setchell D. J. (1984) An investigation of marking materials used in occlusal adjustment. *Br. Dent. J.* **156**,3, 96–102.

Kenedi R. M. and Cowden J. M. (1976) *Bed Sore Biomechanics:* Proceedings of a Seminar on Tissue Viability and Clinical Applications. London, MacMillan.

Kennedy E. (1928) *Partial Denture Construction.* New York, Dental Items of Interest Publishing Co. pp. 3–8.

King G. J. and Fischlschweiger W. (1982) The effect of force magnitude on extractable bone resorptive activity and cemental cratering in orthodontic tooth movement. *J. Dent. Res.* **61,** 775–779.

Knowles J. W., Ramfjord S. P., Burgett F. G., Nissle R. R. and Shick R. A. (1972) Plaque score related to long-term results of periodontal therapy. *J. Periodont. Res.* Suppl. 10, 39–40.

Koivumaa K. K. (1956) Changes in periodontal tissues and supporting structures connected with partial dentures. *Suom. Hammaslääk Toim.* **52,** Suppl. 1.

Koivumaa K. K., Hedegård B. and Carlsson G. E. (1960) Studies in partial dental prosthesis. I. An investigation of dentogingivally supported partial dentures. *Suom. Hammaslääk. Toim.* **56,** 248–306.

Körber K. H. (1971) Electronic registration of tooth movements. *Int. Dent. J.* **21,** 466–477.

Krasse B., Jordan H. V. and Edwardsson S. (1968) The occurrence of certain 'caries-inducing' streptococci in human dental plaque material. *Arch. Oral Biol.* **13,** 911–918.

Kratochvil F. J. (1963) Influence of occlusal rest position and clasp design on movement of abutment teeth. *J. Prosthet. Dent.* **13,** 114–124.

Krol A. J. (1973a) R.P.I. clasp retainer and its modifications. *Dent. Clin. North Am.* **17,** 631–649.

Krol A. J. (1973b) Clasp design for extension base removable partial dentures. *J. Prosthet. Dent.* **29,** 408–415.

Krol A. J. (1981) *Removable Partial Denture Design.* 3rd ed. Univ. Pacific School of Dentistry, California.

Kurrasch M. (1983) I-bar removable partial dentures. In: Stewart K. L., Rudd K. D. and Kuebker W. A. (ed.) *Clinical Removable Partial Prosthodontics.* St Louis, Mosby, pp. 274–282.

Kydd W. L. and Daly C. H. (1982) The biologic and mechanical effects of stress on oral mucosa. *J. Prosthet. Dent.* **47**,3, 317–329.

Kydd W. L., Daly C. H. and Wheeler J. B. (1971) The thickness measurement of masticatory mucosa in vivo. *Int. Dent. J.* **21,** 430–441.

Kydd W. L. and Mandley J. (1967) The stiffness of palatal mucoperiosteum. *J. Prosthet. Dent.* **18,** 116–121.

Kydd W. L., Stroud W., Moffett B. C. and Tamarin A. (1969) The effect of mechanical stress on oral mucoperiosteum of dogs. *Arch. Oral Biol.* **14,** 921–933.

Laird W. R. E., Grant A. A. and Smith G. A. (1981) The use of magnetic forces in prosthetic dentistry. *J. Dent.* **9,** 328–335.

Laster L., Laudenbach K. W. and Stoller M. H. (1975) An evaluation of clinical tooth mobility measurements. *J. Periodontol.* **46,** 603–607.

Ledger E. (1856) On preparing the mouth for the reception of a full set of dentures. *Br. J. Dent. Sci.* **1,** 90.

Lee J. H. (1963) Sectional partial metal dentures incorporating an internal locking bolt. *J. Prosthet. Dent.* **13,** 1067–1075.

Lee J. H. (1964) A new design for removable partial dentures. *Dent. Practit.* **14,** 284–288.

Leof M. (1944) Clamping and grinding habits; their relation to periodontal disease. *J. Am. Dent. Assoc.* **31,** 184–194.

Lewis A. J. (1978) The influence of design and production on the structural integrity of tensile test specimens and stated values for mechanical properties. *Aust. Dent. J.* **23,** 275–278.

Lilja E., Lindskog S. and Hammarström L. (1981) Orthodontic forces and periodontal compression. *Acta Odontol. Scand.* **39,** 367–378.

Linderholm H. and Wennstrom A. (1970) Isometric bite force and its relation to general muscle force and body build. *Acta Odontol. Scand.* **28,** 679–689.

Lindhe J., Hamp S. E. and Loe H. (1973) Experimental periodontitis in the Beagle dog. *J. Periodont. Res.* **8,** 1–10.

Lindhe J. and Nyman S. (1975) The effect of plaque control and surgical pocket elimination on the establishment and maintenance of periodontal health. *J. Clin. Periodontol.* **2,** 67–79.

Lindhe J. and Nyman S. (1977) The role of occlusion in periodontal disease and the biological rationale for splinting in treatment of periodontitis. *Oral Sciences Reviews* **10,** 11–43.

Lindhe J. and Svanberg G. (1974) Influence of trauma from occlusion on progression of experimental periodontitis in the Beagle dog. *J. Clin. Periodontol.* **1,** 3–14.

Ling B. C. (1982) Rare earth magnets as locking devices in sectional dentures. *J. Prosthet. Dent.* **47**,3, 252–255.

Loe H., Theilade E. and Jensen S. R. (1965) Experimental gingivitis in man. *J. Periodontol.* **36,** 177–187.

Lofberg P. G., Ericson G. and Eliasson S. (1982) A clinical and radiographic evaluation of removable partial dentures retained by attachments to alveolar bars. *J. Prosthet. Dent.* **47**,2, 126–132.

Lukyn E. (1859) *A Popular Treatise on the Preservation, Management and Surgical Treatment of the Teeth and Gums.* London, Savill and Edwards, p. 51.

Lundgren D., Nyman S., Heijl L. and Carlsson G. E. (1975) Functional analysis of fixed bridges on abutment teeth with reduced periodontal support. *J. Oral Rehabil.* **2,** 105–116.

McCarron R. and Sharkey S. W. (1977) A posterior milled retained anterior prosthesis. *Br. Dent. J.* **143**,8, 283–285.

McDowell J. A. and Regli C. P. (1961) A quantitative analysis of the decrease in width of the mandibular arch during forced movements of the mandible. *J. Dent. Res.* **40,** 1183–1185.

MacEntee M. I., Goldstein B. M. and Price C. (1982) Submucosal root retention. A two-year clinical observation. *J. Prosthet. Dent.* **47,** 483–487.

MacGregor A. R. (1958) Biting loads on the free-end saddle. *Int. Dent. J.* **8,** 35–37.

MacGregor A. R. (1960) The free-end saddle. *Dent. Practit.* **10,** 267–270.

MacGregor A. R. and Miller T. P. G. (1974) Two modifications of the lower disjunct partial denture. *J. Dent.* **2,** 211–215.

MacGregor A. R., Miller T. P. G. and Farah J. W. (1978) Stress analysis of partial dentures. *J. Dent.* **6,** 125–132.

MacGregor A. R., Miller T. P. G. and Farah J. W. (1983) The support of bounded saddles. *J. Dent.* **11,** 139–150.

MacGregor A. R. and Stafford G. D. (1983) Private communication.

McLean J. W. (1980) *The Science and Art of Dental Ceramics.* Vol. 2. Chicago, Quintessence, p. 332.

Manderson R. D., Wills D. J. and Picton D. C. A. (1979) Biomechanics of denture-supporting tissues. In: Lefkowitz W. (ed.) *Proceedings of the Second International Prosthodontic Congress.* St Louis, Mosby, pp. 98–101.

Martinelli N. and Spinella S. C. (1981) *Dental Laboratory Technology.* 3rd ed. St Louis, Mosby.

Matsumoto M. (1984) In: Bates J. F., Neill D. J. and Preiskel H. W. (ed.) *Restoration of the Partially Dentate Mouth.* Chicago, Quintessence, pp. 282–283.

Matsuo E. and Shimegi S. (1981) *Screw-retained Dental Prostheses,* Chicago, Quintessence.

Matthews E. and Smith D. C. (1955) Nylon as a denture base material. *Br. Dent. J.* **98,**7, 231–237.

Mauk E. H. (1942) Classification of mutilated dental arches requiring treatment by removable partial dentures. *J. Am. Dent. Assoc.* **29,** 2121–2131.

Mensor M. C. (1981) Attachments for overdentures. In: Rudd K. D., Morrow R. M. and Eissmann H. F. (ed.) *Dental Laboratory Procedures.* Vol. 3. St Louis, Mosby, ch. 19.

Miller S. C. (1938) *Textbook of Periodontia.* 1st ed. Philadelphia, Blakiston.

Miller S. C. and Firestone J. M. (1947) Psychosomatic factors in the etiology of periodontal disease. *Am. J. Orthodont.* **33,** 675–686.

Morelli G. (1920) Ueber Kaundruck. *Wiener Vierteljahresschrift fur Zahnheilkunde* **36,**4, 240–248.

Morrow R. M. (1978) *Handbook of Immediate Overdentures.* St Louis, Mosby.

Moss J. P. (1980a) The soft tissue environment of teeth and jaws. An experimental and clinical study: Part 1. *Br. J. Orthodont.* **7,** 127–137.

Moss J. P. (1980b) The soft tissue environment of teeth and jaws. Experimental malocclusion: Parts 2 and 3. *Br. J. Orthodont.* **7,** 205–216.

Moss J. P. and Picton D. C. A. (1974) The effect on approximal drift of cheek teeth of dividing mandibular molars of adult monkeys. *Arch. Oral Biol.* **19,** 1211–1214.

Moyers R. E. and Bauer J. L. (1950) The periodontal response to various tooth movements. *Am. J. Orthodont.* **36,** 572–580.

Mühlemann H. (1967) Tooth mobility: A review of clinical aspects and research findings. *J. Periodontol.* **38,** 686–713.

Nally J. N. (1961) The use of prefabricated precision attachments. *Int. Dent. J.* **11,** 196–216.

Nathanson D. and Moin K. (1980) Metal-reinforced anterior tooth replacement using acid-etch-composite resin technique. *J. Prosthet. Dent.* **43,** 408–412.

Neff D. (1967) Acid production from different carbohydrate sources in human plaque in situ. *Caries Res.* **1,** 78–87.

Neurohr F. G. (1939) *Partial Dentures.* Philadelphia, Lea & Febiger, pp. 122–123.

Norman R. D., Mehra R. V., Swartz M. L. and Phillips R. W. (1972) Effects of restorative materials on plaque composition. *J. Dent. Res.* **51,** 1596–1601.

Nutting P. G. (1921) A new general law of deformation. *J. Frankl. I.* **191,** 679–685.

Nyman S., Lindhe J. and Ericsson I. (1978) The effect of progressive tooth mobility on destructive periodontitis in the dog. *J. Clin. Periodontol.* **5,** 213–225.

Nyman S. and Lundgren D. (1973) Nagra synpunkter pa parodontalbehandling och bettrekonstraktion med fasta broar vid fall av avancerad marginal parodontit. *Tandlakartidningen* **65,** 638–680.

O'Leary T. J. (1970) Oral hygiene agents and procedures. *J. Periodontol.* **41,** 625–629.

Osborne J. and Lammie G. A. (1968) *Partial Dentures.* 3rd ed. Oxford, Blackwell, p. 1.

Osborne J. and Lammie G. A. (1974) *Partial Dentures.* 4th ed. Oxford, Blackwell Scientific Publications, p. 5.

Osborne J. and Tomlin H. R. (1964) Medial convergence of the mandible. *Br. Dent. J.* **117,** 112–114.

Osborne J., Wilson H. J. and Mansfield M. A. (1979) *Dental Technology and Materials for Students.* Oxford, Blackwell Scientific Publications.

Pacer F. J. and Bowman D. C. (1975) Occlusal force discrimination by denture patients. *J. Prosthet. Dent.* **33,** 602–609.

Parfitt G. J. (1960) Measurement of the physiological mobility of individual teeth in an axial direction. *J. Dent. Res.* **39,**3, 608–618.

Parfitt G. J. (1961) The dynamics of a tooth in function. *J. Periodontol.* **32,** 102–107.

Parkinson C. F. (1982) Endodontic abutments and complete dentures. *J. Prosthet. Dent.* **47,** 600–602.

Picton D. C. A. (1962) Distortion of the jaws during biting. *Arch. Oral Biol.* **7,** 573–580.

Picton D. C. A. and Moss J. P. (1973) The part played by a transeptal fibre system in experimental approximal drift of the cheek teeth in adult monkeys. *Arch. Oral. Biol.* **18,** 669–680.

Picton D. C. A. and Wills D. J. (1978) Viscoelastic properties of the periodontal ligament and mucous membrane. *J. Prosthet. Dent.* **40,** 263–272.

Polson A. M. (1980) Interrelationship of inflammation and tooth mobility (trauma) in pathogenesis of periodontal disease. *J. Clin. Periodontol.* **7,** 351–360.

Preiskel H. W. (1979) *Precision Attachments in Dentistry.* 3rd ed. London, Kimpton.

Pryputniewicz R. J. and Burstone C. J. (1979) The effect of time and force magnitude on orthodontic tooth movement. *J. Dent. Res.* **58,** 1754–1764.

Pullen-Warner E. (1964) Sectional partial dentures. *Dent. News (Lond.)* **2,**2, 1–4.

Pullen-Warner E. (1965) Anterior sectional dentures. *Dent. News (Lond.)* **2,**12, 1–2.

Pullen-Warner E. and L'Estrange P. R. (1978) *Sectional Dentures—A Clinical and Technical Manual.* Bristol, Wright.

Ramfjord S. P. (1974) Periodontal aspects of restorative dentistry. *J. Oral Rehabil.* **1,** 107–126.

Ramfjord S. P. and Ash M. M. (1983) *Occlusion.* 3rd ed. Philadelphia, Saunders.

Ramfjord S. P. and Kohler C. A. (1959) Periodontal reaction to functional occlusal stress. *J. Periodontol.* **30,** 95–112.

Reichenbach E. and Kirchner L. (1952) Ein weiterer Beitrag zur partiellen Prothese in der Sozialpraxis. *Dtsch. Zahnarztl. Z.* **7,** 521–524.

Renner R. P. and Foerth D. (1978) The philosophy and technic of the simplified immediate overdenture. CAL 42, 15–22. (Chicago: COE Laboratories Internat. Corp.)

Reschofsky H. (1906) Ueber die Kautüchtigheit der Plattengebisse. *Österreich–Ungarische Viertel-jahresschrift für Zahnheilkunde* **22,**1, 125–137.

Ridge M. D. and Wright V. (1965) The rheology of skin. *Br. J. Dermatol.* **77,** 639–649.

Roach F. E. (1930) Principles and essentials of bar clasp partial dentures. *J. Am. Dent. Assoc.* **17,** 124–138.

Roberts B. W. (1978) A survey of chrome-cobalt partial dentures. *NZ Dent. J.* **74,** 203–209.

Roberts B. W. (1980) The recall system: a necessary part of a partial denture service. *Br. Dent. J.* **149,**2, 46–48.

Rochette A. L. (1973) Attachment of a splint to enamel of lower anterior teeth. *J. Prosthet. Dent.* **30,** 418–423.

Roydhouse R. H. (1960): The retention of dentures. *J. Am. Dent. Assoc.* **60,**1, 159–163.

Rudd K. D., Morrow R. M. and Eissmann H. F. (1981) *Dental Laboratory Procedures: Removable Partial Dentures.* Vol. 3. St Louis, Mosby.

Russell A. L. (1956) A system of classification and scoring for prevalence studies of periodontal disease. *J. Dent. Res.* **35,** 286–293.

Schei O., Waerhaug J., Lovdal A. and Arno A. (1959) Alveolar bone loss as related to oral hygiene and age. *J. Periodontol.* **30,** 7–16.

Schulte J. K. and Smith D. E. (1980) A clinical evaluation of swinglock removable partial dentures. *J. Prosthet. Dent.* **44,** 595–603.

Schulze W. (1921) Ueber Adhäsion und Luftdruck und ihre Verwendung bei der Fixierung Künstlicher Gebisse. *Deutsche Zahnärztliche Zeitschrift* **24,**45, 538–543 and **24,**46, 553–556.

Shillingburg H. T., Hobo S. and Whitsett L. D. (1976) *Fundamentals of Fixed Prosthodontics.* Chicago, Quintessence, p. 21.

Simmons J. J. (1963) Swinglock stabilization and retention. *Texas Dent. J.* **81,** 10–12.

Skinner C. N. (1959) A classification of removable partial dentures based upon the principles of anatomy and physiology. *J. Prosthet. Dent.* **9,** 240–246.

Skinner E. W., Campbell R. L. and Chung P. (1953) A clinical study of the forces required to dislodge maxillary denture bases of various designs. *J. Am. Dent. Assoc.* **47,**6, 671–680.

Smith B. J. and Turner C. H. (1979) The use of crowns to modify abutment teeth of removable partial dentures. 1. Introduction and partial denture design. *J. Dent.* **7,**1, 52–56.

Stefan M. J. (1874) Versuche uber die scheinbare Adhasion. *Sitzungsberichte Akademie Wissenschaften Wien. Math. Natur. Abt.* **2,** v.69, 713–733.

Steiger A. A. and Boitel R. H. (1959) *Precision Work for Partial Dentures.* Zurich, Stebo.

Stewart K. L. Rudd K. D. and Kuebker W. A. (1983) *Clinical Removable Partial Prosthodontics.* St Louis, Mosby.

Stuteville O. H. (1937) Injuries to the teeth and supporting structures caused by various orthodontic appliances, and methods of preventing these injuries. *J. Am. Dent. Assoc.* **24,** 1494–1507.

Suomi J. D. (1971) Prevention and control of periodontal disease. *J. Am. Dent. Assoc.* **83,** 1271–1287.

Suomi J. D., Greene J. C., Vermillion J. R., Doyle J., Change J. J. and Leatherwood E. C. (1971) The effect of controlled oral hygiene procedures on the progression of periodontal disease in adults. *J. Periodontol.* **42,** 152–160.

Svanberg G. and Lindhe J. (1973) Experimental tooth hypermobility in the dog. *Odontologisk Revy* **24,** 269–289.

Swenson M. G. and Terkla L. G. (1955) *Partial Dentures.* Ch. 17. London, Kimpton.

Synge J. L. (1933) The tightness of the teeth considered as a problem concerning the equilibrium of a thin incompressible elastic membrane. *Philos. Trans. R. Soc. Lond. A,* **231,** 435–477.

Tarbet W. J. (1982) Denture plaque: quiet destroyer. *J. Prosthet. Dent.* **48,** 647–652.

Tautin F. S. (1982) The beneficial effects of tissue massage for the edentulous patient. *J. Prosthet. Dent.* **48,** 653–656.

Taylor R. L., Duckmanton N. A. and Boyks G. (1976) Overlay dentures: philosophy and practice. *Aust. Dent. J.* **21,** 430–439, 495–507.

Taylor D. T., Pflughoeft F. A. and McGivney G. P. (1982) Effect of two clasping assemblies on arch integrity as modified by base adaptation. *J. Prosthet. Dent.* **47,**2, 120–125.

Terkla L. G. and Laney W. R. (1963) *Partial Dentures.* 3rd ed. St Louis, Mosby, pp. 40–50.

Theilade E. and Theilade J. (1976) Role of plaque in the etiology of periodontal disease and caries. *Oral Sci. Rev.* **9,** 23–63.

Theilade E., Wright W. H., Jensen S. B. and Loe H. (1966) Experimental gingivitis in man. *J. Periodont. Res.* **1,** 1–13.

Thompson J. H. C. (1933) On the theory of visco-elasticity: a thermodynamical treatment of visco-elasticity, and some problems of the vibrations of visco-elastic solids. *Philos. Trans. R. Soc. Lond. A.* 231, 339–407.

Thompson V. P., Castillo E. D. and Livaditis G. J. (1983) Resin-bonded retainers. Part I: Resin bond to electrolytically etched non-precious alloys. *J. Prosthet. Dent.* **50,** 771–779.

Tomlin H. R. and Osborne J. (1961): Cobalt-chromium partial dentures: a clinical survey. Br. Dent. J. **110,** 307–310.

Toolson L. B., Smith D. E. and Phillips C. (1982) A two-year longitudinal study of overdenture patients. Assessment of the periodontal health of overdenture abutments. *J. Prosthet. Dent.* **47,** 4–11.

Tuerkheim H. J. (1933) *Taschenbuch der klinischen Prothetik.* Berlin, Verlag von Hermann Meusser, pp. 104–105.

Voigt W. (1928) *Lehrbuch der Krystall Physic.* Leipzig, Trubner.

Waerhaug J. (1955) Pathogenesis of pocket formation in traumatic occlusion. *J. Periodontol.* **26,** 107–118.

Wagner A. G. and Traweek F. C. (1982) Comparison of major connectors for removable partial dentures. *J. Prosthet. Dent.* **47**,3. 242–245.

Walter J. D. (1980) Partial denture technique. 5. Connectors. *Br. Dent. J.* **148,** 133–136.

Wannenmacher E. (1954) Die Prothese als schadigender Faktor durch Reizwirkung auf die Schleimhaut. *Dtsch. Zahnarztl. Z.* **9,** K.89.

Waters N. E. (1972) The rigidity of lingual bars. I: Load-deformation characteristics. *Dent. Practit.* **22,** 209–214.

Waters N. E. (1980) Some mechanical and physical properties of teeth. In: Vincent J. F. V. and Curry J. D. (ed.). *The Mechanical Properties of Biological Materials.* London, Cambridge University Press, pp. 99–135.

Waters N. E. and Nairn R. I. (1972) The rigidity of lingual bars. II: Design criteria. *Dent. Practit.* **22,** 254–259.

Watson R. M. (1977) The effect of the provision of partial dentures upon masticatory function studied by cineradiographic investigation of the placement of the food bolus. MDS Thesis, University of London.

Watt D. M. (1955) Clinical assessment of nylon as a partial denture base material. *Br. Dent. J.* **98**,7, 238–244.

Watt D. M. (1960) Morphological changes in the denture bearing area following the extraction of maxillary teeth. PhD Thesis, University of Edinburgh.

Watt D. M. (1972) Dimple hinge attachments for partial dentures. *Dent. Practit.* **22**,12, 474–476.

Watt D. M. (1981) *Gnathosonic Diagnosis and Occlusal Dynamics.* New York, Praeger.

Watt D. M. and MacGregor A. R. (1976) *Designing Complete Dentures.* Philadelphia, Saunders.

Watt D. M., MacGregor A. R., Geddes M., Cockburn A. and Boyd J. L. (1958) A preliminary investigation of the support of partial dentures and its relationship to vertical loads. *Dent. Practit.* **9**,1, 2–15.

Weinstein S., Haack D. C., Morris L. Y., Snyder B. B. and Attaway H. E. (1963) On an equilibrium theory of tooth position. *Angle Orthodont.* **33,** 1–26.

Wentz F. M., Jaraback J. and Orban B. (1958) Experimental occlusal trauma imitating cuspal interferences. *J. Periodontol.* **29,** 117–127.

Wetherell J. D. and Smales R. J. (1980) Partial denture failures: a long-term clinical survey. *J. Dent.* **8,** 333–340.

Wild W. (1949) Ueber die planmassige prothetische Behandlung des Luckengebisses. *Dtsch. Zahnarztl. Z.* **4,** 131–141.

Wills D. J. (1974) A study of some mechanical properties of tooth supporting tissues in monkeys (*Macaca irus*). PhD Thesis, University of London.

Wills D. J. and Manderson R. D. (1977) Biomechanical aspects of the support of partial dentures. *J. Dent.* **5**,4, 310–318.

Wills D. J., Picton D. C. A. and Davies W. I. R. (1976) A study of the fluid systems of the periodontium in macaque monkeys. *Arch Oral Biol.* **21,** 175–185.

Wilson J. H. (1957) *Partial Dentures.* Philadelphia, Lea & Febiger, p. 81.

Witt E. (1981) Retaining and support elements. *Quintessence of Dental Technology* **5**,9, 887–891.

Wolff J. (1884) Das Gesetz der Transformation der innern Architektur der Knochen bei pathologischen Veränderungen der äusseren Knochenform. *Sitzungsb. Preuss. Akad. Wissensch-zu, Berlin.* Vol. 1, 475–496.

Wolff J. (1891) Ueber die Theorie des Knochenschwundes durch vermehrten Druck und der Knochenanbildung durch Druckentlastung. *Arch. Klin. Chir.* **42,** 302–324.

Wolff J. (1892) *Das Gesetz der Transformation der Knochen.* Berlin, Hirschweld.

Wolff J. (1899) Die Lehre von den funktionellen Knochengestalt. *Virchows Arch.* **155,** 256–315.

Worner H. K. and Anderson M. N. (1944) Biting force measurements on children. *Aust. Dent. J.* **48,** 1–12.

Wright P. S. (1981) Wettability of soft lining materials for acrylic dentures. *Proc. Europ. Prosth. Assoc.,* 5th Annual Meeting.

Yemm R. (1979) Neurophysiologic studies of temporomandibular joint dysfunction. In: Zarb G. A. and Carlsson G. E. (ed.) *Temporomandibular Joint Function and Dysfunction.* Copenhagen, Munksgaard, Ch. 8.

Zarb G. A., Bergman B., Clayton J. A. and MacKay H. F. (1978) *Prosthodontic Treatment for Partially Edentulous Patients.* St Louis, Mosby.

Index